COST–OUTCOME
METHODS FOR
MENTAL HEALTH

COST–OUTCOME METHODS FOR MENTAL HEALTH

WILLIAM A. HARGREAVES
MARTHA SHUMWAY
School of Medicine
University of California
San Francisco, California

TEH-WEI HU
School of Public Health
University of California
Berkeley, California

BRIAN CUFFEL
United Behavioral Health
San Francisco, California

ACADEMIC PRESS
San Diego   London   Boston   New York   Sydney   Tokyo   Toronto

This book is printed on acid-free paper. ∞

Copyright © 1998 by ACADEMIC PRESS

All Rights Reserved.
No part of this publication may be reproduced or transmitted in any form or by any
means, electronic or mechanical, including photocopy, recording, or any information
storage and retrieval system, without permission in writing from the publisher.

Academic Press
a division of Harcourt Brace & Company
525 B Street, Suite 1900, San Diego, California 92101-4495, USA
http://www.apnet.com

Academic Press Limited
24-28 Oval Road, London NW1 7DX, UK
http://www.hbuk.co.uk/ap/

Library of Congress Card Catalog Number: 97-80250

International Standard Book Number: 0-12-325155-9

PRINTED IN THE UNITED STATES OF AMERICA
97 98 99 00 01 02 QW 9 8 7 6 5 4 3 2 1

CONTENTS

3

CONCEPTS OF ECONOMIC COST   39

4

MEASURING UTILIZATION   55

5

ESTIMATING ECONOMIC COST   75

6

MEASURING SERVICE PRACTICE   97

7

MEASURING MENTAL HEALTH OUTCOMES   117

8

AGGREGATING OUTCOME MEASURES   147

9

ANALYZING COST-EFFECTIVENESS   165

10

USING COST–OUTCOME DATA TO GUIDE POLICY AND PRACTICE   189

PREFACE

How good are new mental health treatments in everyday practice? Do they improve outcomes? Do they cost more? How useful are new methods of managing mental health services? Choosing the best policy in adopting service innovations requires clear answers to these questions. Cost–outcome studies are designed to answer these questions and are, therefore, a central aspect of mental health services research.

Major reorganization of health care and the increasing application of managed care approaches to mental health services also have spurred interest in cost–outcome research. Government and insurance industry efforts to contain health costs have raised an outcry from consumers and clinicians that access to care and effectiveness of care are threatened. Policy makers attempting to balance cost containment and quality of care have increasingly sought solid evidence to guide policy choices in health care management.

Mental health services are undergoing even more dramatic changes than the general health sector. Mental health care, especially care for the seriously and persistently ill, traditionally has received much greater public sector funding than general health care, primarily from large state-funded mental health systems and federal Medicaid funding. Publicly funded mental health systems were slow to adopt managed care techniques, but recently virtually every state has rushed to apply these techniques to control expenditures. These changes are part of a general rethinking of the funding and management of mental health care throughout the United States.

This book presents economic concepts of cost and discusses the various approaches to cost–outcome studies, especially cost–effectiveness and cost–utility analysis, as they apply to mental health services. It guides the reader through designing cost–outcome studies; measuring costs, interventions, and outcomes; analyzing study results; and using findings to guide policy and practice. It presents principles and application examples in nontechnical language, and it discusses the details of design, measurement, and analysis to guide the application of these methods to problems in mental health services research.

Our goal is to help readers learn a new vocabulary, consider new perspectives in study design, prepare for productive research collaboration with health economists, and become intelligent consumers of cost–outcome research findings. The book will introduce readers without a background in economics to applied economic methods of cost–outcome research, and it will help readers with a background in research design and statistics to expand their knowledge of these methods as they specifically apply to services research in mental health.

The book will interest graduate and postdoctoral students, psychiatric residents and other clinical trainees, faculty in mental health fields and health economics, investigators employed in mental health organizations and in pharmaceutical and other treatment technology firms, and mental health managers and policy makers. It is designed for use as a text for a graduate or postdoctoral course in mental health cost–outcome research.

Chapters 1 and 3 are an accessible introduction to cost–outcome research in mental health for the general reader. The remaining eight chapters present more technical detail and are intended for readers who have a research background or are in research training. Each chapter begins with a case example that features problems that motivate the principles and methods presented in the chapter.

Chapter 1 sets the stage by considering the kinds of information needed by those who make mental health services policy. It clarifies the distinction between efficacy and effectiveness research, and reviews the history of cost–outcome research in mental health. Chapter 1 then discusses the various barriers to meaningful cost–outcome information, and it explains how the succeeding chapters will help the investigator overcome those barriers. Chapter 2 expands on the implications of the efficacy/effectiveness distinction by presenting research design issues that need special attention in mental health cost–outcome research.

Chapter 3 presents elementary concepts of economic cost, including the societal perspective on cost as well as the perspective of specific payers. It explains the four major types of cost–outcome research—cost-efficiency, cost-benefit, cost-effectiveness, and cost-utility—and presents elements of market theory and welfare economic principles that have motivated many of the economic methods applied in cost–outcome research.

Chapter 4 discusses the choice of what costs to measure and the methods for measuring utilization of mental health services, physical health services, social services, and criminal justice services. It also discusses patient and family time costs and patient productivity. Chapter 5 incorporates data discussed in Chapter 4—the utilization of resources—and presents methods for assigning appropriate cost values to each type of utilization. This allows one to estimate the relative economic impact of each treatment condition and to estimate the differences in economic impact as seen from different payer perspectives.

Chapter 6 presents methods for measuring service practice, so that one can understand the nature of the services being compared and examine factors that may account for the superior cost-effectiveness of one over another.

Chapters 7 and 8 cover service outcome. Chapter 7 introduces outcome dimensions and instruments commonly used in mental health services research and discusses their choice or adaptation for particular studies. Chapter 8 discusses alternative methods for aggregating multiple dimensions of outcome, including choosing one key outcome, using a generic or specific health-related quality-of-life measure, averaging across outcome measures, monetizing outcomes, using preference or utility weights, and estimating quality-adjusted life years.

Chapter 9 discusses statistical issues in analyzing treatment effects on cost and on effectiveness and describes the analysis and interpretation of the relationship of cost to effectiveness. This chapter assumes a graduate-level introduction to the general linear model (multiple regression and analysis of variance), although the techniques used in the chapter are reviewed briefly.

Chapter 10 discusses the use of cost–outcome findings to guide policy and practice and the methods for integrating findings from multiple studies: qualitative reviews, meta-analysis, clinical decision analysis and modeling, and cross-design synthesis. While research findings are only one source of information relevant to policy formation, the chapter shows how the integration of findings and their synthesis in the form of practice guidelines is a major pathway to policy impact.

Work on this book was supported by grants R01MH48141, R01MH47056, R01MH51555, K05MH00900, and P50MH43694 from the National Institute of Mental Health. The authors are grateful for the assistance of Suzanne Fares, Ph.D., who provided major editorial assistance; Tandy Chouljian, Fran Rozewicz, Michele Okun, Todd Wagner, and other colleagues, research assistants, and students who read and critiqued many of the chapters; and anonymous reviewers solicited by Academic Press who made helpful comments on drafts of the book. Carole Siegel, Ph.D., made an important contribution to Chapter 9. Scott Bentley at Academic Press was a continuing source of support and encouragement.

William A. Hargreaves
Martha Shumway
Teh-wei Hu
Brian Cuffel

1

COST–OUTCOME RESEARCH

IN MENTAL HEALTH

*Dr. Doe, the county mental health director, is struggling to prepare her an-
nual budget. The county population has increased since last year, as has demand
for mental health services, but the budget allocation has decreased because of
statewide cutbacks. Not only must Dr. Doe attempt to provide existing services
with fewer dollars, she must also respond to numerous proposals for new services. One request asks her to divert inpatient funding to an intensive community
case management program for the severely mentally ill. Another from the county
hospital asks for more inpatient funding to avoid citations and fines for over-
crowding on the inpatient and emergency services. Outpatient clinic directors
are asking the county to pay for an expensive new antipsychotic medication that
most insurance plans do not cover. The local PTA is requesting special mental
health services for at-risk children in the schools, and the sheriff's department
wants mental health services for inmates in the county jail. Homeowners in several new subdivisions have written letters asking for a new community mental
health clinic. A group of administrators is suggesting that the mental health department join other county health services in developing a managed care plan.
Dr. Doe knows the county mental health department should fund services that
provide the greatest benefit to county residents, but which services are those? All
the current services are used; all the new proposals are promising. How should
the mental health budget be allocated?*

Like Dr. Doe, decision makers at all levels of health and mental health care
face difficult choices. Consumers choose between costly fee-for-service insurance plans that offer many health care choices and less expensive managed care
plans that offer fewer choices. Physicians decide whether the added cost of new

medications is justified. Clinic directors decide whether psychiatrists or social workers should provide outpatient psychotherapy. System administrators decide which types of services should be funded. Legislators determine the appropriate level of funding for public health services. These decision makers have much in common. All seek answers to the same core questions about the outcomes and costs of alternative treatment approaches. How well do the treatments work? How much do they cost? Who pays for them? Which treatments yield the greatest health improvement for each dollar invested?

Whether they make decisions at the individual, community, or national level, these decision makers are typically unable to answer these core questions from their personal knowledge and experience. In choosing treatment strategies, they must rely on external sources of information. They need objective, generalizable empirical evidence about the relationships between treatment costs and treatment outcomes. A set of related strategies, which we call "cost–outcome research," informs treatment choices by systematically analyzing the relationships between the costs and outcomes of alternative health care interventions. By examining outcomes in relation to economic cost, decision makers can determine which treatments and services yield the greatest health improvements for each dollar invested.

This book describes the motivation, application, and interpretation of cost–outcome analyses of mental health interventions. It provides a cohesive and comprehensive guide to both the theory and methods of cost–outcome analysis, including special design issues, economic concepts, methods for collecting cost and outcome data, and strategies for integrating and interpreting these data. This initial chapter introduces the issues associated with cost–outcome analysis and presents an overview of how the subsequent chapters address these issues.

1.1 REAL-WORLD INFORMATION
FOR DECISION MAKERS

The literature on mental health services includes many studies that investigate how well different mental health treatments work. Decision makers who peruse this literature initially may think that it contains ample empirical data to inform treatment decisions. A closer inspection, however, reveals crucial distinctions between **efficacy** studies, which compare alternative treatments under tightly controlled research conditions, and **effectiveness** studies, which compare alternative treatments under typical, real-world treatment conditions. Efficacy studies—the randomized clinical trials and other research designs that have long formed the foundation of scientific inquiry in medicine—usually do not provide all the information necessary for treatment and policy decisions. These clinical studies often are conducted in academic research settings, which differ from typical treatment settings. Such research settings usually employ specially trained staff and often treat only a narrow range of patients who may be more motivated and less ill than patients served in typical service settings. Many clinical studies focus on a limited range of short-term outcomes, such as changes in symptoms, and do not explore long-term impact on more global outcomes, such as social and role functioning. Relatively few clinical studies include information on costs associated with studied treatments. Thus, while traditional clinical efficacy research provides essential information about the relative value of alternative treatments, it does not provide the full range of information decision makers need.

Effectiveness studies examine a broader array of outcomes in relation to treatment costs in typical treatment settings. Thus, effectiveness studies yield results that decision makers can use in making treatment and policy choices. The distinctions between efficacy and effectiveness studies and a variety of research designs appropriate for effectiveness studies are explored in detail in Chapter 2. Here, however, we will briefly examine some of the decisions Dr. Doe faces in our case example to illustrate the importance of these design issues.

It is easy to imagine Dr. Doe turning to the library for empirical evidence about the relative value of the various existing and proposed treatment programs. Dr. Doe might start by looking for literature on the new antipsychotic drug that the outpatient clinics want to prescribe. The randomized controlled trials employed in clinical psychopharmacology should yield unambiguous findings that make it easy to decide whether the county should pay for the drug. Since the drug is new, there are only a few published studies. At first, Dr. Doe is reassured by their well-controlled randomized designs and their statistically significant findings that the new drug provides more symptom relief than a standard antipsychotic. She becomes less confident, however, as she reviews the studies more closely.

The new drug did prove superior to a standard antipsychotic, but the statistically significant differences represented differences of only a few points on a symptom measure administered after six weeks of treatment. Dr. Doe isn't sure that this difference is clinically significant and the journal articles don't describe what happened after six weeks of treatment. Also, the patients in the published studies were carefully selected. They had been ill for less than five years, were stable on other medications when they started the new medication, and had no medical illnesses or substance abuse problems. During the study period, they were seen weekly by research psychiatrists in a university clinic. Dr. Doe knows that patients in the county clinics are much more varied than these samples. Some have been chronically ill for many years, others have never responded well to any antipsychotic medications, and others are dually diagnosed with substance abuse disorders or medical illnesses. Most see an outpatient psychiatrist only once a month. It is not clear that the promising published results would generalize to all these patients. Finally, none of the studies include cost data. It seems obvious that the new drug will cost more than standard drugs and there is no way to tell whether the small clinical improvement will justify the added cost. Dr. Doe sees references to "pharmacoeconomic" studies, which examine costs and outcomes associated with drug treatment, but there are no such studies of this particular drug. Thus, even rigorous efficacy studies may not provide the information required to make optimal treatment choices.

Disappointed by her initial search for evidence, Dr. Doe recalls seeing a number of articles over the years on different forms of community case management for the severely mentally ill. She hopes they will help her evaluate the proposal for the new community-based program. She finds many studies of various forms of case management and "assertive community treatment" (ACT) programs. Several of the ACT studies include both costs and a wide range of outcomes and they indicate that these programs are as good or better than inpatient treatment for many severely mentally ill individuals. Although none of the studies was done in her state, results are similar in older and recent studies conducted in urban and rural settings. These studies convince Dr. Doe that the proposed program merits further consideration and that cost–outcome studies can be valuable decision aids.

The experience of the hypothetical Dr. Doe illustrates the two primary factors that prompted this book. First, cost–outcome analysis is extremely useful for comparing alternative mental health treatments to facilitate optimal treatment and policy decisions. Second, cost–outcome analyses are not conducted frequently enough to inform many important decisions. The next sections review the history of cost–outcome research in mental health and explore obstacles to the conduct of these studies.

1.2 MENTAL HEALTH COST–OUTCOME STUDIES: A BRIEF REVIEW

Decision makers and researchers have long recognized the promise of cost–outcome studies and there has been a relatively high level of interest in cost–outcome research in mental health. In 1981, when Hu and Sandifer reviewed 17 disease categories to compile their *Synthesis of Cost of Illness Methodology,* they found 51 economic studies in the mental disorders category, more than in any other disease category, and the frequency of such studies appeared to be increasing with time. Despite this promising start, however, the number of mental health cost–outcome studies has not continued to increase over time. The percentage of mental health outcome studies with cost components gradually increased from approximately 1% in the late 1960s to approximately 5% in 1985. The percentage then stabilized, or even decreased slightly, between 1985 and 1991 (Yates, 1994). Even more disconcerting is the relatively small number of complete and rigorous studies that compute comparative cost–effectiveness or cost–benefit ratios for alternative mental health interventions. The largest number of such studies (eight) was published between 1981 and 1985, decreasing to five studies between 1986 and 1990 and three studies between 1991 and 1995 (Cuffel, unpublished manuscript).

The body of published cost–outcome studies is also limited in scope. The majority of studies examine the costs and outcomes associated with community-based treatments for the severely mentally ill. This group of studies includes early studies, such as those by McCaffree (1969), Cassell and co-workers (1972), Murphy and Datel (1976), Sharfstein and Nafziger (1976), Guillette and co-workers (1978), and Weisbrod and co-workers (1980; Weisbrod, 1981; 1983). The seminal study in this group is the study by Weisbrod and co-workers—a cost–benefit analysis comparing the Stein and Test "training in community living" (TCL) model with standard hospital-based treatment. Weisbrod's comprehensive cost–accounting framework and rigorous analysis confirm the essential findings of earlier studies that community-based alternatives are equally or more cost-effective than traditional hospital-based treatments for a wide range of persons presenting for hospitalization. Subsequent studies maintained this focus on community treatments for the severely mentally ill, including home-based care (Fenton et al., 1984; Burns et al., 1991; 1993; Knapp et al., 1994), residential treatment facilities (Dickey et al., 1986b, c), day treatment (Wiersma et al., 1995), and various forms of case management and adaptations of the TCL or ACT model (Hoult et al., 1983; 1984a, b; Bond et al., 1984; 1988; Franklin et al., 1987; Jerrell and Hu, 1989; 1991; Rosenheck et al., 1995c). Reviews and syntheses of this group of studies uniformly reach the conclusion that community treatment is as or more cost-effective than hospital-based treatment for the severely mentally ill (Olfson, 1990; Goldberg, 1991; 1994; 1995; Dauwalder and Ciompi, 1995).

Cost–outcome analyses of treatments for the severely and persistently mentally ill are clearly a high priority because these treatments are costly, long-term, and largely government funded. The notable lack of cost–outcome research on treatments for other diagnostic groups, however, limits the information available for comprehensive policy decisions about mental health care. Investigators are beginning to study costs and outcomes associated with serious but less disabling and pervasive disorders. Several recent studies examine alternative treatments for major depression through secondary analysis of existing data (Hatziandreu et al., 1994; Kamlet et al., 1995; Sturm and Wells, 1995) and in randomized cost–outcome trials (Rosset and Andreoli, 1995). Another study examines the cost-effectiveness of treatments for the eating disorder bulimia nervosa (Koran et al., 1995). In addition to increased attention to treatments for specific disorders, there is increased interest in specific treatment modalities—particularly psychotherapy (Krupnick and Pincus, 1992; Miller and Magruder, in press). Pharmacoeconomic research on the costs and effects of specific drugs is also gaining momentum (Revicki and Luce, 1995; Hargreaves and Shumway, 1996). Finally, investigators have also begun to conduct cost–outcome evaluations of mental health system innovations, such as capitated provision of mental health services at both local (Reed et al., 1994) and state (Christianson et al., 1995) levels.

The studies mentioned in this brief review form a promising foundation for mental health cost–outcome research, but many important questions remain unanswered. Key issues remain unresolved even in the relatively well-studied area of community care for the severely mentally ill (Attkisson et al., 1992; Mechanic et al., 1992; Steinwachs et al., 1992). The relative cost-effectiveness of the many forms and applications of psychotherapy remains largely unstudied and unknown (Krupnick and Pincus, 1992). The impact of new managed care strategies on the costs and outcomes of mental health services also remains largely unexamined (Wells et al., 1995).

1.3 OVERCOMING OBSTACLES TO COST–OUTCOME RESEARCH IN MENTAL HEALTH

It is not immediately obvious why the pace of mental health cost–outcome research has slowed. There are strong motivations for cost–outcome analysis and both long-standing and emerging issues to address. Existing studies illustrate the value of cost–outcome comparisons. Careful consideration, however, reveals attitudinal and practical obstacles that limit the conduct of such studies. Attitudinal obstacles include concerns about economic approaches and differences in perspective among researchers studying mental health services. Practical obstacles include a lack of standardized methods, difficulties in adapting standard health economic approaches to the study of mental health interventions, and problems in obtaining and integrating accurate data.

1.3.1 ATTITUDINAL OBSTACLES

One major attitudinal obstacle is distrust of economic evaluation. Many people are uneasy at the prospect of putting a price tag on mental health. They often worry that adding cost data to an analysis shifts attention away from clinical outcomes and merely provides a rationale for funding cuts. Others may feel that cost–outcome analyses are unnecessary because they make faulty assumptions about how costs relate to outcomes. Some people assume that higher expenditures automatically buy more services and better outcomes and that more treatment is always better than less (Yates, 1994). The theory and examples presented throughout this book demonstrate that cost–outcome analysis can be used to test these and other assumptions and is a powerful tool for identifying the most beneficial treatment options and optimizing resource allocation so that more effective treatment can be provided.

Decision makers, including clinicians and researchers, are often wary of cost–outcome analyses because they are not familiar with economic terminology. Some concepts such as "market prices" and "discount rates" may be familiar from introductory economics courses, but others, such as "shadow prices" and the difference between "costs" and "charges" are concepts more specific to cost–outcome research. In Chapter 3, we review the economic theories that form the basis for cost–outcome analysis and define key terms relevant to analyses of mental health interventions. With this basic framework in place, readers will be prepared to understand and apply the methods for data collection, analysis, and interpretation presented in later chapters.

Mental health cost–outcome studies are by necessity multidisciplinary efforts, requiring collaboration among investigators from academic and professional disciplines such as psychiatry, economics, psychology, social work, sociology, biostatistics, and public health. Interdisciplinary differences in research training and perspective can be an obstacle to these collaborative endeavors (Phillips and Rosenblatt, 1992). Researchers from different disciplines identify with different research traditions, are accustomed to different study designs, and are familiar with different data analytic techniques. For example, most psychiatrists and psychologists are experienced in the conduct of randomized, experimental studies and the use of standardized measurement instruments. Many sociologists and social workers are more familiar with observational and qualitative research approaches, while many economists specialize in the integration and analysis of large existing data sets. Ideologically, most mental health services researchers view these different perspectives as an advantage that enriches the field rather than as an obstacle. In practice, however, collaboration is often hindered by subtle differences in vocabulary and methodology. In the remaining chapters we try to identify and explore these disciplinary differences to facilitate effective collaboration in cost–outcome studies.

1.3.2 PRACTICAL OBSTACLES

The most significant obstacles to mental health cost–outcome research stem from the lack of a standard, complete, and feasible methodology. Although there are widely accepted standards for general health economic evaluation, they do not fully address many important issues unique to mental health services. A small, but growing, literature focuses on aspects of cost–outcome methodology specifically relevant to mental health care, and a number of existing texts provide valuable insights into the conduct of cost–outcome research in mental health. They include books by McGuire and Weisbrod (1981a), Netten and Beecham (1993), Knapp (1995a), Frank and Manning (1992), Moscarelli et al. (1996), and Yates (1996). The majority of these references are edited volumes, compiling the work of different authors or describing specific research programs. As a result, they do not provide the systematic discussion of methods that investigators need to design and conduct cost–outcome studies. The primary goal of this book is to provide a comprehensive and cohesive guide to methods for cost–outcome analysis of mental health interventions.

The majority of this book, Chapters 4 through 10, is designed to help investigators overcome the practical obstacles that have limited the implementation of cost–outcome research. These chapters build on the background material on research design and economic theory presented in Chapters 2 and 3 to describe specific methods for collecting and analyzing cost and outcome data and decision strategies for choosing among these methods. Chapters 4 through 7 describe methods for obtaining cost and outcome data. Chapters 8 and 9 describe methods for aggregating and analyzing cost and outcome data, and Chapter 10 describes strategies for applying cost–outcome findings. The content of these chapters is described in greater detail below.

Chapters 4 through 7 provide detailed descriptions of the rationale and applied methodologies for acquiring data for mental health cost–outcome analysis. These four chapters describe methods for collecting data on service utilization, economic costs, service practices, and mental health outcomes.

Computing the cost of any intervention involves multiplying the amount of services used by the cost of each service component. Chapter 4 describes methods for measuring resource utilization. This involves identifying the mental health services, such as hospital care and outpatient psychotherapy, and other resources, such as social services and family contributions, associated with an intervention and determining the appropriate unit of measurement for each resource. For example, utilization of inpatient psychiatric services is frequently measured in days, while utilization of psychotherapy services is frequently measured in minutes or hours. This chapter is closely linked to the methods for cost estimation described next in Chapter 5, since cost values must be assigned to each resource unit.

Chapter 5 describes methods for estimating the economic cost of the units of mental health services and other resources. The chapter builds on the economic concepts presented in Chapter 3 and describes sources of cost data and methods for estimating resource costs to suit different analytic goals. Special emphasis is given to cost estimation problems that are particularly common in studies of mental health services, such as estimating the costs of publicly funded services and determining the dollar value of productivity losses associated with mental illnesses. Methods for adjusting costs to permit valid comparison of interventions implemented at different times and different locations are also presented.

Chapter 6 is devoted to methods for measuring program practices, or the actual content of mental health interventions. Cost estimation is complicated by the great variety and complexity of mental health treatments. Common labels for mental health services, such as case management and psychotherapy, do not accurately reflect real variations in treatment content. It is difficult to accurately estimate service costs if treatment content is not adequately described or measured. In the absence of an accurate description of treatment content, it is also difficult to determine whether success or failure of a service model is due to specific, planned features of the model or to other, unintended factors.

Outcome measurement in cost–outcome studies is discussed in Chapter 7. The outcomes targeted by most mental health interventions, such as psychotic or depressive symptoms or general psychological well-being, tend to be more subjective than the outcomes of most physical health interventions. Physical health outcomes often are reflected quite meaningfully by simple indicators such as mortality rate, while many mental health outcomes require more complex and cumbersome psychometric assessment instruments. Not only are mental health outcomes generally more difficult to measure, most mental health interventions have multiple outcomes that must be assessed using different outcome measures. This chapter identifies key outcome domains and characteristics of outcome measures particularly appropriate for cost–outcome research. The strengths and weaknesses of general approaches to outcome measurement and of specific outcome instruments are reviewed to illustrate strategies for selecting measures in different study contexts.

Chapters 8 and 9 describe methods for aggregating and analyzing cost and outcome data after it is collected. Chapter 8 presents strategies for aggregating outcome measurements. As Chapter 6 illustrates, the complexity of mental health outcomes necessitates the use of multiple outcome measures. However, the kind comprehensive cost–outcome analyses that reveal the superiority or inferiority of a particular intervention require a single aggregate outcome indicator that can be examined in relation to total cost. Various strategies for obtaining aggregate outcome indicators are discussed. These strategies include using global measures, weighting outcomes by measures of importance or utility, and converting outcomes into common metrics such as quality-adjusted life years (QALYs).

Methods for analyzing cost and outcome data are presented in Chapter 9. Discussion of statistical inferences in cost–outcome analysis and interpretation of cost–effectiveness ratios is followed by illustrations of regression approaches to analyzing the impact of treatment, subject characteristics, site, and time on cost-effectiveness.

Chapter 10 discusses how research findings are applied to policy and practice. The concept of policy itself is discussed from an economic perspective. Four techniques for reviewing and synthesizing research findings to facilitate choice among policy alternatives are considered: qualitative reviews, meta-analysis, clinical decision making, and cross-design synthesis. Finally, Chapter 10 reviews the recommendations made throughout the book for improving the quality and policy relevance of cost–outcome research on mental health care.

1.4 CHAPTER REVIEW

Cost–outcome research informs treatment practice and policy by examining relationships between the costs and outcomes of alternative health care interventions to determine which treatments and services yield the greatest health improvements for each dollar invested. Cost–outcome research studies "effectiveness" rather than "efficacy." Efficacy studies evaluate the effects of interventions under optimal conditions in which specially trained clinicians treat a highly selected patient population following strict protocols. Effectiveness studies complement the findings of efficacy studies by evaluating interventions in conditions, settings, and target populations that reflect typical conditions for service delivery.

Although cost–outcome analysis has long been recognized as a valuable tool for decision making about mental health services, only 5% of mental health outcome studies include cost components, and very few studies report cost–effectiveness or cost–benefit ratios for alternative interventions. There appears to be a renewed emphasis on cost–outcome analysis, but it is not yet reflected in publications. Published cost–outcome studies are also relatively limited in scope, with most focusing on community-based treatments for the severely mentally ill. A few recent studies address other disorders, such as depression, and specific treatment modalities, such as psychotherapy. Nonetheless, many important questions about mental health services remain to be addressed.

Attitudinal and practical obstacles have limited the application of cost–outcome analyses in the evaluation of mental health services. Attitudinal obstacles include concerns about economic approaches and differences in perspective among researchers studying mental health services. Practical obstacles include a lack of standardized methods, difficulties in adapting standard health economic approaches to the study of mental health interventions, and problems in obtaining and integrating accurate data. This book attempts to overcome these obstacles by presenting economic concepts in a way that is accessible to students and investigators who do not have a background in economics, by presenting currently accepted methods, and by discussing issues encountered in adapting economic methods to the study of mental health services.

2

SPECIAL DESIGN ISSUES IN COST–OUTCOME RESEARCH

A large health maintenance organization (HMO) initiates discussion with an academic research team about the possibility of adopting a brief group psychotherapy intervention for posttraumatic stress disorder (PTSD). The HMO's research director and chief of psychiatry explain that a growing number of trauma victims are seeking repeated emergency medical care even after recovery from the specific injuries caused by the trauma. Their psychiatry service has no specific expertise in the treatment of posttraumatic stress and would welcome assistance in implementing the treatment and in testing its cost-effectiveness. The academic research team has conducted controlled efficacy trials of the intervention with military veterans and the results have been promising. They are interested in understanding the generalizability of their intervention to women and nonmilitary personnel.

Early discussions between the two groups are encouraging. Each agrees that the intervention should be limited to research participants and that assignment to the intervention should be random. Talk stalemates, however, over the criteria for selecting trauma victims for the new intervention. The HMO insists that the new intervention be offered to persons as soon as they are identified as trauma victims with symptoms of anxiety or depression. The academic investigators insist that they enroll only those persons who meet diagnostic criteria for posttraumatic stress disorder. Using diagnostic criteria for PTSD, persons would not be eligible for the intervention until one month following the traumatic event, consistent with the DSM-III-R. The academic investigators state that early intervention would prevent a clear diagnosis and preclude learning whether the intervention "really works for PTSD." They argue that an efficacy trial should first examine intervention effects on true PTSD before testing whether it is effective for a broader population. The HMO thinks it unlikely that strict criteria for PTSD can be implemented in their primary care service and that narrow inclusion criteria will impair the generalizability of the findings to the HMO's typical patient. Both parties come to realize that their disagreements reflect differences in the specific research question each thinks is important and that their differences can be settled only when they agree on whether the study should test the intervention's "efficacy" or "effectiveness."

Investigators studying the costs and outcomes of mental health services face many challenges in designing studies that are valid and generalizable. As the case example illustrates, there is sometimes a divergence between an optimal study design in an "efficacy trial" and an optimal study design in a "effectiveness trial." Drawing on the work of Cook and Campbell (1979), we discuss here four elements of study design as they bear on this divergence: (1) internal validity, (2) external validity, (3) construct validity, and (4) statistical conclusion validity. We discuss internal validity as it pertains to confounding in mental health intervention research, external validity as it pertains to the generalizability of cost–outcome findings, construct validity as it pertains to the specification and measurement of mental health interventions and outcomes, and statistical conclusion validity as it pertains to planning cost–outcome studies, especially the choice of sample size. Statistical analysis of cost–outcome data is more generally presented in Chapter 9.

2.1 INTRODUCTION TO STUDY DESIGN AND TERMINOLOGY

In its simplest terms, experimental research examines the effects of X on Y. X is typically an intervention of interest and is manipulated or controlled in order to determine its influence on a set of outcomes denoted by Y. Readers of this book are probably concerned with one of three types of interventions: (1) a new clinical treatment, (2) a new clinical program, or (3) a new way of organizing or financing mental health care. Published research has examined the effectiveness and cost of all three types of interventions. See for example, Essock et al. (1996a, b) for a cost–effectiveness study of a clinical intervention, Weisbrod (1983) for a cost–benefit study of a clinical program, and Lurie et al. (1992) for a cost–effectiveness study of a change in mental health financing. Y is a set of outcome variables hypothesized to be affected by the intervention and may include both costs and outcomes. Outcomes may be specific signs and symptoms of mental disorder; functional deficits resulting from mental disorder; or broader outcomes, such as health status or quality of life. X is commonly referred to as the independent variable, and Y as the dependent variable or outcome variable.

In this chapter, we discuss many choices regarding the design of studies that will test differences in costs and outcomes across interventions that are commonly encountered in research on mental health services. The reader expecting a catalog of methodological do's and don'ts will undoubtedly be disappointed. Choice of appropriate method is frequently determined by the overall goals of the research and existing or theoretical knowledge of X, Y, and the nature of the relationship between X and Y. In the example at the beginning of this chapter, the most appropriate study design depends on whether the investigator's goal is to examine the effects of an intervention as it might be practiced in a typical practice setting or in a specially constructed scenario assuring diagnostic homogeneity in the study sample.

The example illustrates a methodological distinction that is central to many decisions regarding the design of cost–outcome studies. In this book, we contrast the design of efficacy studies with that of effectiveness studies. Different design choices in efficacy and effectiveness trials stem from differences in their purpose, including differing emphasis on internal and external validity. Efficacy studies evaluate the effects of an intervention under optimal conditions, when implemented by highly skilled practitioners using comprehensive treatment protocols under expert supervision. Effectiveness studies extend the evaluation of interventions to conditions and settings that reflect the usual circumstances of service delivery. Efficacy trials use highly controlled experimental conditions to unambiguously estimate treatment effects. In doing so, the experimental conditions of efficacy trials often do not resemble usual practice conditions and limit the generalizability of study findings. Effectiveness trials do not sacrifice the generalizability of study results by creating artificial intervention conditions although internal validity is still important. Knowing whether one's primary goal is to test an intervention's effectiveness or efficacy is of primary importance in guiding many design choices.

Design choice is also guided by the researcher's knowledge (or conjecture) of how the intervention (X) affects outcomes (Y). The art and craft of study design lies in how the researcher translates insights into the nature of intervention and outcome into study designs that test key aspects of the intervention-outcome connection. Expert knowledge of the intervention will guide decisions about what outcomes to measure, how to measure them, over what periods of time, and in what types of populations. Expert knowledge also will include knowledge of the existing empirical literature for the intervention. Researchers should set the priorities among their own research questions with full knowledge of the findings of prior studies of the same or similar interventions. If an intervention's efficacy has been established in prior research, how does the intervention perform in typical practice settings on a broad range of economic and clinical outcomes? If an intervention's effectiveness has been established in a variety of practice settings, what is known about the intervention's mechanisms of effect and how can these hypothesized mechanisms be measured? As empirical knowledge of an intervention advances, priorities can be tailored more specifically to the remaining gaps in knowledge. Chapter 6 expands on this process of translating theories of interventions into testable hypotheses and measures. The remainder of this chapter will explore some basic principles of study design.

2.2 INTERNAL VALIDITY

The central problem faced in research is that the dependent variable may be affected by factors other than the independent variable. Any variable that affects the dependent variable other than the independent variable is referred to as an extraneous variable. In the case example, the outcomes of brief group therapy for PTSD may be affected by factors other than the intervention, such as the demographic characteristics of those receiving the intervention, whether or not they abuse alcohol, and whether or not they have preexisting anxiety or depressive disorders. If extraneous variables are related to the intervention in a systematic way, they are said to confound, or bias, study results. A confound is any extraneous variable that varies systematically with the intervention and represents a more or less compelling alternative explanation for study findings. That is, for any study in which a confound has been identified, the results could be due to the effects of the intervention, the effects of the confound, or both, and there is no way to disentangle those effects.

Internal validity is the degree to which the study is confound free. An internally valid design minimizes the confounding effects of extraneous factors. In cost–outcome research, internal validity is the degree to which the clinical, programmatic, or system intervention is unconfounded by extraneous factors that might affect study outcomes. The number of possible confounding factors in research on mental health costs and outcomes is large, and the number of valid study designs are relatively few. We review three designs available for studying costs and outcomes: the pretest-posttest design, the randomized groups design, and the nonequivalent groups design. Then we describe threats to internal validity in the pretest-posttest design and describe how the two alternative designs reduce the confounding influence of these threats through the use of control groups.

2.2.1 PRETEST–POSTTEST DESIGNS AND THREATS TO INTERNAL VALIDITY

Sometimes investigators try to estimate the effects of an intervention by comparing the performance of a group following an intervention to their performance prior to an intervention, a so-called "mirror-image" design. Sometimes this design is presented with the hope that the subjects are "serving as their own controls." In the case example, the various outcomes—symptoms, functioning, quality of life, and health care costs—would be compared before and after the brief group treatment. Unfortunately, improvements in any of these outcomes could not be attributed unambiguously to the effects of the intervention. That is, there would exist a number of "threats" to the internal validity of the design

(Cook and Campbell, 1979; Campbell and Stanley, 1966). We will mention three briefly: (1) regression to the mean, (2) testing and instrumentation, and (3) history and maturation.

Regression to the Mean

Extreme scores on any outcome measure tend to return or "regress" to less extreme scores on subsequent administrations of the measure whether or not an intervention takes place. If patients are selected at a high level of symptoms or a low point of functioning, they will tend to improve, returning toward a more moderate level, regardless of treatment. This results from two types of "measurement error." First, selecting those with extreme values at baseline ensures selection of persons who are more symptomatic or poorer functioning than usual. Regression to the mean, reflecting subjects' return to their typical level of symptoms and functioning will artificially appear as improvement in study outcome measures. Second, study outcomes usually are not measured with absolute accuracy. Therefore, some subjects erroneously will score high enough at baseline to qualify for the study. On repeated administration of the outcome measures, such subjects are likely to get lower scores again, reflecting regression to the mean. This change also will appear to be improvement when outcome measures are examined. Regression effects will not be offset by regression to the mean of erroneously healthy baseline scores because those potential subjects have been excluded from the study. A comparison group selected in the same way but not receiving the intervention is necessary to estimate the size of these regression effects. Regression to the mean as a study confound is illustrated by a recent study of clozapine treatment for schizophrenia, as described in Example 1.

EXAMPLE 1

Meltzer et al. (1993) studied 47 patients with schizophrenia receiving the antipsychotic drug clozapine, collecting cost data for two years before and two years after patients started the drug. There was a 23% drop in treatment cost from reduced hospital days and improvement in symptoms and quality of life among a subgroup who continued on clozapine for two years. The authors concluded that clozapine is a cost-effective treatment. Does their study design support their claim?

In a subsequent exchange of letters, critics questioned the study methodology (Essock, 1995; Meltzer and Cola, 1995; Rosenheck et al., 1995a; Schiller and Hargreaves, 1995). They cited evidence that selection for clozapine tends to identify patients at a low point in functioning and a high point in hospital utilization. Therefore, regression to the mean could produce apparently improved outcomes and lower costs regardless of the effect of the drug.

This type of patient selection effect is widespread in studies of innovative treatments. Patients screened on entry to treatment are typically at a bad place in their lives. That may be why they sought treatment, or why others pressured them to get treatment. Similarly, study subjects selected because they are experiencing an acute episode, or are being discharged from the hospital, or are "high-cost" patients will show improvement with time, on average. For patients in continuing treatment, usual practice is to implement an innovative treatment when results of current treatment are unsatisfactory either to the clinician or patient. All of these patient groups, on average, may tend to do better after study entry regardless of subsequent treatment. Thus, information on previous life course and treatment cost can be valuable, but it does not substitute for a design that includes a control or comparison group that is subject to the same regression effects.

Testing and Instrumentation Effects

The act of measuring mental health outcomes may threaten the internal validity of the pretest-posttest study if baseline measures affect responses on follow-up measures. There may be practice effects on measures of cognitive impairment, allowing persons to improve their scores through repeated exposure to the test rather than through improvements in their cognitive functioning. Measures of psychological distress may show improvement on repeated administration because subjects may benefit from talking to a concerned research interviewer about their lives, their symptoms, and inner experiences.

Measurement problems may be compounded if measurement procedures vary over the course of the study. Many mental health outcome measures involve interviewer ratings or observational procedures. Such measurement procedures inevitably involve some judgment on the part of the individual administering the measure, and ratings may "drift" over time as interviewers and observers become more experienced with the measures and adjust their rating standards based on experience with rating prior subjects. In addition, staff turnover may result in different interviewers conducting baseline and follow-up assessments. Finally, ratings requiring observer judgment are affected by subjective factors such as expectancies and interviewer biases. Changes in outcome measures may not reflect real changes in outcomes, but instead reflect changes in how outcome measures are being administered. The effects of baseline measurement on outcomes cannot be estimated without a more complex design.

History and Maturation

Historical events or naturally occurring changes shared by subjects in pretest-posttest studies may account for observed outcomes. Subjects in particular settings may experience beneficial or detrimental life events that affect outcomes but are not due to the intervention. For example, clinical settings are inevitably embedded in a changing mental health and social service environment. Changes to the treatment delivery system and broader social service system may impact outcomes or costs beyond the treatment itself. In addition, factors such as caseload changes and staff turnover during the study may affect treatment outcomes.

The natural progression of mental disorders also may account for improvement or deterioration in outcome. Persons act to alleviate the symptoms of their disorders more or less successfully on their own and independently of the studied intervention. Without appropriate control groups, the effects of these naturally occurring changes cannot be disentangled from the effects of the intervention in simple pretest-posttest designs. Therefore, an important aspect of research design is the creation of control or comparison groups through random assignment and through other mechanisms.

2.2.2 RANDOM ASSIGNMENT OF SUBJECTS TO TREATMENT

Random assignment of subjects to treatment and comparison groups is the most dependable way to avoid the confounds inherent in pretest-posttest designs. With random assignment, all persons enrolled in a study have the same probability of being assigned to the intervention group. Assignment is determined using a randomly generated sequence of treatment assignments. As sample size increases, the distribution of extraneous variables affecting treatment outcome will tend to be equally distributed between treatment and control groups. The real strength of random assignment is that it equalizes the groups, on average, even on unmeasured factors. In effectiveness research, the number of possible extraneous variables is large, difficult to specify ahead of time, and impossible to measure in totality. This is why random assignment is the "gold standard" of cost–outcome study design. This does not mean that the patient groups randomly assigned to each service will always have exactly the same distribution of extraneous variables, since this distribution will vary randomly and only tend toward equality with large sample sizes. One can improve comparability by taking into account known prognostic variables in the randomization procedure, but the randomization process will still balance the groups on unknown factors. Random variation remains, but is taken into account in statistical analyses of group differences in outcome.

Several conditions are necessary for a randomized design to be feasible and ethical. In most situations subjects can only be randomized to treatment after they have been given an adequate explanation of the study and their choices outside of the study. They must be able to understand this explanation, they must consent to participate without coercion, and they must be free to withdraw from the assigned treatment or any study procedures at any time after consent. Investigator compliance with these standards is monitored before and during the study. It is generally considered unethical to randomize subjects to a treatment that is less than the currently accepted local standard of treatment for their condition—that is, what they would receive in the local setting if there were no study. Thus, the cost-effectiveness of the currently accepted and available treatment cannot, in principle, be evaluated in a randomized trial in which a less intensive or substandard treatment forms the comparison condition.

These conditions are not as much of a limitation as they might seem. Most innovations are attempts either to improve effectiveness, or to reduce cost without reducing effectiveness. If the innovation plausibly meets this definition, it can be studied in a randomized trial. Even draconian cuts in services can be evaluated in a controlled trial, if the cuts are made independent of the research, and the research compares the new care standard to an enhanced service condition like the former care standard. Such comparisons are ethical only if access to previously accepted, higher level services is through participation in the study. The incremental funding to restore the previous level is explicitly part of the funding of the study, and the extra funding would not be available if the study were not being conducted. The strong feelings and real ambiguities associated with these ethical issues highlight the value of independent institutional review of study protocols.

2.2.3 THREATS TO INTERNAL VALIDITY IN RANDOMIZED TRIALS

Loss of Subjects from Follow-up

Loss of data on subjects after they are recruited, give consent, and are randomized threatens the internal validity of a randomized trial. Failure to stay in touch with all subjects to the end of the planned follow-up period and failure to complete all outcome assessments can lead to biased loss of subjects. If subjects with poor prognosis are more likely to be lost to follow-up in one service than another, that service will spuriously appear to have better outcomes.

Loss of Subjects from Assigned Service

After randomization, a subject may refuse the assigned service or drop out early. Investigators sometimes feel that such subjects should be excluded from the analysis because they did not get the full treatment. It is important not to drop subjects from outcome assessment because they have stopped the assigned treatment, however, since their loss may destroy the original comparability of the treatment groups produced by randomization. Standard practice is to conduct "intent-to-treat analyses" in which all of the originally assigned subjects are included in statistical analyses, regardless of treatment dropout or crossover, to minimize the introduction of bias from differential subject loss and preserve both internal and external validity (Lavori, 1992a, b; Greenhouse, 1992; Kraemer, 1992; Laska, 1992; DB Rubin, 1992; Shrout, 1992). One can also conduct and report "as-treated" analyses, including only subjects who received a minimum amount of treatment. Confidence in the findings is strengthened if both types of analysis lead to the same conclusion. If findings differ, one must try to understand why, usually by determining the biases in the dropout or crossover process. If the investigator drops from follow-up subjects who leave or never accept their assigned treatment, however, and if this number is large, interpretation of study findings will be seriously compromised, because the effects of dropout biases will be difficult to evaluate.

Improperly Implemented Randomization

Improperly implemented randomization can also jeopardize the internal validity of a randomized trial. The key is to keep the recruitment process absolutely separate from randomization. If anyone knows the assignment of the next subject, there will be opportunities to intentionally or unintentionally corrupt the randomization process. Subjects may be subtly encouraged or discouraged from joining the study depending on the recruiter's view of the suitability of the assigned service to the candidate. Intentional bias is also possible by rearranging the order of recruitment so that assignments match the recruiter's judgment of suitable assignments. Adequate randomization requires an arm's-length procedure, such as one in which the recruiter, having determined that the person is qualified and having obtained written informed consent, contacts a project coordinator to log in the subject and get the assignment.

2.2.4 NONRANDOMIZED COMPARISON GROUP DESIGNS

Sometimes randomization is not an option. This is often true in studies of service system innovations. If the innovation is introduced in all sites, there may be no alternative to a simple pre-post design, which may not allow a meaningful cost–outcome investigation. A "pilot program" process is sometimes used, however, to stage the introduction of an innovation. This has been true in several states as they have introduced capitation and other managed care innovations into the delivery of publicly funded mental health care. Investigators working with these states have been able to mount comparison designs that take advantage of the experiment-like staging of the innovation, even when randomization has not been the method used to determine the sequence in which sites must adopt the innovation (e.g., Bloom et al., 1997). Such "natural experiments" are often sufficiently important and informative that they are undertaken even though baseline site differences are a constant threat to the interpretation of findings. Studies that use natural variation or any other nonrandom method of assigning subjects to the experimental and comparison groups are referred to as "nonrandomized," "nonequivalent," or "quasi-experimental" comparison designs.

In nonrandomized designs, the equivalence of the experimental and comparison groups cannot be assured, and investigators use various strategies to counter these threats, such as studying subareas of sites to obtain better cross-site matching on demographic and socioeconomic characteristics. Even in nonrandomized studies there are usually some variables—such as severity of illness and prior utilization of services—that can serve as a proxy for baseline prognosis. When baseline prognostic variables differ across treatment groups, it is common to use regression techniques to adjust statistically for the association of these baseline variables with effectiveness and cost, but such adjustments can be suspect for several reasons. Observed baseline differences may not accurately measure prognostic differences. Some methods of statistical adjustment, such as analysis of covariance, involve assumptions that may be unrealistic in particular situations. Finally, unreliable baseline variables can induce spurious apparent group differences in outcomes if relatively simple, common analysis methods are employed. In spite of these shortcomings, careful interpretation of nonexperimental comparative studies can generate useful hypotheses and establish the range of variation for key variables.

When one is planning a study in which randomization is feasible and ethically justifiable, one almost always should choose a randomized design, but there are exceptions. If a very inexpensive trial can be carried out that takes advantage of an existing situation (a "natural experiment"), sometimes this is worth doing rather than a randomized trial, just as Drake et al. (1994; Example 2) took advantage of a planned conversion of a day treatment program into a supported employment program for the same clients. They used a nonrandomized design and dealt with threats to internal validity by using relatively simple statistical analyses. Results were convincing despite the nonequivalent character of the comparison group.

EXAMPLE 2

Drake et al. (1994) compared the effectiveness of supported employment and day treatment in improving vocational outcomes in persons with severe mental illness. Their design was a nonrandomized design that took advantage of a natural experiment occurring in two similar New England communities. Their study design and findings nicely illustrate the advantages and limitations of nonrandomized designs.

In one community, a new supported employment program was being substituted for an existing day treatment program, creating the opportunity to study changes in outcomes for persons in this new program relative to outcomes for persons in the day treatment program of a neighboring community. Clients in both programs were assessed for one year prior to the program change and for one year following implementation of the program.

In the supported employment program, the percentage of persons with some competitive employment increased from 25% to 39% in the follow-up year, while day treatment clients stayed at 13%. No increase in negative outcomes such as suicide attempts, rehospitilization, homelessness, or dropout were observed in the new program.

The investigators discuss potential confounds in their design, noting that baseline rates of competitive employment were higher in the experimental program. To test the effects of this confound, they analyzed only persons without competitive employment during the baseline year. Even with this group, the remodeled program led to greater employment, suggesting that baseline differences in employment did not bias study findings. Staffing and cost were reduced in the remodeled program, so the superior performance was attained in spite of fewer resources.

2.3 EXTERNAL VALIDITY

External validity refers to the extent to which the study results can be generalized beyond the specific circumstances of the experiment. We can think of three broad domains of generalizability that are of particular interest in policy research on mental health costs and outcomes: generalizability to other samples, environments, and times. External validity receives only limited attention in most efficacy studies, but in policy-oriented cost–effectiveness studies external validity is a central issue. To draw policy implications from study findings one must know to whom and to what set of circumstances the findings can be generalized.

2.3.1 THREATS TO THE EXTERNAL VALIDITY OF THE SAMPLE

There are four serious threats to the external validity of the study sample. These four threats occur sequentially in the route from the relevant target group in the population to the analyzed sample of study subjects. Threats to external validity include: (1) systematic exclusion of part of the relevant target group, (2) biased procedures for selecting persons to be approached for consent, (3) biased refusal of consent to the study, and (4) biased loss of subjects from follow-up and outcome assessment. The last is also a threat to internal validity.

Threat 1: Systematic Exclusion

If we consider that the relevant target population for most interventions can be found in communities across the country or across the world, a large portion of any target population is excluded from study because samples are drawn from a limited number of sites. The social, demographic, and economic characteristics of communities from which samples are drawn affect the characteristics of samples and potentially reduce the generalizability of study results to the target population. Generalizability of the sample is further limited if study sites are university settings or any other types of clinical settings in which the study sample is likely to be an unusual subset of the population in some respects.

Rarely does one have a wide choice of study sites and regions except in large multisite trials. For this reason, a unique site may provide an important opportunity to replicate or qualify previously reported findings. The external validity of a single study is rarely adequate to establish generalizability of study results to the target population. Several replications may be needed to obtain confidence in the generalizability of the conclusions.

Investigators moving from efficacy to effectiveness studies often carry with them subject selection habits designed to produce a homogeneous subject population thought to increase study power by removing extraneous sources of variability. Such habits need to be questioned carefully in effectiveness research. Intentional exclusion of subgroups of the target population limits the external validity of the study. A larger study sample, selected with less restrictive criteria, may be more consistent with the objectives of an effectiveness study. The supply of eligible study candidates will be greater when the criteria are less restrictive making larger samples more feasible.

Examples of questionable restrictions easily come to mind. Is the treatment really not applicable to pregnant or lactating women or does it just need to be applied with appropriate caution? Is the service not relevant to persons who refuse it upon first learning about it or is the real world one where clinicians and patients have ongoing conversations about intervention trade-offs and opportunities? Is a new oral antipsychotic not relevant for patients with schizophrenia who are receiving injections of long-acting ("depot") antipsychotic medication and have a history of violence when they go off medication, or would one consider tapering the depot medication slowly while adding the innovative oral agent? Is a psychosocial intervention not applicable to persons who are not fluent in the dominant language of a region, or should intervention staff (and research interviewers) be recruited who can work in the language of a locally numerous ethnic minority? As can be seen, it may be necessary to modify the nature of the service itself to provide effective access to some part of the relevant target group. Thus the service definition and the relevant target group definition should often be considered together in planning a study.

Threat 2: Nonrepresentative Sample Asked to Consent

The second threat to generalizability comes from the procedure used to identify potential study subjects. The traditional efficacy study procedure is to make known the study entry criteria and depend on local clinical facilities to refer or identify potential study subjects. Research staff also may review admissions or other clinical records to identify eligible subjects. In epidemiology this sampling strategy is called a "convenience sample," which has no logical or inferential link to the population. This is the reason many efficacy studies have limited external validity and therefore limited policy relevance.

The direct and ideal route to external validity is to employ epidemiologic screening of the intended target population. This is particularly valuable in the study of innovative treatments for which no tradition of referral and eligibility determination exists, or where referral practices can be assumed to evolve during the course of introduction of the service innovation. A direct screening of eligible participants is always desirable if usual referral practices are unlikely to identify a representative sample of the relevant target group (Essock et al., 1996a).

One needs to be careful that an epidemiological eligibility survey that bypasses current referral practices does not also bypass current wisdom or previous findings about the nature of the relevant target group. For example, the California legislature mandated a cost–outcome study of a capitated full-service community service model for persons with severe and persistent mental illness (Hargreaves, 1992). Selection criteria set by the state legislature required subjects to be a representative sample of persons with severe and persistent mental illness living in the local community of each test site. Design of the intervention and setting of the capitation rates targeted a "high user" subset of persons with severe and persistent mental illness. This mismatch severely crippled the study, since most study subjects were stable community residents who received few services in usual care and were not at great risk of rehospitalization. The expensive innovative model showed little relative advantage except in cases in which interventions heavily focused on vocational rehabilitation (Chandler et al., 1996).

Threat 3: Refusal of Consent

Biased refusal to consent to study participation is the third major threat to external validity. It is important to organize and record the consent process so that reasons for refusal are clear and refusal of study procedures can be distinguished from refusal of treatment. When possible, characteristics of subjects who refuse should be recorded to determine whether refusers and participants differ on demographics or other clinical characteristics. In many situations, these data may not be available to the investigators. When subjects are selected from existing data, however, such as intake admission records or service information systems, basic information about refusing subjects usually can be obtained.

In some situations, one may retain treatment refusers in a study. In this type of design, subjects are randomized only to a *recommendation* about treatment assignment. Subjects randomized to an innovative service are encouraged throughout the study period to accept it, whether they ever do so or not. This design is relevant for interventions such as intensive case management, vocational rehabilitation, and substance abuse treatment, whose success may depend in part on their success at engaging users.

Randomizing subjects to a treatment recommendation has both advantages and disadvantages. While conceptually appealing, this approach may lengthen the study period and reduce power through continued refusal by some subjects. It is relevant to evaluate an intervention by including the cost of engaging users.

Since refusers do not use the innovative intervention, they cause little increase in the marginal cost of *offering* the intervention, so study power may be limited less than one would suppose. Not only does one gain an estimate of the acceptability of the innovation, one may be able to identify a subgroup that is very likely to refuse, and even examine whether such people, when they do accept the innovation, benefit as much as other subgroups. As with the other four sources of unrepresentativeness, one must analyze this biased loss and present findings with appropriate cautions about the limits of generalizability.

Threat 4: Loss of Subjects from Follow-up

The fourth threat to external validity is biased loss of subjects of particular kinds from follow-up data collection. Such biased losses weaken generalization to the kinds of target population members who were selectively lost from follow-up. One must determine whether biased losses have occurred and discuss one's findings with appropriate caution if the relative cost-effectiveness of the innovation is different for the kind of subject who is frequently lost compared with the kind of subject who is rarely lost.

2.3.2 PRESERVING THE EXTERNAL VALIDITY OF THE SAMPLE

Clear definition of the relevant target population is a key design step in any cost–outcome study. The target population is all persons for whom the innovative service model is intended. In defining the relevant target population, it is important not to equate who is usually selected to receive innovative services with the broader group of persons who might benefit from the service. In fact, cost–outcome studies often seek to influence the service selection process. Therefore, the definition of the relevant target group may need to take into account all those situations in which, by hypothesis, a person should consider or be considered for receiving the innovative service. For example, one usually would not study a single diagnostic group as a relevant target group in services research. Usually a relevant target group is defined by a combination of illness characteristics, disability characteristics, personal strengths, and current service situation. An example might be a target group relevant to offer treatment with the antipsychotic medication clozapine (see Example 3).

EXAMPLE 3. ELIGIBILITY FOR CLOZAPINE

INCLUSION CRITERIA:
- Age 16 or above
- Schizophrenia or schizoaffective diagnosis
- Has experienced no period of 3 months during past year with adequate functioning (GAF rating of 60)

- Two documented adequate antipsychotic medication trials with inadequate clinical response or intolerance of the medicaiton due to side effects; each trial must have included 6 weeks at a dose equivalent to 600 mg/day of chlorpromazine or unacceptable side effects

EXCLUSION CRITERIA:
- Current myeloproliferative disorder
- Current severe CNS depression or coma
- Current WBC less than 3500
- Current granulocyte count below 1500
- Current debilitated physical state
- Pregnant or producing breast milk
- Needs a concurrent medication that also tends to suppress bone marrow
- Has failed a previous clozapine trial due to inadequate response, agranulocytosis, severe leukopenia, or unmanageable side effects

The ideal way to assure that study subjects represent the relevant target group is to randomly select potential subjects from the population. In practice, one often needs to use less direct methods for estimating the relationship of the subject group to the relevant target group, but epidemiological methods set the standard and clarify the inference issues.

2.3.3 THREATS TO THE EXTERNAL VALIDITY OF THE INTERVENTION

Investigators often worry that striving for external validity risks giving up the safeguards of internal validity that are the hallmarks of efficacy studies. While there is some truth to this, this feeling sometimes reflects a confusion about the nature of the interventions studied in cost–outcome studies. Efficacy studies determine the effects of specific drugs, types of psychotherapy, or other treatment interventions, by ruling out effects other than the "pure" effects of the treatment. By contrast, effectiveness studies are concerned with the entire, realistic context of interventions as encountered in usual treatment conditions. Thus the "effectiveness" of a treatment may result from a combination of influences that are associated in everyday practice with that treatment.

Threat 1: Atypical Site Characteristics

Mental health systems are embedded in communities with particular social, demographic, and economic characteristics. Just as the external validity of a sample is dependent upon the population characteristics of communities from which it is drawn, the external validity of an intervention is dependent on the characteristics of mental health systems in which it is embedded. An intervention that appears effective in one community may not be effective when implemented in another because of community differences in the size, funding, and organization of their mental health systems and the size, funding, and organization of the health care and social services agencies that work in concert with their mental health systems. For this reason, the external validity of a single-site study is rarely adequate to establish that the intervention is effective across communities. Several replications of a study in systematically different mental health care systems may be needed to obtain enough confidence in the generalizability of the conclusions to justify dissemination of the intervention to all communities.

Threat 2: Atypical Treatment Conditions

The varying nature of the conditions under which treatment is provided in cost–outcome research may also limit the generalizability of study findings. Treatment conditions include such characteristics as the skill with which specific treatments are provided; the degree to which patients and clinicians form a productive working alliance; the difficulty or inconvenience of receiving the treatment; the cumulative consequences of treatment side effects; and regional differences in the background, training, and practice patterns of clinicians. These factors usually are controlled or optimized in efficacy studies but may be allowed to vary in cost–outcome studies to approximate typical treatment conditions. This means that the implementation and delivery of interventions in effectiveness studies will be more variable and less homogeneous than in efficacy studies. Some level of treatment heterogeneity is necessary to study the effects of treatments in the context of usual care, but increased heterogeneity increases the likelihood that extraneous factors related to broader service delivery conditions may also affect treatment outcomes. Thus, treatment implementation and other service delivery conditions are sometimes confounded in effectiveness trials. This is not necessarily problematic because efficacy studies will often have shown a treatment to be efficacious when delivered under optimal conditions and the effectiveness study is being conducted to determine whether it is effective under usual care conditions.

The confounding of service delivery effects with pure treatment effects can lead to a finding that an efficacious treatment is not effective under usual treatment conditions. When confronted with such findings, it may be necessary to pursue the question using more complex studies in which patient selection and treatment delivery factors are varied systematically within one design. It may be that the treatment is effective only with particular patient subgroups or with particular methods of delivery.

Threat 3: Blind versus Open Designs

Examining the pharmacologic effects of a new psychotropic medication on the symptoms of a psychiatric disorder requires not only a randomized trial, but a carefully blinded design. In a double-blind drug trial, neither the patient, the prescribing physician, nor anyone who provides ratings of outcomes knows the patient's treatment assignment. Blind conditions are important because unblinded ratings of symptoms (and the symptoms themselves) can be influenced by the participants' expectations. Thus the double-blind design is standard in studies of the short-term effects of drugs on symptoms. Indeed, the "triple-blind" design, in which all study (and funded) personnel are kept blind until a complete, edited data set is ready for final analysis, is now standard in industry-sponsored drug development trials (Laska et al., 1994; Kartzinel et al., 1994). When one or more arms of a study cannot be blinded, as in studies of psychosocial treatments, some writers recommend the use of blind evaluator ratings (Rush et al., 1994).

Once there is adequate evidence that a new compound is more efficacious than placebo and of equal or greater efficacy than standard medications, studies of its effectiveness and cost become relevant. The effect under study is no longer the pharmacologic effect of the compound but the broader clinical and social effect of using that compound to treat a mental disorder. That broader effect includes the pharmacological effect of the drug on symptoms and side effects, but also the acceptability of the drug to patients, clinicians, and family members, and the long-term consequences for instrumental functioning and quality of life that result from the use of that drug.

In effectiveness studies, completely blind designs may reduce the generalizability of the findings because the required restrictions on dosing practice and drug choice are not typical of usual care. It is also desirable to study effectiveness over relatively long periods, beyond the six to twelve months that experience has shown is the limit of feasibility in a blinded study. Therefore many effectiveness studies use open designs.

Open designs compromise the meaning of outcomes that require subtle judgments by raters or by patients (e.g., symptom severity and global functioning), since such judgments are easily influenced by expectations. It is not usually practical, however, to measure subtle, fluctuating symptoms in most long-term effectiveness studies. Therefore, it makes sense to focus effectiveness measurement on relatively concrete variables such as cost, instrumental functioning, and quality of life. This does not mean that we should ignore mechanisms of effect, but that we should make wise choices about the priority and timing of research questions, including when to mount fully developed studies of mechanisms of effect that can test assumptions about issues such as the importance of symptom control for long-term rehabilitative cost-effectiveness.

2.3.4 PRESERVING THE EXTERNAL VALIDITY OF THE INTERVENTION

Just as in evaluating the external validity of the sample, evaluating the external validity of the intervention and intervention sites means determining whether the interventions studied in a cost–outcome trial are representative of the conditions in which these interventions usually are implemented. Estimates of costs and outcomes can be generalized only when study conditions approximate those in routine clinical care. Although routine care conditions imply variability in implementation, this variability can be systematically measured and controlled by the investigator. Ideally, study sites and intervention conditions will be thoroughly specified and measured to understand and account for differences that might affect the external validity of the intervention. Needless to say, characterizing complex clinical treatments, programs, and service interventions is extremely difficult and the methodology for doing so is in its infancy. In the next section, we will describe general issues involved in specifying and measuring the implementation of a mental health intervention. In Chapter 6, we describe measuring program implementation in more detail.

2.4 SPECIFYING AND MEASURING IMPORTANT DESIGN CONSTRUCTS

Observations are the building blocks of science and hinge on reliable and valid measures of theoretical constructs (Cook and Campbell, 1979). As we have stated already, the theoretical constructs relevant to most effectiveness studies are mental health interventions and outcomes. Specifying and measuring interventions and outcomes in effectiveness research is of such importance that we have devoted separate chapters to each (Chapters 6 and 7). A few words pertaining to construct validity, however, are appropriate in the context of research design.

2.4.1 SPECIFYING AND MEASURING THE INTERVENTION

As in the specification of any independent variable, specification of a mental health intervention starts with an initial concept and proceeds through a global description of goals to a detailed description of principles, objectives, and practices that lend themselves to measurement. The difficulty of an adequate specification of the intervention depends on its novelty and complexity. The nature and intensity of an intervention can be measured only if the intervention has been appropriately specified. Intervention measures prevent the intervention from being an unknown system, or "black box," of variables. Intervention measures allow study investigators to check the adequacy of the independent variable they have spent so much time and energy studying. In addition, specification and measurement of the intervention aids investigators in understanding the conditions to which results can be generalized (external validity) and gives policy makers information about the conditions they need to maintain to replicate study findings in other settings (Hargreaves and Shumway, 1995). Effectiveness research in mental health has reached the point in its development in which random assignment of subjects to ill specified and unmeasured treatment conditions is no longer "state-of-the art." Chapter 6 deals with the specification and measurement of mental health interventions in the conduct of effectiveness research.

2.4.2 MEASURING COSTS AND OUTCOMES

The variables of interest in cost–outcome studies are economic cost and individual consumer status. Conceptualization and measurement of these two extremely broad constructs is critical to the design of cost–outcome research. In this book, we conceptualize mental health outcomes to encompass disorder- specific outcomes, such as symptoms and morbidity; functioning in major roles; general health status; quality of life; and public safety and welfare. Chapter 7 discusses the issues related to measuring mental health outcomes and the most prominent measures within each outcome domain. Measuring economic outcomes involves two processes: measuring resources used or lost as a result of mental illness and its treatment (Chapter 4) and valuing those resources (Chapter 5).

2.5 STATISTICAL CONCLUSION VALIDITY IN COST–OUTCOME STUDIES

An important part of drawing valid inferences from the data collected in cost–outcome research is the appropriate application of statistical analyses (Cook and Campbell, 1979). The statistics used to test study hypotheses should be considered carefully in the planning phase of a project. Appropriate inferences using statistical tests depends on the adequacy of a very basic element of study design: the size of the study sample. In this section, we focus on one aspect of statistical conclusion validity, determining an appropriate sample size, which is essential for valid inference from statistical tests in cost–outcome research.

2.5.1 STATISTICAL POWER AND ERRORS IN INFERENCE

After cost and outcome data are collected, statistical analyses are used to make inferences about the effects of the intervention. In some cases, we hope to infer that average costs, outcomes, or both, are statistically different for two or more interventions. In other cases, we hope to infer from the data that costs, outcomes, or both, are statistically equivalent. Probability theory states that errors in inference will occur with a known likelihood in the statistical analysis of data. Sample size is set to control two types of errors in inference: concluding that outcomes are different when in fact they are not ("Type I error"), and concluding that outcomes are not different when in fact they are ("Type II error").

In this chapter, we have been concerned with the cost and effectiveness of an intervention group relative to a comparison group. In this context, statistical tests estimate the probability that group differences in costs and outcomes as large as those observed in the data occurred by chance alone. If the probability (p) that an observed difference is due to chance is small (p<.05), group differences in costs and outcomes are usually attributed to factors other than chance, such as the effects of the intervention. Of course, this means that 5 times out of 100 we incorrectly will attribute chance differences between groups to the effects of the intervention. The probability that chance differences (i.e., differences due to sampling error) between groups are large enough in any sample to be considered statistically significant is referred to as the Type I error rate and is symbolized by α.

Statistical tests may also fail to detect real group differences in costs or outcome. That is, group differences in costs and outcomes observed in the study may fail to exceed that expected by chance (α). The rate at which real differences between groups will be small enough to be statistically nonsignificant is referred to as the Type II error rate and is symbolized by β. Power is equal to 1-β and is the probability that a statistical test will correctly detect real differences in costs or outcomes between interventions. Sample size usually is set so that power is at least .80 while maintaining α at .05. That is, we hope to have enough subjects to have an 80% chance of finding a true difference between interventions given that we will erroneously conclude there is a difference no more than 5% of the time.

Estimating statistical power is a crucial part of planning a study. Grant application reviewers and funding agencies require evidence that sample sizes are sufficiently large to justify the resources the proposed study will consume. It also should be of interest to the research group who could spend years carrying out a study that has little chance of detecting an effect. Kraemer and Pruyn (1990) state the ideal: "A proposal for [a randomized clinical trial] should present explicit power calculations based on the preliminary evidence for the magnitude of the effect size for *each* outcome measure to be used. No proposal for [a randomized clinical trial] should be funded unless such power calculations indicate that there is a good chance of an unambiguous and convincing result" (p. 1164).

Power is a function of four quantities: (1) sample size, (2) the sample standard deviation or other estimate of standard error for a specific outcome measure, (3) the size of the true intervention differences (the "effect size") in the population, and (4) the acceptable Type I error rate. If we set power = .80 and α = .05, then sample size is a function of two quantities: the size of differences that we expect between the intervention and control group in the population and the magnitude of the sample standard error on a given outcome measure. Once these quantities are specified, many statistical packages are available for estimating the needed sample size (Goldstein, 1989).

It is easy to observe in any table of statistical power that as the true population difference in costs and effectiveness between interventions increases, the number of subjects needed to achieve a power of .80 decreases, regardless of the test statistic used. For sample size estimates to have meaning for planning purposes, the population difference between groups for each of the outcome variables must be estimated accurately. Similarly, it is easy to observe that as the estimated standard error of the difference between the groups increases, so does the number of subjects needed to achieve a power of .80 using any test statistic. The reader who is planning a cost–outcome study may be dismayed at this point, wondering how one can estimate population differences and standard errors *before* conducting the study!

Three methods of specifying population differences and standard errors are employed. First, previous studies of similar interventions using similar outcome measures can be used to estimate the likely differences in group means that might be expected and to give estimates of the standard error of group differences. Such data are extremely valuable in the planning of sample size, but they may not be available to aid investigators planning studies of previously untested interventions. Second, data from pilot studies using the relevant outcome measures can be used to generate estimates of group differences and standard errors. Such data may lead to the most relevant estimates of statistical power, because they are derived from the population from which the larger study will sample. With pilot studies, however, sample size will usually be very small, and so the precision of the estimates will be poor. Finally, group differences can be specified *a priori*. Clinical and policy considerations may provide thresholds above which group differences become meaningful. On outcome measures, judgments of clinicians and consumers may suggest when reductions in clinical symptoms and improvements in functioning represent meaningful change in an individual's life. Group differences below the threshold of clinical importance may not be of interest to investigators. Therefore, sample size usually will not be set to detect group differences below this threshold with adequate power. Policy makers may be able to suggest how large a difference in costs is relevant to policy decisions.

We illustrate the estimation of sample size for a very simple and common study design: a group-comparison, repeated-measures design. Assume that the purpose of the study is to compare the cost-effectiveness of a new case management intervention to usual care for persons with severe mental illness. Thus, two groups of subjects (case-managed or usual care) are measured before the intervention (Time 1) and then again after some follow-up interval (Time 2). Change computed as the difference between Time 1 and Time 2 measures will be compared between the two groups, to determine whether case management leads to greater improvement. For the sake of this example, we will calculate sample size estimates for commonly used outcome measures, including total service cost, the Brief Psychiatric Rating Scale (BPRS), and the Global Assessment Scale (GAS). Chapter 7 describes the BPRS and GAS.

One way to estimate sample size for a simple 2 × 2 (groups × time) design is by comparing the magnitude of change between the intervention and control groups. Let us say that estimates of change will be obtained by obtaining cost and outcome measures at baseline and later at 6-month follow-up. Outcomes will be defined as change from Time 1 to Time 2 in costs, BPRS, and GAS. The sample size needed is in part a function of the acceptable Type I error rate and the desired power. For this example, assume that the acceptable α is .05 and the desired power is .80. At this point, we must estimate the magnitude of the group difference in outcomes. Let us say that policy considerations suggest that the intervention can only be considered a success if the intervention saves at least $3,000 per individual and that individuals improve at least 4 more BPRS total score points and 8 more GAS points than the control group over the 6-month period.

Finally, we need an estimate of standard error. In this example, and for others involving repeated measures, some estimate of the amount of variability in change over time must be used as an estimate of standard error. In this example, we use the standard deviation of change scores obtained from previous research using the outcome measures of our proposed study. In data collected in an earlier study of treatment costs for the severely mentally ill, the standard deviation in cost change scores over 6-month intervals was $9,571. The standard deviation of BPRS change scores has been estimated at approximately 8 total score points. Finally, the standard deviation of GAS change scores have been estimated to be approximately 9 over a 6-month interval. When estimates of the standard deviation of change are not available they can be estimated from cross-sectional data (Overall and Starbuck, 1979).

Equation (1) is the power function in standard score units for comparing two groups of a given sample size (n), population group difference (δ), standard error (σ), and α rate.

$$Z_{1-\beta} = \frac{\delta}{\sigma\sqrt{\frac{2}{n}}} - Z_{1-\alpha/2} \tag{1}$$

Once $Z_{1-\beta}$ is computed, statistical power $(1-\beta)$ can be obtained by looking up the value obtained for $Z_{1-\beta}$ in a probability table of the normal distribution. When estimating sample size, rather than power, Equation (1) can be solved for n. For longitudinal studies, n should be adjusted for the rate of attrition expected during the follow-up interval. Equation (2) expresses the recruited sample size per group as a function of the desired power, the acceptable α rate, the population group difference (δ), and standard error (σ).

$$N_{recruited} = 2\sigma^2 \frac{(Z_{1-\beta} + Z_{1-\alpha/2})^2}{\delta^2(1-r)} \tag{2}$$

In Equation (2), where r is equal to the attrition rate expected in the sample, $Z_{1-\beta}$ is usually .85, representing the standard score associated with a statistical power of .80. $Z_{1-\alpha/2}$ is usually 1.96, representing the standard score associated with a Type I error rate of .05. When these values are substituted, Equation (2) simplifies further and easily is used to estimate sample size for a variety of standard error estimates (σ) and effect size estimates (δ). Because standard error may vary from sample to sample, it is useful to examine several scenarios of statistical power assuming different standard error estimates. A conservative estimate of standard error can be created by increasing standard error estimates by 10 or 15%.

Equation (2) assumes that sample size (n) and the standard error estimate (σ) are identical across groups within a study. A more general formula exists for statistical power when the planned sample size and standard error estimates are not equal:

$$Z_{1-\beta} = \frac{\delta}{\sigma_{\text{pooled}} \sqrt{\dfrac{1}{n_1} + \dfrac{1}{n_2}}} - Z_{\alpha} \tag{3}$$

Where σ_{pooled} is computed according to Equation 4:

$$\sigma_{\text{pooled}} = \frac{(n_1 - 1)\sigma_1^2 + (n_2 - 1)\sigma_2^2}{n_1 + n_2 - 2} \tag{4}$$

Equations (3) and (4) cannot be simplified or rearranged to solve for sample size. This usually is not a hindrance because statistical power analysis and sample size estimation are made considerably easier by widely available computer packages for desktop computers. The use of such programs greatly facilitates exploration of factors that affect statistical power such as unequal sample sizes and heterogeneity in standard error estimates, and the reader is referred to a recent review of these statistical packages (Goldstein, 1989).

The power analysis computer program PowerPak was used to estimate the sample size necessary to detect group differences in pre-post changes in mental health costs, the BPRS, and the GAS (Lenth, 1987). Figure 2.1 displays statistical power for each measure under two different estimates of standard error and for a variety of study sample sizes. For the smaller standard error estimates, Figure 2.1 shows that a sample size of about 175 is needed to attain statistical power of .80 to detect a cost difference of $3,000, compared to a sample size of 75 to detect a mean difference of 4 on the BPRS, and a sample size of only about 25 to detect a mean difference of 8 on the GAS. The greater sample size requirement to detect the cost difference results from the size of the group difference that we are interested in, $3,000, relative to the magnitude of the standard error of estimation, more than $9,000. In contrast, we only need 25 subjects to detect a GAS difference that is almost as large as its standard error.

Sample size estimation, especially for complicated hypotheses, is best done in collaboration with a skilled biostatistician. Biostatistical consultation is also helpful in improving study design and analysis to optimize power.

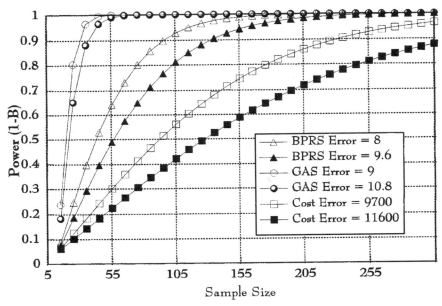

FIGURE 2.1   Statistical power curves for the BPRS, GAS, and treatment costs.

2.5.2 EQUIVALENCE TESTING

Many important policy implications flow from a conclusion that two interventions have equivalent outcomes, or equivalent societal cost, or equivalent cost to the policy maker. It is widely recognized that the mere failure to find a significant difference does not establish population equivalence. What is needed is a clear understanding of the evidence necessary to conclude that two groups are sufficiently similar to be considered equivalent. Methods for establishing that two interventions are equivalent in terms of their effects have been developed and are now widely accepted (Rogers et al., 1993; Stegner et al., 1996). Equivalence is an issue, for example, when a drug manufacturer proposes to the U.S. Food and Drug Administration that it be allowed to market a generic substitute as equivalent to a brand name drug.

Equivalence testing is relatively straightforward. It differs from traditional hypothesis testing in how it specifies the null and alternative hypotheses for the particular test statistic. In traditional hypothesis testing, the null hypothesis is that differences among group means are zero. The alternative hypothesis is that differences among groups are not zero. The reverse is true in equivalence testing. Here, the null hypothesis is that the difference in group means is greater than some minimum difference defining practical equivalence, and the alternative hypothesis is that the difference in group means is not greater than this minimum difference. This approach can be applied with any test statistic, including means, proportions, and any other statistic on which one can construct a confidence interval.

To examine the equivalence of intervention conditions in terms of costs and outcomes, one first must pick a boundary that defines how small the mean population difference must be to consider interventions equivalent. For example, one might want evidence that the experimental treatment produces a result within 10% of the control result *in the population,* if one is to conclude that the two treatments are equivalent. One then wishes to decide from one's experiment whether this is true, and do so with, say, the conventional 5% risk of Type 1 error. The somewhat counterintuitive method is that one computes a *90%* confidence interval on the difference in population means, and if this confidence interval falls entirely within the range of ±10% of the control mean, one can conclude with *95%* confidence that the treatments are equivalent. This difference between 90 and 95% confidence reflects something of the reverse of a two-tailed probability logic. The upper or lower limit of the 90% confidence interval nearest to the *a priori* equivalence boundary determines the entire result, and therefore one only has a 5% risk of an erroneous conclusion. Empirical work has established that indeed the obtained error rate is less than or equal to 5% using this method (Makuch and Simon, 1978; Anderson and Hauck, 1983).

Equivalence testing has major implications for sample size planning. The formula for estimating power (Equation 1) is modified to estimate the appropriate sample sizes for traditional tests of the difference in two means and of the equivalence of two means based on independent groups t-test. In traditional difference testing, δ in Equation 1 is set to a difference in group means that is large enough to be important based on clinical and policy considerations. In equivalence testing, δ is set to a relatively small difference that is small enough to be considered equivalent based on clinical and policy considerations. In traditional difference testing $Z_{1-\alpha}$ is two tailed (or 1.96 for alpha = .05). In equivalence testing $Z_{1-\alpha}$ is one tailed (1.65 for alpha = .05).

Examination of Figure 2.2 indicates a dramatic difference in the sample size required to conclude that two means are equivalent rather than to conclude that two means are different. Using cost data from the above example, we compare estimates of the sample size necessary to test for group differences and estimates of the sample size necessary to test for group equivalence. In the group difference scenario, described above, we were interested in the power to detect group differences larger than $3,000. In the group equivalence scenario, we are interested in detecting group differences within 10% of the estimated control group mean. If the expected average cost of treating severe mental illness is $10,000, then the group equivalence boundaries would be set at ±$1,000. As can be seen in both Figures 2.1 and 2.2, the power to test for a group difference of $3,000 (given the larger standard error estimate of $11,600) is .80 with a sample size of about 475. In contrast, power to test for group equivalence within $1,000 with the same standard error is .80 only with a sample size of about 3,300.

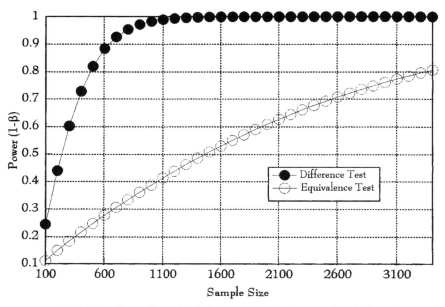

FIGURE 2.2   Comparison of statistical power for difference and equivalence tests.

There are several implications of the difference in power associated with tests of differences and tests of equivalence. First, these results have major implications for understanding the cost–outcome literature. It is unlikely that the majority of published cost–outcome studies of mental health treatments and services have had adequate statistical power to establish equivalence. Among studies that have failed to reject the null hypothesis of no difference in costs and outcomes, conclusions about the equivalence of intervention and control groups cannot be made without first understanding whether the sample size allowed adequate power to determine group equivalence. Because these studies in all likelihood have set their sample sizes using traditional power estimates, the ability to conclude equivalence may be extremely limited. Second, sample size estimates must be congruent with the study purpose. If the purpose of the study is to determine whether a treatment innovation is equivalent to an established standard of care in terms of costs and outcomes, then the sample size necessary to achieve adequate power for an equivalence test should be estimated.

2.6 CHAPTER REVIEW

Cost–outcome research typically examines the effects of a treatment (the independent variable) on costs and outcomes (the dependent variables). In cost–outcome research, both internal validity and external validity are important.

Internal validity is the ability to infer that outcomes like clinical improvement or cost reduction are an effect of the treatment, and could not be the effect of other factors. When other factors could account for the effect, that means they were "confounded" with the treatment effect. For example, confounding occurs when groups in different treatment or service assignments differ in average prognosis at baseline.

External validity is the ability to infer that study findings apply to the intended target population under the usual conditions of mental health care. In efficacy studies the traditional emphasis has been on internal validity. In effectiveness studies the emphasis is on adequate external validity, while preserving internal validity.

Random assignment to treatment is the most dependable way to avoid confounding and enhance internal validity, since randomization tends to balance treatment groups on all confounding factors at baseline, even those not measured or not thought to be important. When randomization is not possible, second best procedures include matching groups on some potential confounding variables at baseline and examining baseline differences and trying to take into account their effects. Pretest-posttest (or "mirror-image") designs with no control or comparison group are extremely vulnerable to confounding, since one rarely knows what the time course of outcomes or costs would have been without the intervention.

Even in randomized designs, baseline prognostic balance can be lost, although there are countermeasures for each type of loss. Balance can be lost when there is loss of subjects from follow-up. The primary countermeasure is to successfully follow up every subject over all of the planned assessment times, even if they drop out of other aspects of the study. If follow-up is not complete, one needs to analyze the baseline differences in the prognosis of subjects lost versus retained in each treatment group. Balance can also be lost when subjects drop out of their assigned service, and one should always use a conservative "intent-to-treat" analysis that compares outcomes as assigned, regardless of actual treatment or service received. Even randomization itself can be corrupted if it is not properly designed and executed, resulting in nonequivalent groups. The primary safeguard is that the person determining the qualifications of potential subjects and obtaining consent must not know what the random assignment will be.

External validity is impaired if the subjects are not representative of the intended target population or the service setting and service execution are not typical of usual service conditions.

Recruited study subjects can be unrepresentative of the intended target population for many reasons. A common reason is that investigators intentionally exclude subjects who are thought to be less likely to respond well to the treatment, such as those with concurrent substance abuse. The circumstances of recruitment also may cause an unrepresentative sample to be invited into the study, such as only inpatients or only those who are likely to appear consistently for scheduled outpatient appointments. Even requiring that subjects complete a baseline assessment can sometimes cause this type of biased loss from a study. A third loss of representativeness occurs if particular types of potential subjects refuse to consent to the study (e.g., those who are less "compliant," or who are better informed about the treatment alternatives and will not accept the possibility of being randomized to a condition other than the one they desire). Subjects who are lost from follow-up assessments and cannot be included in key data analysis also may be unrepresentative of the total group. Finally, persons who drop out of service also may be unrepresentative. These threats to external validity are all countered by two strategies: first, a design that obtains a representative study sample, and second, analyses of losses to detect the degree of bias the losses have induced in the analyzed study sample.

Representativeness of study treatments and services is enhanced to the extent that the study site or sites represent the full array of usual care settings with regard to factors that may affect outcomes or costs, such as the skill of service providers, the quality of the management of services, and freedom from research procedures that might influence the cost or effectiveness of services. The measurement of study services, as discussed in Chapter 6, is an aid to characterizing the services actually compared and determining the conditions to which study findings can be generalized.

3

CONCEPTS OF ECONOMIC COST

Mary Jones and John Smith, faculty members in Middle America University's social work program, were very pleased to receive state funding to do a comparative study of their innovative in-school intervention for emotionally disturbed children. They were a bit apprehensive, however, because the state made the funding contingent upon their studying the costs, as well as the outcomes, associated with their intervention. They had both read published cost–outcome studies and could see how valuable such studies could be in the evaluation and selection of publicly funded programs such as theirs. Being social workers, and not economists, however, they found many of the technical terms in the published studies quite unfamiliar and confusing, and they had a lot of questions about how to conduct such a study. What is the difference between a "cost–benefit" study and a "cost–effectiveness" study? Which is best suited to their intervention? How should they measure costs? Bills are generated for some services, like the outpatient therapy children receive outside of school, but they don't bill anyone for their experimental therapy. Also, many parents devote extensive amounts of time to caring for their children and participating in treatment with them. Should they include the costs of parents' time? How do they determine the cost of that time? Should they convert their study outcomes, such as social functioning and school performance, into dollars? How would they make that conversion? After pondering these questions and reviewing published studies several times, John and Mary agreed that they needed to know more about economic theory before they could design and implement their cost–outcome study.

As Chapter 1 illustrates, cost–outcome analyses of mental health treatments can help a wide variety of decision makers make informed treatment choices.

But, as this case study shows, no matter how obvious the practical motivations, it is difficult to conduct cost–outcome studies or interpret cost–outcome findings without an understanding of the underlying theoretical and economic basis of cost–outcome research. The three main sections of this chapter acquaint the non-economist with the broad economic concepts that form the foundation of cost–outcome analysis. The first section introduces the four types of analytic models used in cost–outcome analysis; the second section gives an overview of the economic theories that motivate and support cost–outcome analysis; and the third section provides introductory illustrations of how key theoretical concepts are applied in cost–outcome analysis and defines specific terms that will be used throughout the book.

3.1 MODELS FOR COST–OUTCOME ANALYSIS

Four related approaches to cost–outcome analysis are used to evaluate a wide range of programs: cost–efficiency analysis, cost–benefit analysis, cost–effectiveness analysis, and cost–utility analysis. For reasons outlined below, the latter two models—cost–effectiveness analysis and cost–utility analysis—are generally preferred in evaluations of health and mental health programs. It is important, however, to understand the full range of models. It is easier to see why certain models are preferred when their similarities and differences are well delineated. In addition, clear definitions are useful in interpreting study findings, since some authors blur the distinctions between different analytic models. Readers desiring a more in-depth discussion of these models may refer to a general text (e.g., Mishan, 1988; Layard and Glaister, 1994; Merkhofer, 1987), or to texts that focus on cost–outcome analyses of health programs (e.g., Warner and Luce, 1982; Drummond and co-workers, 1987; Gold and co-workers, 1996).

3.1.1 COST–EFFICIENCY STUDIES

Cost–efficiency, or cost–minimization, studies are conducted when there is conclusive evidence that interventions are equally effective. There is no need to evaluate outcomes if alternative interventions are known to achieve equivalent outcomes. In such situations, decision makers only need to know which intervention achieves the desired outcome at the lowest cost. For example, imagine that the investigators in the case study at the beginning of this chapter were comparing two interventions shown to be equivalent in efficacy studies. One intervention for emotionally disturbed children is conducted in the school while the other is conducted at a separate free-standing clinic. A cost–efficiency study could be a useful strategy to determine which intervention achieves the common outcome at the lowest cost. Cost–efficiency studies are appealing because collecting cost data is less complicated than collecting both cost and outcome data. Cost–efficiency studies are usually not practical, however, because there is rarely sufficient evidence to demonstrate that treatment alternatives have equivalent outcomes.

3.1.2 COST–BENEFIT STUDIES

Cost–benefit studies are conducted when both costs and outcomes are expected to differ and when all outcomes can be expressed in dollar values. This approach is desirable because expressing both costs and outcomes in monetary terms facilitates integration of costs and outcomes as well as comparison of disparate programs. When results are expressed in the common metric of dollars, decision makers can compare two alternative programs for a mental illness, compare a mental health program to a cancer treatment program, or compare a public health program to a public transit program.

Theoretically, a common monetary metric is extremely flexible and useful. Practically, however, it may not yield meaningful comparisons because it is very difficult to assign valid dollar values to all outcomes. Cost–benefit analysis has been most widely applied in the evaluation of public works projects, such as bridge building or dam construction. It is easy to see how many of the outcomes of such projects can be expressed in monetary terms. For example, the costs of a dam constructed to produce hydroelectric power can be compared to the value of the electricity that will be generated. Even a project like this, however, has less tangible effects that are difficult to monetize, such as effects on the aesthetic quality of the area surrounding the dam, effects on wildlife, and effects on recreational opportunities (Kelman, 1992). This limitation is particularly evident in the evaluation of mental health programs, which have many outcomes with no obvious monetary value, such as changes in psychiatric symptoms, medication side effects, and social functioning. As a result, cost–benefit analysis is not widely applied in the evaluation of mental health programs.

3.1.3 COST–EFFECTIVENESS ANALYSIS

Cost–effectiveness analysis, like cost–benefit analysis, is used when both outcomes and costs are expected to differ. In cost–effectiveness analysis, however, outcomes, or "effectiveness," are measured in units that seem more natural than dollars. In some health care applications, the units might come from specific laboratory values, such as cholesterol levels, or broad indicators of mortality, such as lives saved. Most mental health outcomes, such as psychiatric symptoms, are more complex and subjective and are typically measured using rating scales and other measures developed in clinical research. (Outcome measurement is discussed in detail in Chapter 7.)

Measuring outcomes in more natural or intuitive units makes cost–outcome comparisons more valid and interpretable to most decision makers, but it is not without limitations. Most mental health interventions have multiple relevant outcomes that cannot be measured using a common metric. Analysts and decision makers alike are challenged to integrate the different outcomes in some way to assess overall treatment effectiveness. Consider a comparison of two interventions for emotionally disturbed children in which one is superior in improving social functioning, while the other is more effective in improving academic performance. It is not obvious which intervention is most effective, or how social functioning and academic performance should be combined to represent overall effectiveness. The standard approach is to analyze cost-effectiveness separately for each outcome and let readers and decision makers decide for themselves which treatment is most effective overall. This strategy obviously introduces unstated individual valuations of the multiple outcomes into each interpretation and fails to identify one universally superior intervention. Furthermore, while natural effectiveness units increase the interpretability of a single study evaluated in isolation, they tend to make cost–effectiveness findings less comparable than cost–benefit findings, because outcomes of treatments for different illnesses, or even different treatments for the same illness, are not measured in a common metric.

Despite these limitations, most mental health researchers are more comfortable with cost–effectiveness analysis than with cost–benefit analysis, and some evidence suggests that the two approaches typically yield similar conclusions (Phelps and Mushlin, 1991; Garber and Phelps, 1992). In addition, as the next section describes, the extension of cost–effectiveness analysis to cost–utility analysis allows the conversion of health units to a common metric expressed in terms of quality-adjusted life years.

3.1.4 COST–UTILITY ANALYSIS

Cost–utility analysis extends cost–effectiveness analysis by incorporating measures of the relative importance of the multiple outcome domains. A variety of methods have been developed for quantifying preferences for, or the "utility" of, different health outcomes. These methods yield numeric weights that can be combined with the original outcome measures to compute a single, comprehensive outcome indicator. Incorporating outcome utilities is particularly important when there are value trade-offs between outcomes, such as beneficial treatment effects versus harmful side effects, or when benefits and side effects are valued differently by different segments of society. Most utility measurement approaches facilitate conversion of the aggregative effectiveness indicator into common units expressed in terms of quality-adjusted life years (QALYs). This common unit permits comparison of the cost–effectiveness of different interventions with different outcomes. Cost–utility methods generally are viewed as a desirable extension of cost–effectiveness methods, but their implementation is limited by the feasibility and credibility of the methods for measuring preferences for treatment outcomes and obtaining empirical importance weights. (Utility-based methods and other methods for aggregating outcomes are discussed in greater detail in Chapter 8.)

3.1.5 SIMILARITIES AND DIFFERENCES
AMONG ANALYTIC MODELS

As this overview indicates, the four analytic approaches to cost–outcome analysis differ in the way they deal with outcomes. With the simplest approach, cost–efficiency analysis, all outcomes are assumed to be equivalent and are not included in the analysis. In cost–benefit analysis, outcomes are expressed in monetary terms. This approach facilitates comparisons between both similar and disparate programs, but is limited by difficulties in determining the dollar value of all outcomes. Cost–effectiveness analysis is currently favored in analyses of mental health interventions because outcomes are measured in meaningful health units. Cost–utility analysis builds on the cost–effectiveness approach by weighting outcomes by their importance to compute an aggregate measure of effectiveness.

Although these four analytic models approach outcome measurement in different ways, they rely on common approaches to cost measurement. Cost measurement typically involves identification of the types of resources used in an intervention, measurement of the quantity of resources used, and the assignment of a dollar value to each resource. Practical strategies for implementing these steps are the topics of Chapters 4 and 5. These cost–estimation strategies cannot be implemented consistently, however, without a firm theoretical foundation. The next sections introduce the major concepts of economic cost used in cost–outcome analysis.

3.2 ECONOMIC THEORY AND COST–OUTCOME ANALYSIS

This section discusses the characteristics of health and mental health services in the context of economic theories of competitive markets and social welfare. A brief overview of these theories illustrates that estimating costs in cost–outcome analyses of health programs is complicated because we cannot rely on competitive markets to readily identify which services provide the greatest health benefit for each dollar invested. We can use welfare economic principles, however, to estimate and compare the social value of different services.

3.2.1 MARKET THEORY AND HEALTH CARE

The most familiar economic theories are those related to free, competitive market economies. These theories, however, do not adequately explain the economics of health and health care. In the ideal free-market economy, neither consumers nor producers dominate. Consumers are well informed about the nature of the products or services they would like to buy, and they try to maximize their satisfaction by buying the most desirable goods at the lowest possible price. Producers, on the other hand, want to maximize their profits, but must set prices that are acceptable to consumers.

These competitive market conditions rarely prevail for health and mental health care (Cullis and West, 1979; Feldstein, 1988; Drummond, 1993). The market for health care differs from the ideal competitive market in several important ways. These differences can lead to market failure because they disrupt the supply and demand relationships that allow producers and consumers to arrive at market prices. Two types of market failures are common in health care markets: imperfect information and limited competition. The presence of third-party payers, such as insurance companies, and government intervention in response to market failure further complicate health care markets.

Imperfect Information

Standard market theory assumes that consumers have sufficient information to make rational choices among available goods and services. As consumers, however, patients are often unable to obtain the information required to make optimal, rational choices about health care. Patients seeking health care cannot typically obtain comparative price and quality data in the same way that they can when they are shopping for a car or a television. Data are generally not available, and most patients lack the special knowledge necessary to interpret data that are available. Furthermore, many medical interventions occur in emergent situations when patients do not have time to gather or evaluate information on procedures or providers. Individuals in need of mental health services may be even less able than consumers of other medical services to find and use information. Without adequate information, consumers cannot make health care decisions based on service cost and quality and cannot play their vital role in setting market prices.

Limited Competition

Competition among medical care providers is limited in a number of ways. Market theory assumes that multiple, profit-maximizing producers compete to provide goods that consumers desire at the lowest possible cost. The behavior of health care providers is not typically consistent with these assumptions. First, in some instances there are few competing producers from which to choose. This is especially true of specialty providers, such as free-standing psychiatric hospitals, because there is not enough demand in most localities to support multiple, competing providers. Second, even when there are multiple providers, as in the case of general hospitals, patients may not be able to choose among them because the choice is made by their doctor or insurance carrier. Third, many health care providers do not seek to maximize profits, and a large number operate on a not-for-profit basis. Elimination of a profit motive does not necessarily decrease prices because many nonprofit providers sponsor educational or charitable programs that increase the costs of services. When competition is limited, providers do not have sufficient incentives to reduce service cost and increase service quality.

Third-Party Payers

The involvement of third parties, such as insurance companies, further discourages competition. Health insurance tends to eliminate incentives for either producers or consumers to make treatment choices based on prices. Consumers with insurance that pays for their health care may become more focused on the price of insurance than on the price of the actual services they receive. Providers may become more focused on providing services that insurance will cover than on providing the most appropriate, cost-effective services.

Government Intervention

Governments often intervene in production or distribution when competitive markets fail and needed goods are not produced in adequate quantities or sold at prices consumers will pay. Government intervention is very common in health care for two reasons. First, society benefits from maintaining and improving the health of its members, and second, there are ethical concerns about denying basic medical care on economic grounds. Government response to market failure is evident in the high level of federal, state, and local government funds allocated for treatment of the severely mentally ill. There is no competitive market for many treatments for severe mental illness because most individuals disabled by these illnesses cannot pay for the treatments they need. As a result, those treatments are largely provided or funded by government agencies. Government involvement in health care is necessary, if not desirable, but it does not restore a competitive market for the services it provides and may affect markets for related services, by setting artificial prices for services or otherwise altering supply and demand relationships.

The relatively abstract concept of market failure has direct practical implications for decisions about the delivery of health and mental health care. Since there is not a true competitive market for health care, market forces do not identify the most desirable services, and decision makers must somehow evaluate the costs and outcomes of alternative services to determine the optimal allocation of resources. It is not obvious, however, how to calculate and compare costs in the absence of market prices. The subdiscipline of welfare economics provides a theoretical basis for estimating the costs of public and social programs in the absence of ideal market conditions.

3.2.2 WELFARE ECONOMICS

Welfare economics addresses questions about social welfare, or the aggregate well-being of a society. It provides a framework for evaluating public programs, including public health programs, in terms of how they better society. Typically, governments sponsor public programs in response to market failures, and their performance cannot be evaluated using normal market criteria. Cost–outcome analysis is a strategy for systematically applying welfare economic principles to compare the societal value of alternative programs. These principles do not provide the sole justification for cost–outcome analysis, nor are all cost–outcome analyses completely consistent with these principles. However, welfare economics provides a framework for determining the societal value of resources, which is essential in the absence of competitive markets and market prices (Feldstein, 1988; Garber and Phelps, 1992).

A complete exploration of welfare economics is beyond the scope of this chapter. For more complete and technical presentations of the welfare foundation of cost–outcome analysis, readers may consult the texts by O'Connell (1982), Mishan (1988), and Johansson (1991) as well as reviews by Battiato (1993), Williams (1993), and Garber and Phelps (1992). The following sections describe the specific ways in which the welfare economic concept of societal value is applied to estimate the economic cost of resources associated with provision of mental health treatments.

3.3 DEFINITIONS OF ECONOMIC COST

This section illustrates how the broad economic theories introduced above are linked to practical cost estimation. We begin with a conceptual definition of cost and discuss how economic concepts are used to arrive at estimates.

3.3.1 WHAT IS A COST?

In the context of health and mental health care, a cost is conceptually equivalent to the value of a resource consumed or lost as a result of illness. Thus, the cost of a mental illness is equivalent to the value of resources consumed or lost by ill individuals, treatment providers, government entities, or other segments of society as a direct or indirect result of the illness. It is often useful to divide costs into two categories: direct and indirect costs (Rice, 1966; Hu and Jerrell, 1991). **Direct costs** are incurred when resources are used directly to provide treatment, services, or other assistance. Psychiatric inpatient and residential care, outpatient and medication management visits, emergency and crisis services, case management, legal and correctional services, and travel expenses incurred to obtain treatment are direct costs. In contrast, **indirect costs,** are defined as resources lost due to illness. Most indirect costs involve the value of time that could be devoted to other activities in the absence of illness, such as the cost of lost employment or productivity by patients or their family members.

The terms "resources" and "value" are central to the definition and calculation of cost. **Resources** include time inputs by clinicians and others required to provide treatment and services, medication, supplies, and space. **Value** is the worth of one unit of a specific resource. The task of cost estimation is to identify the types of resources associated with illness and its treatment, to enumerate the quantities of those resources used or lost, and to assign appropriate monetary values to each resource. The unit value of each resource is then multiplied by the number of units used, and the total cost is calculated as the sum of all resource costs.

These basic definitions are fine in principle, but they do not provide a practical basis for determining resource value and estimating cost. Our review of market theory and market failure demonstrated that we cannot rely on market forces to determine prices for health services that accurately reflect resource value. We may find that there are no market prices for some resources because there are no markets. Other resources may have market prices, but those prices may be distorted, inaccurately reflecting true value, as a result of market imperfections. In the absence of valid market prices, we turn to two concepts from welfare economics, societal value and opportunity cost, for guidance in the estimation of true resource value.

3.3.2 OPPORTUNITY COST

One of the central welfare economic concepts applied in cost–outcome analysis is opportunity cost. The opportunity cost of any resource is its value in its best alternative use. When we use a resource to provide a specific mental health service, we give up the opportunity to use that resource in another way. Thus, the opportunity cost of that resource is the value, or societal cost, of the same resource if it were used for the next best purpose. Cost estimates based on opportunity cost are called "shadow prices." The opportunity cost concept is often easier to define than to apply. It is rarely possible or practical to employ the opportunity cost principle in its strictest sense because it is virtually impossible for an analyst to enumerate all the possible alternative uses of even a single resource (Jacobs, 1991).

While the concept of opportunity cost does not provide a strict algorithm for determining resource value, it provides a valuable standard for evaluating price and cost data available for cost–outcome analysis. For example, if a mental health intervention employs nurses to deliver treatment in an area in which a variety of other nursing jobs exist, it is typically assumed that the prevailing market wage for those existing nursing jobs is an accurate estimate of the opportunity cost for the nursing activities in the studied intervention. In contrast, if a state hospital operates in a building fully owned by a public agency, it initially may appear that there are no costs associated with the use of the building. However, if we consider the value of the building from an opportunity cost perspective, and try to determine its best alternative use, we can see that if the state hospital were not using the building, it could be rented or sold. Thus, we could estimate its value as the rental cost or sale price of similar buildings in the same locality. In Chapter 5, we describe specific methods for determining the opportunity costs of a variety of resources associated with mental health services. In preparation for that detailed discussion, we give two broadly applicable examples of how the concept of opportunity cost is applied to estimate the value of resources that have distorted, or nonexistent, market prices.

Costs and Charges

The distinction between costs and charges illustrates the use of opportunity costs when market prices are distorted. In conversation, the terms "price," "cost," and "charge" are essentially identical. They would also be identical in a well-functioning, competitive economic market, in which they reflected buyers' and sellers' consensus about the value of a good or service. As discussed in earlier sections, however, there is not a well-functioning, competitive market for health care. As a result, charges—the amounts providers bill patients and insurers—are not equivalent to costs—the actual value of the resources used to provide those services. Charges look like costs because they are carefully recorded in dollars and cents on numerous claim forms and bills. Appearances are misleading, however, because charges reflect the price distortion prevalent in health care markets and are not typically reliable or accurate proxies for true resource value. Charges often do not represent the opportunity cost of services because they commonly reflect cost shifting between different service types and different client or payer groups. For example, if a hospital increased the cost of laboratory services to subsidize the emergency room, the charges billed for laboratory services would be higher than the true cost, and the charges for emergency services would be lower than the true cost. Similarly, if an outpatient clinic negotiated a special low rate for office visits with one health insurance plan and made up for this reduction in income by charging other patients a higher rate for office visits, then the charges appearing on the bills of both groups of patients inaccurately would reflect the value of the office visits.

Given the potential for price distortion in markets for health and mental health care, analysts must recognize that charges do not represent the opportunity costs of most services. It is not always necessary to calculate directly the opportunity cost of each service examined in a cost–outcome study. In many cases, combining the market prices of the inputs used in providing a service, such as staff time and office space, provides an acceptable estimate of opportunity cost. These estimation techniques are described in detail in Chapter 5.

Time Costs

The concept of opportunity cost is also applied extensively in valuing the time costs associated with interventions. Time costs are incurred when patients spend time in treatment, when patients are unable to work as a result of illness, and when family members or other non–health-care providers spend time caring for ill individuals. These costs differ in important ways from the health care service costs discussed in previous sections. Those services are associated with prices, even though those prices tend to be distorted and not representative of true resource value. In contrast, many time costs are not associated with any prices at all, and considerable thought and effort are necessary to determine their value. Specific methods for estimating the value of different time costs associated with mental illness and its treatment are presented in Chapter 5. Here, we focus on general issues that arise in determining the opportunity cost of time and discuss the two primary methods for valuing time costs. The first method, the human capital approach, clearly reflects the opportunity cost perspective. The second method, the willingness to pay approach, is more associated with competitive market theory.

The **human capital** (HC) approach equates the value of an individual's time with his or her economic productivity. This is essentially equivalent to proposing that the best alternative use of any individual's time is competitive employment and the opportunity cost of his or her time is equivalent to the prevailing wage rate for competitive employment or an imputed wage rate for noncompetitive productive activity, such as household work (Rice, 1966; Rice et al., 1990). This focus on economic productivity reflects a broad societal perspective, and the use of prevailing wage rates yields reliable and internally consistent estimates (Robinson, 1986). Recent methodological advances promise to improve the accuracy of HC estimates by accounting for labor market conditions, such as unemployment (Koopmanschap and van Ineveld, 1992).

On a theoretical level, the HC approach is problematic because market wages do not fairly represent individual productivity, and reliance on aggregate wage rates tends to overvalue some groups (employed white men) in relation to other groups (the young, the elderly, women, and nonwhite men) (Luft, 1975; Chirikos and Nestel, 1985). Furthermore, HC estimates represent only the economic impact of disease, not the comprehensive value of life, which would include psychosocial costs such as pain and suffering. As such, the HC approach has been criticized for lacking appropriate conceptual foundation in economic theory.

On a practical level, problems arise in determining which, if any, wage rate appropriately reflects the true opportunity costs of different kinds of time. There have been attempts to distinguish work time, defined as hours spent in competitive employment, from nonwork or leisure time, defined as time not spent in competitive employment. These distinctions do not prove useful in practice (Sharp, 1981). First, many nonwork hours are not devoted to the kinds of pleasurable activities associated with leisure. Many hours are devoted to relatively nondiscretionary activities, such as eating and sleeping, which are essential to productive work. Second, many individuals find common nonpaid activities, such as household work, less enjoyable than their paid work activities. Third, many people would spend additional time in paid employment if they had the opportunity to do so. As a result, even if it were possible to correctly classify hours devoted to leisure, it would be very difficult to assign these hours a meaningful value. Given the difficulty of distinguishing work from nonwork time, wage rates provide the most reliable estimate of time costs.

Although wage rates provide the most reliable estimate of the value of an individual's time, it is not always clear which rate provides the most valid estimate of the real opportunity cost. If an individual takes time off from paid employment to receive mental health treatment, then the wage he or she receives from that employment is equivalent to the opportunity cost of his or her time. If an individual is too disabled to engage in competitive employment, however, assigning a wage rate to the time he or she spends in treatment may inaccurately inflate the cost of treatment. Similar concerns arise in estimating the value of time that patients' family members spend in treatment or providing various kinds of informal care, such as help with household tasks, transportation to treatment, or other kinds of assistance. Family members' competitive wages may be accurate estimates of their opportunity cost if they forego employment to provide informal care. As discussed in detail in Chapter 5, however, the wage rate of a home health worker may provide a better estimate of treatment cost.

An alternative approach to valuing time, the **willingness to pay** (WTP) approach, is designed to remedy the deficits of the HC approach. In concept, it is more consistent with both welfare economics and market theory because it attempts to estimate the dollar amount that consumers would pay to improve their individual welfare by avoiding illness or disability. These estimates are more comprehensive than HC estimates because they combine intangible costs such as pain and suffering with monetary costs. WTP estimates are based on either indirect evidence of individuals' revealed preferences or on direct evidence of individuals' stated preferences. Indirect estimates are obtained through analyses of market data, by calculating the increment in wages employees require to assume risky jobs, or the price consumers pay for safety devices such as smoke detectors (Dardis, 1980). Direct estimates are obtained through surveys in which respondents are asked directly how much they would pay to achieve a certain health change or outcome (Viscusi, 1992).

Despite their theoretical consistency, WTP estimates are likely to be no less biased and are potentially more variable than HC estimates. Although WTP is designed to avoid HC's reliance on biased aggregate wage rates and prevailing income distributions, external factors, particularly income, influence responses and willingness to pay cannot be separated from ability to pay (Lubeck and Yelin, 1988; Thompson, 1986; Evans and Viscusi, 1993). Furthermore, valuations tend to covary with severity of illness, with sicker individuals stating a greater willingness to pay to avoid illness (Lubeck and Yelin, 1988).

Significant measurement problems limit the use of both indirect and direct WTP estimates in cost–outcome studies of health and mental health services. Indirect WTP estimates derived from market data typically reflect societal preferences related to the discrete health events, such as death or loss of a limb. Market data do not readily yield estimates of individual consumers' willingness to pay for more subtle or short-term increments in health status or treatment effectiveness.

There are also problems with survey and interview techniques used to obtain direct WTP estimates. Individuals' hypothetical survey responses may not be consistent with their true actions. In particular, value estimates may vary depending on whether respondents would need to be "willing to pay" with their own funds. For example, individuals who assume they will be assessed in proportion to their WTP may understate their valuations. Conversely, individuals asked to value a publicly supported program may overstate their valuations in an attempt to encourage public funding (Landefeld and Seskin, 1982). Survey and interview procedures also can be sensitive to relatively subtle changes in question and word order (Green et al., 1994).

Individuals may have difficulty quantifying their willingness to pay for very costly treatments or major changes in health status because they either do not pay all of their own health care expenses or do not typically make lump sum payments for changes in their health. Successful implementations of direct WTP assessment strategies have involved small expenditures similar to those that consumers encounter on a daily basis, such as the incremental cost of safer household cleansers and pesticides (Viscusi, 1992).

In cost of illness studies that measure the comprehensive, societal cost of particular illnesses, the HC and WTP approaches provide different, though complementary, results. In comparative cost–outcome studies, however, the HC approach is much more appropriate and practical. WTP estimates are traditionally quite global, addressing broadly defined, long-term outcomes, such as probability of a cure or death, that are not specific to a particular intervention and encompassing both monetary costs and nonmonetary outcomes. Both of these characteristics are problematic in most cost–outcome studies. WTP methods have been adapted to focus on specific interventions in a number of studies, such as Johannesson and co-workers (1991) and Appel and co-workers (1990). These adaptations, however, pose problems with appropriate question formulation, are limited by respondents' difficulties in dealing with probability values reflecting the likelihood of different health outcomes (Gafni, 1991), and are likely to increase considerably data collection expenses. In addition, WTP valuations are difficult to apply to small time increments, such as time spent in treatment. Most importantly, however, the comingling of costs and outcomes in a comprehensive WTP estimate is inconsistent with the primary goal of most cost–outcome studies, which is to understand the nature of the relationship between costs and outcomes.

In view of these limitations with the WTP approach to valuing time, the HC approach is the preferred method in cost–outcome studies of mental health services. Specific examples of ways in which the opportunity cost perspective is used to estimate the value of different kinds of time costs are presented in Chapter 5.

3.4 ANALYTIC PERSPECTIVE

3.4.1 SOCIETAL PERSPECTIVE

When we apply welfare economic principles, such as opportunity cost, in the conduct of cost–outcome analysis, we implicitly adopt a societal perspective. An analysis conducted from a societal perspective includes all the costs incurred and effects experienced by all segments of society—patients, family members, citizens at large—as a result of illness or treatment. The societal cost associated with a mental health intervention would include all costs associated with mental health treatment, medical treatment costs, other social service costs, law enforcement and legal costs, and the costs of informal care provided by patients' family or friends. The societal effect of an intervention includes the intended impact on patients' symptoms and quality of life, but also includes unwanted side effects of treatment, and any other effects associated with the intervention. Some interventions can have positive and/or negative effects on individuals who are not directly involved. For example, a new halfway house for homeless mentally ill persons could have a positive effect on the surrounding community by helping disturbed individuals get off the streets. Those members of the community living adjacent to the new halfway house, however, might feel that it had a negative impact on their quality of life. The comprehensive societal cost perspective is a powerful tool for shaping public policy because it permits examination of the distribution of costs and benefits among multiple payer and beneficiary groups, revealing which segments of society pay for an intervention and which segments benefit.

The societal perspective generally is considered the "gold standard" for cost–outcome analysis and is particularly valuable in the study of mental illnesses that have widespread economic and psychosocial impact. The complete and generalizable data that a societal cost analysis yields, however, are extremely expensive and time-consuming to obtain. It may be difficult for investigators studying one intervention, such as inpatient treatment, to obtain utilization data for all other treatments and services that their patients receive. Valuing family members' and friends' contributions of money and time to the treatment and care of ill individuals requires painstaking interviewing and record keeping on the part of both investigators and contributors. The effort and expense that societal cost analysis demands may not be feasible or necessary in all circumstances.

3.4.2 OTHER PERSPECTIVES

Cost studies may be conducted from perspectives more narrowly focused than a societal perspective. Some studies include only costs incurred by a single public program or a single employer-paid health plan. Others may include all mental health treatment costs while excluding other costs, such as physical health care, social services, legal, and family costs. Although these narrower perspectives are less comprehensive than the societal cost perspective, they can yield useful information in many situations in which the time and resources required for a societal cost study are unavailable.

When a full-scale societal cost study is not possible, more modest studies can be quite valuable as long as cost estimation methods are appropriately matched to the goals and conclusions of the study. For example, if a state psychiatric hospital succeeded in closing a ward because a new medication enabled patients to return to the community, they might well find a significant decrease in their in-patient treatment costs. This might be very useful information for the state hospital, but this finding could not be interpreted as a cost savings for the state as a whole and could even have caused an increase in costs for other mental health agencies that had to provide care for patients discharged from the state hospital, as well as for other patients who could not be admitted to the closed ward. Thus, focused cost studies can be useful ventures, but they cannot address large-scale generalizability or policy questions.

3.5 CHAPTER REVIEW

There are four approaches to comparing the costs and outcomes of different interventions. They treat costs similarly, but deal with outcomes in different ways. Cost–efficiency studies only examine costs and are used when one can assume equal effectiveness. Cost–efficiency studies often are not practical because evidence of equal treatment effectiveness is rare. Cost–benefit studies are done when effectiveness can be converted to monetary values, allowing input cost to be compared to monetary return. Cost–benefit studies of mental health treatments usually are difficult to conduct because it is difficult to determine the monetary value of key outcomes. Cost–effectiveness studies measure effectiveness using natural outcome units or scales. The multidimensional nature of outcomes in most mental health research requires some method for integrating multiple outcome dimensions to make meaningful cost–effectiveness ratios possible. Cost–utility studies extend the cost–effectiveness approach, integrating outcomes using value judgments of the relative importance of the multiple outcomes. Cost–effectiveness and cost–utility studies are the primary focus of this book.

Economic theory provides the conceptual underpinning of cost–outcome methods. Competitive markets operate to identify the most desirable, cost-effective services and products. Such markets require well-informed consumers and multiple, competing producers. However, competitive market conditions rarely exist for health and mental health services because consumers cannot obtain good comparative information on the price and quality of health care and competition among producers is limited because consumers commonly lack a choice of providers for health care. The involvement of third-party payers, such as insurance carriers, and government intervention further distort the market. Thus, cost–outcome analyses of alternative health and mental health services are necessary because we cannot rely on competitive markets to readily identify the services that provide the greatest health benefit for each dollar invested.

The theory of welfare economics provides a framework for determining the societal value of resources, which is essential in the absence of competitive markets and market prices. The societal cost of an illness is equal to the value of resources consumed or lost as a result of the illness. Resources consumed are called direct costs; resources lost are called indirect costs. In most cases, the quantity of resources used is measured and subsequently assigned a monetary value. Use of resources such as clinician time, medication, supplies, and space are counted in their natural units (e.g., hours of clinician time) and their value is estimated (e.g., cost per hour of clinician time). Since market prices do not provide accurate estimates of the cost of units of resources, the welfare economic concepts of opportunity cost and societal value are used to provide a substitute estimate of value, or a "shadow price." The opportunity cost of a resource is the value of a resource if it were used for its next best purpose.

Economic cost may differ from the price charged when market prices are distorted. Therefore, charges should not be used uncritically to estimate the value of a resource. Charges billed for services often reflect cost shifting between different types of service or different payer groups.

A market does not exist for time costs, such as the time a patient spends in treatment, so we apply the opportunity cost concept to estimate its value. There are two competing theories about the opportunity cost of such time, the human capital approach and the willingness to pay approach. The human capital approach proposes that the next best use of a person's time is his or her usual productive work, and the opportunity cost of this work is the prevailing wage rate for competitive employment or an imputed wage rate for noncompetitive productive activity. The willingness to pay approach, by contrast, bases value either on indirect evidence or direct ratings of individuals' preferences. Both human capital and willingness to pay approaches have major flaws and limitations. On balance, in comparative cost–outcome studies the human capital approach is more appropriate.

The costs and benefits of an intervention may look different to different members of society. The societal perspective examines all the costs incurred and all the benefits received as a result of an intervention, even those that are unintended. It is generally considered the gold standard for cost–outcome analysis because it reveals which segments of society pay for an intervention and which segments benefit. It is especially appropriate for studying mental health services that have widespread economic and social impact. Studies of societal cost are expensive, however, and sometimes studies include only costs incurred by a single payer, or only mental health service costs but not other health care, social service, and criminal justice costs.

4

Measuring Utilization

The Mental Health Outpatient Department of HealthPlus, a large health maintenance organization, is faced with the challenge of serving a growing caseload while containing treatment costs. The department has developed a plan to encourage clients seeking individual outpatient treatment to accept diagnosis-specific group treatment instead. The HMO would like to evaluate the cost-effectiveness of the new approach before fully implementing it; specifically, whether the new service model is cost-effective for two costly disorders, schizophrenia and major depression. They plan to do this by carrying out a randomized cost–outcome study. As the members of the research team develop their research strategy, they wonder what costs they should measure. How should they measure them? Should they measure the same costs for both diagnostic groups? Can they use the same cost measurement protocol they used for last year's study of inpatient care?

A crucial design step in cost–outcome research is selecting the proper costs to measure. These cost variables correspond to mental health services and other resources used in connection with the mental health phenomena under investigation. Once cost variables are selected, measuring them involves two steps: (1) counting the utilization of each of these types of cost and (2) assigning value to each cost variable. This chapter addresses the first of these two steps; Chapter 5 addresses the second. In particular, this chapter discusses decisions about which costs to measure; various sources of utilization and cost data; and strategies for measuring resource utilization with sufficient precision and accuracy. The next chapter presents strategies for estimating the monetary value of each cost variable.

4.1 CHOOSING THE TYPES OF COSTS
TO INCLUDE

Seven broad types of services and other costs usually are considered in planning any study comparing mental health interventions. These include mental health treatment, physical health care, criminal justice services, social services, time and productivity (not only of the patient, but perhaps other family members as well), other family costs, and transfers and other income. Deciding which costs to include and how much emphasis each should receive involves both art and science.

The selection of cost variables is driven by the nature of the study questions and what might be called "the importance principle." The study questions tell you which costs are more important in your study and which are less important. A resource cost that is central to one study of mental health treatment might be peripheral to another. In the case example above, where investigators wish to compare individual to group outpatient treatment for persons with either schizophrenia or depression, the investigators might emphasize the assessment of inpatient care more heavily for the persons with schizophrenia than for those with depression, since persons with schizophrenia are in general at higher risk for hospitalization. In addition, since the study subjects are to be recruited when initially seeking outpatient care, it can be anticipated that outpatient mental health services will be prominent in both groups. General health services probably should be studied also, since mental health services are being provided in an integrated general health care setting, and the two mental health outpatient interventions being compared may have different effects on the use of other health care.

In planning a study, investigators must consider the costs and benefits of measuring each of the many types of costs potentially affected by a mental health intervention. They must seek an efficient selection that will not omit costs that might compromise the study findings or the policy implications of the study. Once the costs have been selected, a unit of measure must be specified for each cost, so that costs deemed most important to the study findings—the most expensive or the most frequently used services and resources—are measured with the greatest precision and accuracy. The following sections give specific guidance about the range of choices, units of measure, and data sources for each of the seven types of mental health services and other resource costs.

4.2 MENTAL HEALTH TREATMENT COSTS

Mental health treatment costs are the primary focus of most mental health cost–outcome studies. Therefore, investigators enumerate mental health treatment costs in greater detail than other types of costs. Mental health treatments include inpatient care, skilled nursing care, residential treatment, emergency room contacts, outpatient sessions, case management hours, day treatment services, partial hospitalization, social skills training, vocational rehabilitation, medication, and laboratory procedures. As described in Chapter 3, all of these services will be enumerated in a societal cost study. Frequently used treatments generally must be measured more carefully than rarely used treatments. More focused cost–outcome studies may include only a subset of these services. An experimental treatment usually is assessed in greater detail than other treatments (Knapp and Beecham, 1993). Studies that compare different approaches to providing the same kind of treatment also usually require detailed measurement of the component resources used in treatment.

Investigators must define and count units of services with sufficient accuracy to answer the study questions. The main components of mental health treatment are staff time, medication, and laboratory and other ancillary services. In some studies these components are measured individually, while in other studies they are combined into "units" of a specific treatment modality, such as a day of inpatient hospitalization or an hour of outpatient therapy.

4.2.1 STAFF TIME COSTS

Staff time represents the bulk of the cost of most health interventions. Counts of outpatient visits, hospital days, and emergency service contacts all implicitly include measures of staff time. In comparisons of treatments that use different staff mixes, it may be necessary to count specific quantities of time inputs by different staff disciplines to accurately distinguish competing treatment approaches and to determine their true cost. For example, outpatient psychotherapy provided by physicians may need to be distinguished from therapy provided by social workers.

Detailed measurement of staff activities may also be necessary in studies of interventions that may indirectly affect the use of staff time. For example, a new drug treatment could alter the way inpatient treatment is provided. Increased monitoring of side effects may take up more staff time, while reduced psychotic symptoms and decreased seclusion and restraint may take less staff time, and both effects may be important in evaluating the cost-effectiveness of the new medication. Such differences between the experimental and comparison treatments can only be detected if the duration and nature of staff activities are examined. If these differences could have important cost or policy implications (e.g., altering ward staffing), it may be valuable to devise a method for recording staff activities at this level of detail. It may be sufficient to time-sample staff activities rather than institute routine recording of all such activities, but then one must take care to consider how the time sampling can be devised to cover the times most likely to be sensitive to the treatment comparison. For example, day shifts and night shifts typically have very different levels of ward staffing and might respond differently to changes in workload.

In some situations, it may not be necessary to estimate all of the staff time resources that comprise a treatment. An intermediate level of disaggregation may
permit examination of specific components that an intervention is likely to impact. Partial disaggregation may be difficult to implement because of problems
with double-counting of resource use. For example, it is difficult to separate the
costs of seclusion and restraint use in inpatient treatment because staff integrate
observation of patients in seclusion or restraint with other clinical activities,
such as providing therapy and dispensing medication. Thus, it may be problematic to estimate the incremental or component cost of seclusion or restraint without observing and valuing the full range of staff activities.

Institutional statistical reporting systems usually disaggregate outpatient visits into initial evaluations, individual psychotherapy sessions with a single therapist, group or family sessions with more than one consumer and perhaps more
than one clinician (perhaps with number and type of participants recorded in
each instance), medication evaluation and prescription, and so forth. Aspects of
services that are not enumerated (telephone contact with a consumer or on be-
half of a consumer, supervision and training, the composition of group sessions,
case planning conferences, etc.) will then be considered as a "time overhead" of
providing these services. Institutional accounting reports or study-specific cost
estimation will distribute such staff time overhead in some systematic way
across all units of service. One needs to consider whether these approximations
will seriously distort the meaning of the findings of a particular study. For treatments or services that are the primary focus of the study, investigators often
supplement institutional statistical data with more detailed staff time logs either
gathered routinely or time-sampled, in order to help interpret the meaning of
standard units of service in each treatment group (e.g., Brekke, 1988).

4.2.2 MEDICATION COSTS

Medication is an important aspect of many mental health treatments, and
medication cost is of particular interest in studies of newly introduced and more
expensive antipsychotic and antidepressant drugs. Drug prescription, dispensing,
and consumption can involve immensely detailed data collection, and one needs
to tailor the level of detail to the purpose of the study. From a cost perspective,
the resources used to prescribe and dispense a drug are usually consumed
whether the patient takes the drug or not, but it may also be important to know
whether the patient took the drugs as intended. The amount of drugs prescribed
may also help the investigator to evaluate whether the quality of medication
management was adequate in each treatment condition. These questions must be
considered during study design so the method for enumerating medication aspects of study treatments will adequately serve all important study purposes.

Typically, the amount and type of medication prescribed and/or dispensed is
recorded for those medications that are central to the treatment, as in drug stud-

ies of antipsychotic, antidepressant, or anxiolytic medications, or studies of psychosocial interventions in which concurrent medication is expected to be a frequent accompaniment or component. For these primary medications, amounts prescribed or dispensed, or both, may be recorded for each day, week, or month in the study, depending on study goals. The detail with which medication adherence is monitored also may vary from periodic patient reports during an assessment interview to more intensive measures, such as pill counts in returned containers, use of containers that record the number of times they have been opened, or assays of drug levels in blood. During inpatient care, if each medication dose is dispensed personally, detailed drug consumption can be obtained from required nursing dispensing records (e.g., see Hargreaves et al., 1987). However, the method of recording medication use is usually limited to the method that is feasible in the least restrictive setting experienced by most subjects. For inpatients, this may be the amount of medication that is dispensed, which is relatively close to the amounts consumed. For outpatients, it may be the amount of medication that is prescribed, augmented with interview data on what medications were consumed.

It may not be necessary to measure use of ancillary medications, such as antidepressants in the treatment of schizophrenia and drugs used to manage side effects of other medications, in as much detail, especially if the ancillary medications are relatively inexpensive or infrequently used. Utilization may be represented more simply, such as by recording whether the particular class of medication was used at all during a particular week or month. It may be sufficient to determine that treatment groups did not differ in the frequency of use of particular types of ancillary medications, without including these medications in the cost estimation.

4.2.3 COSTS OF LABORATORY AND OTHER ANCILLARY SERVICES

While most laboratory and other ancillary services, such as imaging studies, are appropriately treated as medical services, some services, particularly drug level assays and tests used to monitor potential drug side effects, may be a central part of mental health treatment. Some of these services, such as the weekly blood monitoring required during clozapine treatment, may have a significant impact on treatment cost. In some settings, there will be utilization databases or billing records that can be used to enumerate this type of utilization; in other settings, they will need to be enumerated by abstracting clinical records. In many cases ancillary service use will represent too small a proportion of treatment cost to justify data collection at the individual patient level, and costs of other treatment units, such as hospital days, will be adjusted as described in Chapter 5 to incorporate the average amount of these costs.

4.2.4 RESEARCH COSTS

In studies of research-funded innovative services, it is important to exclude the costs of research activities—including staffing, supply, and space costs—that would not be necessary in a real-world implementation of the same service model (Rosenheck, Neale, and Frisman, 1995b). Careful consideration is necessary because including research costs can overstate total costs, while overzealous elimination of research-related costs can understate costs. Some research activities, such as research interviews, while they may have a clinical impact, are always treated as a research cost. Other activities, such as reminder calls, may serve both treatment and research purposes. Many staff members will have both research and clinical or administrative duties, making it more difficult to identify research costs. Methods for identifying research activities and excluding them from cost analyses should be devised during the design phase of a project.

4.3 PHYSICAL HEALTH CARE COSTS

In analyses of the full societal cost of mental illness and its treatment, it is desirable to collect and examine data on medical services as well as on mental health services. Mental illness and its treatment may be associated with physical health and utilization of medical services in a number of ways. Some individuals may seek out medical care providers for help with mental health problems because they may not recognize a specific need for mental health services, may not know how to obtain such services, or may not want to risk the potential stigma of seeking mental health care. Recent epidemiological studies have shown that a large portion of mental health care is provided by primary care physicians. If such persons obtain appropriate mental health treatment, they may use fewer medical services, or they may use them more appropriately (Shemo, 1985). In contrast, persons with severe and disabling mental illnesses may be unable to obtain needed health care services without the assistance they receive in mental health treatment.

In studies carried out in specialty mental health settings, however, a relatively small proportion of subjects' health services may be provided by the general health sector. While investigators are rightly concerned to detect potential cost offsets between the specialty mental health sector and general health care, utilization of general health care is usually measured using one of two fairly approximate methods. One approach is to interview patients about their utilization of general health care, getting consent to obtain more complete data by requesting copies of bills from providers. The second method, available in some studies, such as studies of veterans, members of health maintenance organizations, or persons eligible for Medicaid or Medicare funding of their health care, involves cross-matching individual patient identifiers to large public or private reimbursement databases.

Local billing data on medical care is available in some form from providers and from public or private insurance claims databases. Provider bills may be an adequate source of services utilization data, but as discussed in Chapter 5, billing data often are not closely related to economic cost. In addition, since services typically are billed periodically until payment is received, repeated billing for the same services may introduce errors if uncorrected billing records are used to estimate utilization. Medicaid and private insurance databases are more limited because they tend to include only reimbursed care and do not include continuously well-defined populations of individuals (Lave et al., 1994). Some of these database limitations may be less of a problem for care provided by health maintenance organizations or the Veterans Administration.

4.4 CRIMINAL JUSTICE COSTS

Criminal justice activities are particularly challenging to enumerate. First, the criminal justice system has multiple components, including police protection, legal and judicial services, and federal and local correctional facilities. Second, interactions with the criminal justice system can involve one or more of many types of contacts, including citations, arrests, hearings, court trials, sentencing, jail or prison time, probation and conservatorship. Third, many of the contacts that mentally ill individuals have with law enforcement—such as dispute resolution and transportation to a hospital—do not result in citations or arrests and may not be formally recorded in law enforcement data systems. Fourth, law enforcement contacts may involve one or more agencies, each with its own organizational structure and official mandates. Jurisdictional and confidentiality concerns complicate collection and integration of data from different agencies. In most localities the criminal justice databases are limited to arrest and conviction data. Other data need to be collected from subject interviews, with details filled in through a hand search of paper criminal justice records, with subject consent.

4.5 SOCIAL SERVICE COSTS

Social services include free meal programs, homeless shelters, physical or vocational rehabilitation services, developmental disabilities services, money management services, and evaluation of income support eligibility and other aspects of administering transfer payments. Many of these services are provided independently by local charitable organizations or in partnership with local government agencies and tend to vary considerably in organization and scope.

For research in which social services are not the primary intervention under study, it is often adequate to gather utilization data from patient interview, perhaps supplemented by interview data from a key family member or other primary caregiver. When it is expected that social services will be an important aspect of total cost, more precision usually will be desired, so that interview data is supplemented with information from agency utilization databases or search of paper agency records. This will most often be relevant in studies of services to very disabled populations.

4.6 TIME AND PRODUCTIVITY COSTS

The total cost of mental illness and its treatment includes a variety of time costs incurred by patients, and in many cases, patients' relatives. Time costs typically include the value of time patients and their relatives spend in treatment and traveling to and from treatment as well as the value of productive time lost by patients as a result of their illness or lost by relatives who forgo productive activity to care for ill individuals. The different types of time costs need to be clearly understood and may require different data collection methods. In Chapter 5 we discuss different methods of valuing time as well. The issues raised in both this chapter and Chapter 5 are grounded in theoretical considerations presented in Chapter 3. There, we contrasted the two primary theoretical viewpoints in estimating time costs, the "human capital" approach and the "willingness to pay" approach, and we discussed the theoretical problems in distinguishing work time from leisure time. Time costs usually are more difficult to estimate than more discretely defined treatment or service costs, and multiple considerations are involved in deciding how to characterize these costs, which costs to include in an analysis, and (as discussed in Chapter 5) how to estimate those costs.

4.6.1 PRODUCTIVITY COSTS

There is little question that the value of lost productivity is an important component of the societal cost of illness and that it should be included in societal cost analyses. In studies of employer-paid health services the employer may also be very interested in the effects of alternative services on the insured person's productivity.

Data gathering procedures vary, depending on the level of work force participation of most of the study subjects and whether vocational rehabilitation interventions are the primary focus of the study. When vocational performance is not the primary service focus, it is often adequate to gather employment data from patient interviews. A common structure of interview protocols is to use a "time-line follow-back" method to reconstruct periods of up to several months before the current interview during which the subject was employed, was experiencing more illness-related absences from work, was seeking employment, was receiving work-related training or rehabilitation, was out of the labor force, and so forth. This is a particularly efficient interview structure if the time-line follow-back method is being used to gather other retrospective data as well. When vocational performance is a primary outcome, it is common to gather more detailed data, even including job coach and supervisor ratings of the quality of performance. In studies focused on a particular employer's workforce, company records of work absences and turnover may be available and can be accessed with methods that are both unobtrusive and appropriately confidential.

4.6.2 TREATMENT COST OF PATIENTS' TIME

Time that people spend in, or traveling to, treatment is appropriately considered a cost of treatment from a societal perspective. The value the investigator assigns to the person's time, however, is affected by the person's other life circumstances, as discussed in Chapter 5. Time spent in treatment can be viewed from the perspectives of different payers. For example, time consumed participating in treatment can be considered a cost to the patient, or the patient's employer if the patient is given time off with pay from work. Alternatively, the value of the productivity lost while a person was in treatment can be considered an indirect cost to society. Both perspectives are valid in different analytic contexts. However, time spent in treatment should be considered either a direct treatment cost or an indirect cost of lost productivity. "Double-counting" the time as both a direct and indirect cost will overstate total cost.

4.6.3 FAMILY MEMBERS' TIME COSTS

Family members of mentally ill persons, especially family members of persons with severe and disabling mental illness, may experience a significant burden as a result of the family member's illness (Grad and Sainsbury, 1963; 1968; Alterman et al., 1980; Bernheim and Lehman, 1985; Lefley, 1987; Gubman and Tessler, 1987; Noh and Avison, 1988; Tessler et al., 1987; Carpentier et al., 1992; Tessler and Gamache, 1995). This burden includes psychological stress, financial burden, and the time costs of providing a wide range of informal care to ill relatives. This informal care can range from occasional assistance with transportation or shopping to constant supervision and assistance with basic activities of daily living. Well family members may also participate in family treatments related to a relative's illness.

For gathering data on treatment participation, treatment contact records may include data on whether one or more family members participated in the contact. Beyond this, gathering data on family burden requires interviews with a key family member (e.g., see Tessler and Gamache, 1995).

4.7 OTHER FAMILY COSTS

Families also often make direct cash contributions to the support of an ill family member (Franks, 1990; Carpentier et al., 1992; Clark and Drake, 1994).

Gathering data on cash and in-kind contributions to an ill family member usually involves periodic interviews with key family caregivers, but is sometimes gathered in interviews with the ill persons themselves, as part of questions on the amount and sources of their income.

4.8 TRANSFERS AND OTHER INCOME

Transfers include payments from entitlement programs such as Old Age, Survivors, and Disability Insurance (OASDI); unemployment insurance; workers compensation; public assistance; supplemental security income (SSI); food stamps; veterans benefits; and other disability insurance. Transfers are not true societal costs because they reflect only a shift of existing resources rather than creation or consumption of resources. Data on transfer payments commonly are obtained by asking clients or proxy respondents the type and amount of payments received. These benefits are so central to disabled clients' well-being that they usually are able to report the amount of their monthly payment accurately. Clients could also be asked to bring in a check stub to verify the amount. One drawback in obtaining transfer payment data in interviews is that the client may be reluctant to reveal the amount of their welfare or disability payments. This problem is most likely when clients are not well acquainted with the research interviewer. It is possible to obtain individual client records from entitlement programs. Accessing program records however, requires special consent from recipients, and considerable effort to establish relationships with local entitlement program offices.

The subject's income may be derived from such sources as earned wages, pensions, investment income, public transfer payments, illegal activities, and private transfers such as family support, trust income, and alimony. In cost–outcome studies in which the subject is interviewed, data usually are gathered on the amounts and sources of income during the study period. The emphasis in such data collection is on income that reflects productivity, such as competitive employment, or income that reflects transfers. Investigators should not expend great effort measuring other kinds of income, such as income from investment activities. The economic meaning of income varies with its source. Earned wages are of special interest because wages are a marketplace estimate of the value of resources created by the subject's work. As discussed above, some investigators analyze lost wages as a cost of the illness or of its treatment, and improved wage income as a valued outcome that can offset treatment costs. Even when productivity effects are not analyzed in monetary terms, it is useful to report data on earned wages for readers who would like to estimate resulting monetary benefits to society from improved treatment effectiveness.

4.9 SOURCES OF DATA
ON RESOURCE UTILIZATION

The primary methods of collecting data on utilization are: (1) analyzing administrative data bases; (2) carrying out interviews of patients or family members; and (3) study-specific methods, such as abstracting service records and requesting copies of billing records. The second method is familiar to clinical investigators experienced in efficacy or effectiveness studies, and indeed one often simply adds questions about service utilization to outcome instruments such as those discussed in Chapter 7. The principal burden is a modest increase in the length and time of interviews. Unfortunately, only selected aspects of utilization data are best gathered through interview. Other methods will absorb most of the research effort devoted to utilization measurement in the typical prospective cost–outcome study.

4.9.1 ADMINISTRATIVE DATABASES

Administrative databases are huge and cumbersome compared to the research data files with which most clinical investigators have experience. There is increasing consistency of content among mental health utilization databases in the United States, reflecting the impact of the Mental Health Statistics Improvement Program coordinated by the federal government (Leginski et al., 1989). Nevertheless, each local mental health system implements its own database somewhat differently to meet its own state reporting requirements and other local needs. Furthermore, a research programmer or data analyst can rarely, if ever, directly extract research data from an agency database. To maintain database security, agencies often insist that their own programmers extract the required data and investigators may need to pay agencies for this service.

To use data from an administrative database, the investigator must accomplish at least six tasks: (1) understand the structure of the database; (2) identify the information to extract from the database (which fields in which records in which files); (3) negotiate permission for access to the database and determine the cost that must be reimbursed to the agency for programming time; (4) obtain all needed human subjects approvals; (5) understand the physical steps to get these very large files to the investigator's computer; and finally (6) work with agency programmers to obtain the analysis files.

If one needs to merge data on the same subjects from separate databases (e.g., mental health, substance abuse, social services, criminal justice, Medicaid), one not only has to accomplish these six steps with each of the separate agencies, but obtain sufficient identifier information from each agency to merge the files with reasonable accuracy in spite of data errors in all of the source databases. First and last name, social security number, date of birth, and gender are reasonably adequate, but even these are not available in many databases. Laws governing research access to such identifier data vary by state and type of agency, and the laws are interpreted cautiously by many agency administrators.

One needs to take seriously the risk to subject confidentiality one may create by assembling such files, and construct more layers of safeguards than one's intuition initially might suggest. Locked data cabinets and signed oaths of confidentiality by each research staff member are only the starting point. Data analysis computers should not be accessible from the Internet and perhaps not even from local area networks. Names and social security numbers should only be retained in data files until the files have been successfully merged and a unique study identifier assigned. If one needs an identifier file after this, it best may be limited to two copies, both kept personally by the project director at secure sites away from the blinded data files. A useful exercise in planning security precautions is to assume that someone who is highly motivated, intelligent, and knowledgeable will try to penetrate the research operation and obtain sensitive data on some specific research subject. For federally funded research projects the investigator should also obtain a "certificate of confidentiality" that helps when attempting to protect research files from subpoena.

In planning how to extract research data from an agency database, the first task is to understand the structure and content of the database. One must learn what files the system contains and obtain the codebook for each relevant file, which lists each variable's name, format, meaning, possible values, and value labels for categorical variables. It is not uncommon for the usage or coding of the same variable to change over time or to be used inconsistently by different programs in the same mental health system, so one needs to be alert to such possibilities.

Since the primary goal of acquiring administrative data is to obtain counts of units of service used by study subjects, it is necessary to understand how units of service are recorded. For example, a mental health database might consist of three hierarchical files: a client file, an episode file, and a visit file. These three types are of increasing size. A client file may have one record for each client ever seen in the system, and contain key identifying and demographic variables. An episode file might have a record for each treatment episode, including a provider code, entry and exit date, entry and exit diagnosis, referral source, and disposition codes. One needs to know how an episode is defined in practice. For example, if a patient is seen in an emergency room, then hospitalized, then transferred to another ward in the same hospital, there might be three episode records, one for each stage in this sequence. If one wishes to analyze this sequence as one hospital episode, the three records would need to be linked during data analysis. If the same patient was being seen in an outpatient clinic prior to this hospitalization, there would be an outpatient episode that began some time before hospital admission and might continue until many months after discharge from the hospital. One needs to know whether the end of an outpatient episode has any relationship to the last date the person was actually seen. For example, an outpatient episode record might have a variable called "last date seen," while the episode ending date might only reflect the date when the closing information was recorded. In some systems an open episode is reflected in an episode record with a missing end date, while other systems may have a separate file of open episodes, and records are not added to the historical episode file until they are closed. Finally, a visit file will have a record for every occasion on which a person was seen, along with billing information such as type of contact, amount of time, a clinician identifier, and so forth. These huge visit files are difficult and expensive to manipulate. Visit information summarized in episode files may or may not be sufficient for research needs. Episode files are smaller, but still large by microcomputer standards, and client files are relatively compact. However, even client files may contain records for more than 10% of the residents of the service area.

Medicaid data files provide an attractive source of information on mental health and other medical care provided in the private sector. This source is valuable for persons with schizophrenia served in the public sector, since most of them are eligible for Medicaid coverage. In each state, Medicaid bills and payments are processed by a company that serves as the Medicaid fiscal intermediary. The fiscal intermediary is required to convey complete files to a common federal repository. The state fiscal intermediary usually can provide data more quickly than the federal government. In order to link patients with their Medicaid bills one needs to collect the patient's social security number and other identifying information during the consent process. As states experiment with capitated contract funding for Medicaid recipients, the current relative uniformity of Medicaid databases may not be maintained.

The Department of Veterans Affairs maintains centralized units-of-service data for individual veterans, linked to an accounting cost–center system that provides a reasonable way to estimate the cost of each unit in each facility. Methods for analyzing these data have been developed by VA's Northeast Program Evaluation Center (Rosenheck et al., 1993), and by the Health Services Research and Development Center at the Palo Alto Veterans Affairs Hospital (Beattie et al., 1992).

4.9.2 INTERVIEW SOURCES OF UTILIZATION DATA

In prospective cost–outcome experiments each subject typically is interviewed at baseline and periodically during the study using an instrument that contains scales to measure symptoms, functioning, quality of life, and satisfaction with services, as discussed in Chapter 7. These interviews can also serve as a source of data on services utilization, although interviews usually will not yield the complete coverage of mental health services obtainable from local administrative databases. Interview data is especially useful in identifying additional service providers seen by the patient. When an agency that was not included in the original consent process is reported, it also provides an occasion to obtain a signed release from the subject to access information directly from this agency. Utilization data from interviews cannot be assumed to provide accurate counts of units of service, which few respondents can recall accurately over several months, but can identify providers from whom direct utilization data should be sought. Subjects also may report types of utilization that may not be available from any other source. These may include contacts with self-help programs, police, mental health services in other communities, homeless shelters, and so forth. Interviews are also a convenient source of information on income sources and amounts, including earned wages.

Interviews of a key family caregiver are also discussed in Chapter 7. Such interviews can provide information on the psychological, financial, and time burden of the family in caring for its ill member, and family members' views about the quality of services and the way that service providers related to family members. In addition to being a source of information on financial and time costs experienced by the family, the family informant also can identify services used by the subject that may not have been identified in other sources of information, so that detailed information on utilization can be sought.

4.9.3 OTHER METHODS FOR GATHERING UTILIZATION DATA

Certain utilization data that is central to the study aims may not be available except in clinical or other agency records. In such cases, investigators must develop a method for abstracting the data of interest from the records. An example is provided by a form, called Medication and Ancillary Treatments, that was developed by Essock et al. (1996b) for a cost–effectiveness study of a novel antipsychotic medication, clozapine, among persons with schizophrenia who were long-stay state hospital patients at study entry. The form was designed to record clinical record information for successive 30-day periods throughout each subject's 24 months in the study. It was completed by research staff using clinical records in whatever facility was currently managing the subject's medication. This was initially an inpatient ward, but the same form was used when a subject was discharged to the community. Abstracted data served multiple purposes, and contributed to checking the implementation of study treatments (as discussed in Chapter 6) and assessing effectiveness (e.g., restrictiveness of care, disruptive behavior) as well as counting units of service. Antipsychotic medication was measured in total daily dose of each antipsychotic agent, since in this study cost results might have been sensitive to choice and dosage of antipsychotic drug. Ancillary and side-effect medications were measured more globally (days on a particular class of drug), since cost effects were not expected to relate to specific agents or dose levels within classes. The day-by-day location of the medication management responsibility revealed the number of days each subject was on particular wards of a hospital or in different community settings, which might have different staffing costs. The form included specific data on each subject's time in seclusion, restraint, or close observation, and on specific clinical laboratory tests, both of which were expected to reflect cost differences between the two treatment regimens and would therefore be disaggregated from overall daily hospital costs. The form was also the only source of data on utilization of other services received while in the hospital, such as other mental health care, medical, dental, and social services, legal system contacts, and psychiatric hearings. Those same items used when the subject was out of the hospital were intended to function like interview data on services, providing clues rather than primary data regarding these units of service.

Another common strategy in medical care cost–outcome studies is to seek interview reports of medical care received, obtain a signed release, and then mail requests to providers for copies of bills for medical services that identify the specific procedures that were performed.

4.10 IDENTIFYING AND SELECTING RESOURCE UNITS

As Chapter 5 will discuss, a common method for estimating the value of a service unit is required to determine the cost of staff time and other resources used to deliver a particular service. Accounting systems usually are designed to aggregate the costs of the components of a particular service, such as staff time and space, to calculate the average cost of an individual unit of that service, such as a day of inpatient hospitalization or an hour of psychotherapy. The resulting unit costs usually are accurate enough for services that are not the primary focus of a study. It is frequently important, however, to examine the costs of key interventions, particularly experimental interventions in finer detail by measuring actual utilization of the different resources that comprise the intervention.

Consider the example at the beginning of this chapter, in which the investigators plan to compare individual outpatient treatment to diagnosis-specific group treatment for two disorders—schizophrenia and major depression—in a randomized cost–effectiveness study. Suppose the staff now providing individual treatment are to be trained also to provide the specialized group treatments. Existing unit cost data may be sufficient if separate unit costs are calculated for group and individual treatment. However, existing unit costs will not be sufficient if both services are combined in the calculation of a single unit cost for outpatient mental health care. If existing unit costs are not calculated separately for the two treatments, the investigators need a way to calculate the cost of the actual resources (including staff time, space, equipment, supplies) used to provide individual and group therapy.

Staff time is the most variable and expensive component of many services, particularly outpatient treatments. In such cases, the emphasis is on determining the amount of staff time used. It may be possible to estimate the utilization of other resources as a proportion of the staff time used. Other study designs will present different problems. In order to plan adequately, the cost estimation procedure for each type of unit of service needs to be planned in advance and the relevant data collection funded and completed in a timely way.

Usually the most important data is information on the way clinical staff allocate their time among their many duties. There are five common ways to gather such data, with different trade-offs between expense and accuracy: subjective evaluation, analysis of utilization statistics, staff time logs, work sampling, and time-motion analysis (Nickman et al., 1990; Sittig, 1993).

Subjective evaluation requires each worker to estimate the time typically spent in each of several types of activities. This might be accomplished by reviewing their appointment records, or done totally impressionistically. This is the least expensive approach, and the least accurate (Roberts et al., 1982).

Utilization statistics can solve the entire problem if one can assume that each type of service involves the same combination of activities, or the statistical system already includes records of time spent. This is an inexpensive method but has its own limitations (Feinstein, 1988) and investigators may wish to use work sampling or time-motion methods to test the adequacy of the existing utilization database.

A staff time log is any method in which each staff member records the duration, type, and recipient of each activity in their work day, including time not spent in service delivery (supervision, education, break time, administration, etc.). This method can be sufficiently accurate if recording is done concurrently and not reconstructed from memory at the end of a shift or work week. Accuracy may tend to degrade during periods of intense work activity (Abdellah and Levine, 1954). This method has been used in studies of assertive community treatment (Brekke, 1988).

Work sampling, a work measurement technique commonly used in industrial engineering, allows the indirect measurement of the proportion of time spent by staff on various activities (Richardson, 1976; Aft, 1983; Nickman et al., 1990). Many instantaneous observations are taken at predetermined intervals or at random, and the current activity recorded at each observation. Both observer and self-report methods have been used, and self-report methods are less expensive and more acceptable in most settings. A small timer about the size of a pager that emits a signal at random intervals can be carried by the worker, who tallies the current activity category at each signal. The steps in developing a work-sampling study are described by Nickman and co-workers (1990). The accuracy of work sampling falls rapidly with increasing numbers of activity categories. However, work sampling is used fairly widely in health services research. Oddone and co-workers (1993b) report that self-report work-sampling data by medical service house staff showed quite different, and presumably more accurate, distributions of work activities than subjective self report. Oddone and coworkers (1995) report an application of work sampling in a primary care clinical trial to aid in cost–effectiveness analysis and measurement of the intervention.

Time-motion analysis is the most expensive and accurate method for measuring work content, in that an observer follows each worker and makes a complete record of the starting and ending times of each type of activity. It is the only practical way to get accurate data on large numbers of categories of activities, most of which take up only a small percentage of the worker's time. Finkler and co-workers (1993) simulated a work-sampling design using complete data from a time-motion study in which observers recorded activities of medical house staff into 67 categories, the most common of which only occupied 8.1% of work time. Quarter-hour work samples varied greatly from the percentages observed in the complete time-motion analysis. One could get greater accuracy by sampling more frequently, but that would require essentially full-time observation, be impossible to accomplish by self-report, and therefore equal in cost to time-motion analysis. If one desired to record activities into only two or three categories, work sampling is reasonably accurate with workable sample sizes and sampling frequency, and can be done by self report.

4.11 PRACTICAL STEPS TO IMPROVE
DATA QUALITY

Utilization data obtained from different sources may not yield identical information about the occurrence or nature of resources used. One needs to develop decision rules for resolving conflicting data and estimating missing data. Records made at the time an event occurs are probably the most reliable, and might be accepted even when other sources do not report the event. On the other hand, when a respondent suggests from memory that an event occurred but it cannot be confirmed, then further checking of alternate providers or times is desirable.

After exhausting consistency checking and other analysis approaches, one is left with a residue of missing or conflicting data. Here one needs rules for estimating missing or conflicting data using average values from similar situations, or other decision rules. As Clark and co-workers (1994) remind us, decision rules are needed that strike a balance between failing to identify resource use and wrongly attributing consumption to study participants. Decision rules that set unrealistically high standards for verifying events may underrepresent resource use, while unquestioningly accepting all reports may exaggerate resource use.

One needs to guard against estimation procedures that may bias utilization data on the service groups being compared. One can explore the effects of decision rules using sensitivity analyses. In a sensitivity analysis one uses alternatively high and low values to see whether the difference affects the findings. Estimation procedures should be reviewed and critiqued by the research team, and careful records kept of the methods used. Estimation procedures should be reported in study publications, or in a manuscript available on request and noted in study publications.

This approach leaves considerable room for variation in methods for gathering the data to estimate social cost. Wolff and colleagues (1997) have shown that variations in research question formulation, data source choice, service use definition, and value calculation method can lead to widely different estimates of social cost. They propose that investigators reach a consensus on data collection, analysis, and reporting standards to reduce this variation. Drummond and co-workers (1993) have made some specific standardization proposals, while Clark and co-workers (1994) and Udvarhelyi and co-workers (1992) have suggested more general principles to guide the application of cost methods. Clark and co-workers (1994) have cautioned that some data collection, especially for nontreatment resource use, requires careful, inventive work and may be hindered by premature standardization. The reader who is initiating a study of cost-effectiveness might like to review these sources and monitor any developing consensus on standards.

Clark and co-workers (1994) suggest several ways to improve the validity of data on resources used. We have already noted the value of interviews in prompting a search of primary data sources. Recall is also a problem when interviewing about frequent events. Infrequent but prominent events like a hospitalization or an arrest will be remembered over several months, but frequent events are best recorded with a time-sampling technique rather than trying to recall the entire interval since the last interview. It is preferable to ask only about the past two weeks on such items as family assistance with transportation and total hours of care. Clark and co-workers (1994) found that asking about the "typical" level leads to reports of fewer hours of care than does asking about the past two weeks.

When resource use occurs in episodes, such as involuntary hospitalization or arrest, it is important to learn the typical patterns of resource use in each site. Police involvement, transportation, legal hearings, and other events may be common events associated with involuntary hospitalization. Similarly, an arrest may lead to much later court costs and incarceration. In some studies it may be very important to ensure that costs associated with a preintervention law enforcement or legal event do not artifactually increase the costs of an intervention. In such situations it may be desirable to attribute events such as postintervention court appearances resulting from preintervention arrests to the time of the arrest or illegal behavior.

In conclusion, one might reflect a moment on the perspective implied by the methods for measuring resource utilization. As this chapter described how to develop a balanced view of costs, the reader may have noticed a disciplinary difference in data collection traditions between clinical and economic research (Phillips and Rosenblatt, 1992). Clinical investigators are accustomed to using multi-item rating scales to obtain adequate reliability and validity in measuring psychological characteristics such as symptoms, attitudes, and opinions. This tradition is dominant in our discussion of measuring service practices (Chapter 6) and outcomes (Chapter 7). When economists measure costs, they emphasize accuracy in counting utilization events that either did or did not occur. These facts are obtained by sleuthing out the truth from multiple sources, then organizing the data and assigning value according to the theoretically grounded cost principles outlined in Chapter 3, a process that requires expert judgment at every step. Thus the most fundamental data gathering steps in the two traditions often focus on somewhat different threats to meaningfulness and validity, which leads to occasional confusion about research methods. In practice, however, the commonalities are much greater than the differences. Furthermore, the two research traditions interact in interesting ways in attempting to integrate outcome trade-offs into utilities (Chapter 8), choosing the most powerful and appropriate statistical analyses (Chapter 9), and reviewing, integrating, and evaluating research findings to maximize their policy usefulness (Chapter 10).

4.12 CHAPTER REVIEW

Chapter 4 discussed the types of services to include in a cost study, and how to measure resource utilization and define units of service. Chapter 5 discusses the valuation of resource units.

Seven services and other cost elements are considered in planning mental health studies: mental health treatment, physical health care, criminal justice services, social services, time and productivity of the patient and family members, other family costs, and transfers and other patient income. How much emphasis is given to each cost element varies with the nature of the study.

Mental health services are typically the primary focus and their utilization is measured with the greatest detail. The main components of mental health services are staff time, medication, and laboratory and other ancillary components. Institutional accounting and reporting systems often provide most of the information about service utilization, the more detailed units of resource may need to be defined and measured to adequately differentiate alternative treatments.

Physical health care, criminal justice services, and social services are included in cost studies when subjects are likely to use these services and use may be affected by the mental health services being studied.

The total cost of mental illness and its treatment includes a variety of time costs incurred by patients and their relatives, such as time patients and relatives spend in treatment and traveling to treatment. Lost productivity due to illness and the rehabilitative effects of study treatments are also important. Sometimes productivity is counted as resources created, offsetting treatment costs, and sometimes productive work is treated as an outcome rather than as part of the cost equation. When family caregivers lose work time to care for the patient or participate in treatment, this may be considered a cost. Family members also support the patient or the patient's treatment, and these costs are relevant for many studies. Transfer payments are not a societal cost but they are a cost to the taxpayer, and the cost of administering transfer payments is a societal cost.

Transfer payments, wages, and other sources and amounts of the patient's income are relevant types of information to gather in many studies.

Three types of sources of utilization data were discussed: administrative databases, interviews, and other study-specific methods. The steps in accessing administrative databases were discussed. Questions about service utilization and other cost information can be incorporated into the kinds of patient and family outcome interviews discussed in Chapter 7. Study-specific data collection may include abstracting clinical records or obtaining bills from medical providers.

Identifying and selecting appropriate units for measuring resource utilization is an important aspect of any cost–outcome study. Accounting and other data systems created for administrative purposes can be a valuable source of utilization data, but these systems may not provide unit costs at the level of detail needed to differentiate alternative treatment programs. Furthermore, experimental, research-funded programs may not be included in existing databases. Investigators may need to devise study-specific methods for measuring utilization when existing systems do not generate unit costs at the appropriate level of detail.

Different sources of utilization information often do not agree, yet triangulation using multiple sources is an aid to accuracy. After consistency checking one is left with a residue of missing or conflicting data. Here one must apply decision rules based on the knowledge of how various services ordinarily work. Sensitivity analyses will be needed to test whether these decision rules could have distorted findings. The expert judgment of a participating health economist often will be needed.

5

ESTIMATING ECONOMIC COST

The Mental Health Department of HealthPlus HMO is moving ahead on the design of their cost–effectiveness study that will compare individual psychotherapy with diagnosis-specific group treatment for schizophrenia and major depression. They have realized that the costs they measured in last year's study of inpatient care are not well focused on this new question. So, they plan to count in detail all of the outpatient intervention activities provided to study patients by the HMO, using staff time logs developed for the study. They plan to use their standard utilization data to count other HMO mental health and medical care. As part of baseline and follow-up interviews with each study patient and a key family member, they plan to ask about use of non-HMO health services, social services, patient contact with the criminal justice system, sources and amount of patient income, and family costs related to the patient's illness. Now they are wondering how to assign dollar values to these costs. It would be most convenient to use the prices the HMO charges for its services when it provides them to nonmembers. Is this appropriate? What if the prices go up during the study, or the wages and benefits of the staff who provide the services change? How will they cost services not provided by the HMO? What about patients' or family members' time taking part in treatment? That is not a cost, is it? If patients are employed more, does that matter? It certainly matters to the employers who contract for service for their employees. Does employment affect the economy in general, or is employment and improved job functioning really an outcome and not a cost issue?

The goal of any cost–outcome study is to identify interventions that provide the best outcomes for the costs incurred. This goal can be achieved only if costs are estimated accurately. The theoretical principles introduced in Chapter 3 guide the process of estimating economic costs, but they do not provide ironclad rules applicable to every study. Estimating the true cost of all resources is extremely expensive and time consuming, especially if the opportunity-cost principle of determining the best alternative use of every resource is applied strictly. As a result, most cost–outcome studies require compromises between accuracy and practicality. As with utilization measurement, investigators must weigh the costs and benefits of the cost–estimation strategy for each study to ensure that effort is allocated in proportion to the overall importance of each resource. The costs of expensive and frequently used resources must be estimated most carefully and accurately.

Choosing appropriate cost estimation procedures for every resource is central to the development of a cost–outcome study. Since cost data are usually collected separately from the utilization and effectiveness data for each study subject, it may be tempting to postpone selection of cost estimation methods until utilization data have been collected. Separating these tasks can be extremely detrimental to a study because utilization and cost must be measured in compatible units so that they can be multiplied together to calculate total cost. Thus, it is essential to specify methods for measuring both utilization and cost at the outset of a study.

In this chapter, we begin by describing three broadly defined sources of cost data. We then work through the list of resources described in Chapter 4 and describe methods for estimating their costs. The strengths and weaknesses of various data sources for different types of studies are discussed.

5.1 SOURCES OF COST DATA

There are three general ways to obtain cost data. They vary in accuracy, detail, and difficulty. The most detailed, specific, and difficult approach is to estimate directly actual costs incurred during the conduct of a study. A simpler, but less accurate, approach is to use local, program-specific, accounting data for resources under study. The simplest, but least accurate, approach is to use existing aggregate or survey data on the costs of resources similar to those under study. All three approaches to estimating resource costs—using study-specific cost data, local accounting data, or existing aggregate data—are appropriate under different circumstances in the conduct of cost–outcome studies of mental health services.

5.1.1 ACTUAL STUDY COSTS

Actual study cost estimates are the most accurate and detailed. Investigators using this approach apply economic valuation procedures to determine the cost of each individual resource related to the provision or receipt of treatment. This involves identifying the individual component parts of each treatment and determining the opportunity cost of each component. For example, the components of outpatient therapy would include space, time inputs by staff, medication, and other supplies. This kind of detailed cost estimation requires measurement of resource utilization at the component level using one of the methods discussed in Chapter 4.

5.1.2 LOCAL ACCOUNTING DATA

Local accounting reports are a common and useful source of unit cost data for mental health and medical services. Most treatment programs routinely calculate unit costs for accounting, budgeting, and reporting purposes. These calculations integrate costs of all resources used to provide services. Existing accounting data frequently are used in cost–outcome research because they are widely available and relatively easy to obtain. Accounting data are particularly desirable when they are stored in computerized databases, which facilitate searching and matching individual client records.

When using accounting data, it is essential that study resource utilization be measured in the same units used in calculating the unit cost. For example, if the available inpatient unit cost is calculated per day of inpatient treatment, then study utilization data should measure inpatient care in days. Incompatibility of resource units can have a major impact on the accuracy of cost estimates. For example, if the accounting unit cost for emergency services was computed for a one-hour unit, and research data included only counts of emergency service visits, it would be virtually impossible to estimate accurately the costs of emergency services in the study sample. These kinds of compatibility issues should be resolved during the design phase of any study.

The obvious advantages of accounting data are its availability and affordability; in most instances it is readily accessible, and researchers do not need to expend the effort necessary to calculate the cost of all treatment resources. Its disadvantages are potential limitations in comparability and accuracy. Health care providers can employ a variety of standard and legitimate cost accounting procedures (Cleverley, 1986). Comparability becomes a concern when different service agencies use different accounting methods to calculate costs; variations can obscure true cost difference or induce spurious differences (Zelman et al., 1982). For example, a program that includes the value of its building and the overhead costs associated with building maintenance will have higher unit costs than a similar program that does not include these items in its unit cost calculation. In many situations, providers use common accounting and reporting methods mandated by a government agency, third-party payer, or corporate entity, and comparability is less of a concern when all studied agencies report to the same authority. Even when common, standard procedures are in place, accuracy may be a problem if agencies do not correctly implement the standard procedures (Copley-Merriman and Lair, 1994). When using accounting data, investigators should make every effort to use costs calculated after the fact based on actual expenditures. Budgets, which provide advance estimates of expenditures and unit costs, are often more readily available, but are much more speculative and less accurate than records of expenditures.

Concerns about comparability may also arise in regard to client characteristics. Accounting costs are calculated on all clients receiving a particular service from a provider and may not apply equally to all patient subgroups. In most cases, the unit cost for a service at a particular agency is an average of all clients' costs. The actual cost of treating a severely ill client requiring ongoing medication management is likely to be higher than the cost of treating a less ill client requiring only supportive psychotherapy. Usually, this kind of variability will be reflected in the amount of service units used by different clients. However, variation in treatment intensity is possible even when the same number of service units are reported. In a study focusing on only one type of client, the average cost over all types of clients may not be an accurate estimate of the true cost of those clients' treatment. It may be unwise to use a program's average unit costs in cost estimation if the case mix of the study sample is not representative of a program's total caseload.

5.1.3 AGGREGATE DATA

Aggregate or survey data are obtained from regional or national databases or from previous cost studies that include unit costs for resources similar to those used in a cost–outcome study. Ease of access is the primary strength of such data. Data collected by government agencies are increasingly accessible through online computer resources.

Existing aggregate or survey data are problematic because it is usually difficult for investigators to determine how similar the valued resources are to the resources in their own study. For example, a survey estimate of outpatient treatment costs based on a varied sample of programs in different locales would be likely to underestimate the cost of outpatient treatment provided in a densely populated urban area by highly paid doctoral-level therapists, but would be likely to overestimate the cost of outpatient treatment provided by masters-level therapists in a rural area. It is often impossible to assess the accounting methods used to determine costs, and it may be difficult to determine the effect of regional cost variation on aggregate costs.

In most cost–outcome studies, aggregate and survey data are only appropriate for relatively low-volume resources that represent a modest proportion of total cost, especially those for which actual study costs or study-specific or local-cost data are not readily available. Law enforcement and justice system services are examples of resources for which aggregate cost data are useful. Local law enforcement and justice agencies rarely calculate unit costs for their services, nor is it typically practical for mental health researchers to conduct time and motion studies of such services when they represent only a small proportion of total costs. Regional or national costs estimated with methodologic rigor are likely to be more accurate than haphazard estimates of local costs. Regional or national data also may be used to estimate the impact of large scale implementation of a program, regardless of how costs of the original treatment alternatives were estimated.

5.2 ESTIMATING RESOURCE COSTS

The next sections are devoted to detailed discussion of estimating the value of resources used because of mental health problems. The discussion is organized around the same list of resources presented in Chapter 4 on measuring resource utilization: mental health treatment, physical health care, criminal justice activities, social services, time and productivity, other family costs, and transfers and other income. In this section we discuss theoretical and practical considerations in assigning dollar values to resource units. For each type of unit we discuss advantages and disadvantages of using different types of data sources, specific data sources that may be available, and principles for selecting valuation methods appropriate to particular research conditions.

5.2.1 MENTAL HEALTH TREATMENT

Mental health treatment costs are the primary focus of most mental health cost–outcome studies. As such, mental health treatment services usually are measured in greatest detail, and the value of the measured service units is estimated most accurately. Therefore, we will discuss mental health treatment in the greatest detail, and other costs more briefly. As discussed in Chapter 4, mental health treatments include inpatient care, skilled nursing care, residential treatment, emergency room contacts, outpatient sessions, case management hours, day treatment services, partial hospitalization, social skills training, vocational rehabilitation, medication, and laboratory procedures. In a societal cost study, all of these treatment resources will be enumerated and valued, although a specific type of treatment, such as an experimental treatment, may be assessed in greater detail than other treatments. The following sections discuss estimating costs of mental health treatment using the three data sources described in Section 5.2.

The extensive effort required to estimate actual study costs for components of mental health treatment is necessary or desirable when those treatments are the primary focus of a cost–outcome study (Knapp and Beecham, 1993). Calculation of actual study costs is often unavoidable in studies of innovative, experimental treatments that are developed and delivered solely in a research context, because accounting cost data usually are not available for these novel treatments. Even when accounting data are available, study-specific cost estimates may be desirable. As discussed in Chapter 4, studies that compare different approaches to the provision of the same kind of treatment usually require examination and valuation of the component resources used in treatment. Identifying the specific quantities of time inputs by different staff disciplines and other resources is necessary to distinguish accurately the competing treatment approaches and to determine their true cost. Use of an average unit cost would obscure the comparison.

In Chapter 4 we discussed the main components of mental health treatment that need to be enumerated in cost–effectiveness studies: staff time, medication, and ancillary services. We now describe approaches to estimating the cost of these enumerated resources, including estimating capital and overhead costs.

Staff Time

Staff time costs typically are estimated using wage and benefit rates for the staff that actually provide the services being studied. It is rarely necessary to assign costs at the level of the individual staff member. Instead, unit costs usually are expressed as an average of the wage and benefit costs of individuals who share a common professional discipline or who provide a common service. The structure of a particular treatment typically determines the method of aggregation. In a setting in which members of different disciplines have well-defined, distinct roles, it would be logical to calculate the average hourly cost of a psychiatrist, a nurse, a social worker, and so forth. In a setting in which members of different disciplines have similar roles, such as outpatient therapist or case manager, average hourly cost could be calculated by role, rather than by discipline. In some contexts, it is useful to conduct multiple analyses using different levels of aggregation. For example, it may be informative to determine whether higher cost staff, such as psychiatrists, are more cost–effective outpatient therapists than lower cost staff, such as social workers. If social workers appear more cost-effective than psychiatrists, it might be a useful modeling exercise to reexamine cost-effectiveness using the lower staff cost for all outpatient therapy contacts.

It is useful to examine the range of wage and benefit rates that contribute to an aggregate staff cost estimate to check for outlying low or high rates, and to look for artifactual wage differentials between different treatment programs. In some cases there may be large differences in wages paid to similarly educated and experienced employees who have similar roles at different treatment agencies. Differences in compensation may reflect real differences in staff competence, but more often reflect artifactual differences, such as agency ownership. For example, civil service employees working in public mental agencies may have markedly different salary scales than similar employees working in private, not-for-profit agencies. It is important to examine carefully the distribution of actual staff wages and construct a wage rate estimate that prevents artifactual differences in wage rates from spuriously affecting study findings.

Medication

Medication is an important aspect of many mental health treatments and is of particular interest in studies of new and more expensive drugs. The price of a single medication can vary dramatically depending on the quantity ordered and the point of distribution. The per-dose price of a medication purchased by a hospital pharmacy can be a small fraction of the price of the same medication purchased by a patient at a local pharmacy. Some of these differences may reflect previously discussed distinctions between costs and charges, but other differences may reflect inclusion or exclusion of labor costs involved in packaging and dispensing medication. For example, the price the hospital pharmacy pays for a medication does not reflect the labor inputs required to label, deliver, and dispense each dose to a patient. The price the patient pays at the pharmacy does incorporate these costs. Obtaining wholesale drug prices from commercial databases such as Medi-span and First Databank can reduce some artifactual variation in drug costs (Copley-Merriman and Lair, 1994). In determining study specific medication costs, however, it is important to ensure that related labor costs are included in estimates of either staff time costs or in estimates of medication costs.

Laboratory and Other Ancillary Services

Most laboratory and other ancillary services, such as imaging studies, are considered to be medical services (see Section 5.2.2). The method for determining resource cost varies with treatment setting.

A broad range of laboratory and other diagnostic studies may be conducted during inpatient treatment. These costs may be estimated using charge data on individual study subjects adjusted using the appropriate charge-to-cost ratio from a hospital's Medicare Cost Report, as discussed at the end of this section. In many cases, ancillary service use will represent too small a proportion of treatment cost to justify data collection at the individual patient level. In such cases, the average cost of ancillary treatment can be calculated as a proportion of total inpatient treatment cost using charge data for a sample of patients. Ancillary costs for all patients then can be calculated using this standard estimate. For example, in a study of 200 patients, an investigator might determine the true ancillary costs associated with inpatient treatment for 20 patients, finding ancillary costs equal to 3% of inpatient per diem costs. Ancillary costs for all inpatient care then could be calculated as 3% of per diem costs.

Capital Costs

The complex process of valuing very visible and obvious treatment components, such as staff time and medication, often draws attention away from valuing the space in which treatment is provided. Capital costs of buildings and land often are neglected, even though they may represent a significant proportion of treatment cost in some circumstances (Weisbrod, 1983; McGuire, 1991). The difficulty of estimating capital costs can vary considerably from setting to setting. The capital costs of a program operating in rental space are equivalent to the rent paid, providing that the space is rented at a fair market rate. Estimating the capital costs of programs operating in publicly owned buildings is considerably more difficult. Most older buildings are fully depreciated, and accounting records do not provide estimates of capital costs.

Rosenheck, Frisman, and Neale (1994) described and tested two methods for estimating the capital costs of mental health programs that were used previously by Dickey et al. (1986b, c). The first method estimates the opportunity cost of capital using the prevailing local rental rate for similar space. The second method uses construction cost estimates and property asset reports to calculate the replacement cost of buildings and land. These authors also presented a method for allocating capital costs to different types of services, such as inpatient and outpatient services, that operate in the same building. Rental estimates were consistently lower than replacement cost estimates, but estimates were similar in nine different VA hospitals. Capital costs accounted for approximately 6% of inpatient costs and 4% of outpatient costs. This relatively low level of capital expense is similar to that seen in other studies of medical care providers. Thus, Rosenheck and his colleagues conclude that calculating capital costs as a fixed percentage of other treatment costs may be reasonable when study-specific capital costs are not available.

Overhead Costs

In calculating actual study treatment costs, it is important to consider overhead costs such as housekeeping, maintenance, and management activities. In small facilities, housing a single program or several similar programs, overhead costs can be determined from accounting records. In large multifunction organizations, such as hospitals, these costs are allocated to each department or program in proportion to level of consumption. The cost accounting procedures used to allocate these costs can be quite complex (Cleverley, 1986; Goldschmidt and Gafni, 1990). Overhead costs typically are allocated to different units or programs in proportion to their consumption of a particular resource, such as square feet of space used, pounds of laundry done, number of admissions processed. Given the complexity of these allocation procedures, investigators are advised to consult program accountants for assistance in determining overhead costs.

Sources of Data for Valuing Mental Health Treatment Costs

Experimental treatments are valued through study-specific estimation. The most common source of cost estimates for other mental health services, however, is local accounting data. Accounting data typically include unit costs, which incorporate the costs of the component resources such as staff time, space, and supplies. Several kinds of accounting data may be used.

Program accounting data is prepared by an individual program for internal planning and budgeting. These data may include calculations of unit costs. This kind of accounting data may be the most detailed and can be the most useful in studies that involve only a small number of programs because study staff can improve the accuracy of cost estimates by discussing cost accounting procedures with program accountants.

In studies that involve a wide variety of programs, variation in accounting procedures can limit the comparability of unit cost calculations across programs and limit researchers' ability to review each program's accounting methods. When many programs are involved, standardized cost reports, such as those submitted to local or regional government agencies or corporate entities, may provide more comparable cost data, since all agencies are required to use common reporting procedures. The computerized databases typically used to store accounting data facilitate access to data on multiple programs and matching of cost data to other research data.

Even when provider organizations accurately calculate unit costs using standard procedures, some legitimate accounting methods may not yield the kinds of cost values desired for economic analysis. For example, the capital costs of fully depreciated buildings typically are absent from accounting records, but may represent a large enough proportion of treatment to affect the relationship between cost and outcome (McGuire, 1991; Wolff and Helminiak, 1996). The ideal approach is for investigators to review the accounting methods used to calculate unit costs and to adjust these costs as appropriate, such as by adding an estimate of capital costs. It may be difficult to adjust costs in studies involving a large number of programs, however, because of the effort involved in reviewing the accounting procedures at multiple sites.

When accounting cost data are not available, it is sometimes possible to calculate costs from data on charges. As noted in Chapter 3, charges are not accurate or reliable proxies for costs. Charges commonly include a share of the cost of uncompensated care for other patients or reflect cost-shifting among different departments in a hospital or service agency. Charges also may reflect profits to private sector providers as well as price discrimination among different client groups if a provider has negotiated special rates with a government program or private insurance plan (Dranove, 1988; Copley-Merriman and Lair, 1994). Despite these inherent limitations, charges sometimes can be used to calculate costs.

Many U.S. institutions prepare a Medicare Cost Report for the Health Care Financing Administration (HCFA) for reimbursement purposes. Data from these reports is maintained in Medicare's Health Care Provider Cost Report Information System (HCRIS) (Lave et al., 1994). These reports contain calculations of institution-specific charge-to-cost ratios, which reflect cost-shifting among departments. For example, if the charge for a day of inpatient hospitalization is $900 and the hospital's charge-to-cost ratio for inpatient psychiatric care is 1.44, the actual cost would be $625. The costs of other services, such as laboratory assays and imaging studies, also can be calculated using these charge-to-cost ratios. Other HCVA indices, such as the Relative Value Unit (RVU) for physician procedures and services, can be used to calculate the costs of physician fees and medications (Dove, 1994; Lave et al.,1994; Morton et al., 1994). Medicare Cost

Reports and other standard reports can be especially useful in multisite studies because the required standard reporting procedures will yield more comparable cost data than costs calculated using site-specific accounting procedures.

If neither cost data nor charge-to-cost ratios are available, administrative payment data provide a better estimate of costs than do charge data alone. Payments are likely to reflect negotiation of an amount closer to actual cost than the original charge (Copley-Merriman and Lair, 1994; Lave et al., 1994).

In most cases, aggregate or survey data that is not specific to studied treatments is not the optimal source of cost data on costly or widely used mental health treatments. National or regional cost data, however, or cost estimates from previous cost studies may be useful in the valuation of resources that are used infrequently. Similarly, aggregate or survey data may be used to estimate costs of services provided at infrequently used or out of area facilities for which local accounting cost data is unavailable.

5.2.2 PHYSICAL HEALTH CARE

While potential links to medical illness and medical care utilization exist in virtually all mental health treatments, the level and importance of medical care utilization should be considered in the design of each study. The wide variety of providers, insurance plans, and payment options makes it more difficult to estimate the cost of medical care than mental health care, and these costs may not be crucial to every cost–outcome study.

It is possible to calculate actual study costs for all types of medical care, and many health economic studies do so. In most studies of mental health treatment, however, medical care represents a relatively small proportion of total cost, and study subjects receive too wide a range of medical services to justify this level of effort.

Charge data is often used to enumerate utilization of general health care, but these data present special problems as a way to estimate the economic cost of medical services. Charges may reflect subsidies of one type of medical service to another, and they may include the cost of uncollected bills or free care.

Charge data from provider and insurer databases may be difficult to link to the kind of utilization data collected in a cost–outcome study. In addition they may not contain data on appropriately representative patient populations. For example, Medicare costs and claims databases provide uniform data on all covered health care services for almost all Americans over age 65. Although these databases are very complete, they include only older and disabled persons, whose patterns of disease and treatment are likely to be different from those of other patient groups. Medicaid databases may provide relatively complete payment data on persons disabled by serious and persistent mental illness.

National or regional aggregate data from surveys or claims databases also can be used to assign costs to medical services. Data from rigorously designed surveys, such as the National Medical Expenditure Survey (Hahn and Lefkowitz,

1992), are widely representative of patient groups, insurance plans, geographic area, and payment sources. Survey data are limited, however, by their reliance on patient reports. Aggregate data from insurance claims databases, like the claims data discussed in the previous section, may not be representative of all patient groups. In mental health studies in which medical care utilization represents a modest proportion of overall cost, the ease of using published, accessible, aggregate data easily may outweigh the costs of using complex payment or claims data to compute medical care costs.

5.2.3 CRIMINAL JUSTICE ACTIVITIES

In Chapter 4 we noted how challenging it is to estimate criminal justice activities. It is equally difficult to estimate actual study costs for each type of criminal justice activity. Actual study cost estimates are largely impractical in studies that do not involve mental health treatments provided within or in cooperation with the criminal justice system. Confidentiality concerns at all levels of the criminal justice system generally will prevent outside researchers from observing activities closely enough to identify and value component resources.

Local accounting data are typically available, though extensive effort is required to obtain access to criminal justice data and link data from disparate data systems. Even when accounting data are available, it may be very difficult to estimate the costs of all component resources, since many criminal justice services are nonmarket resources and providers may not think in terms of service units or unit costs. Some systems routinely may compute cost reports and calculate unit costs for discrete service units, but data quality and availability and the number of relevant independent agencies varies considerably across jurisdictions.

Existing aggregate data may provide the best source of criminal justice cost estimates when local data are not readily available. One example of a rigorously conducted study of criminal justice costs is the National Institute of Justice study of offender processing costs in 1983 and 1984 (Jacoby et al., 1987; Wayson and Funke, 1989). This study computed component costs for five categories of crime (violent crimes, property crimes, drug crimes, other felonies, and misdemeanors) in four sites (Ventura County, California; Mecklenburg County, North Carolina; Allegheny County, Pennsylvania; and Alexandria, Virginia). Unit costs were calculated for law enforcement (e.g., response, arrest, investigation), prosecution and defense costs (hearings, pleas, court appearances, and other attorney services), pretrial release agency activities, court activities (arraignments, hearings, trials), jail and prison incarceration, and probation field services. These cost estimates, adjusted for inflation and regional cost differences, can be used as estimates of local criminal justice costs. The major limitation of these cost data is that specific cost estimates are not available for services that may be particularly relevant to mentally ill populations, such as conservatorship costs and interventions in which no arrest is made (e.g., transportation to an emergency service).

5.2.4 SOCIAL SERVICES

As described in Chapter 4, social services include a variety of supportive and rehabilitative activities provided by local charitable organizations independently or in partnership with local government. The emphasis on data collection regarding social services depends on the study population, but these costs may be important when studying very disabled populations.

Actual study cost data obtained through observation or staff record keeping is likely to be practical only in studies in which a particular social service is central to the study and research funds are available for data collection. Small budgets and limited staffing are common in social service agencies and agency staff generally lack the time and resources to collect cost data on their own.

Similarly, many agencies, particularly those run by charitable organizations that do not have contracts with local government, have limited administrative capacity and are unable to provide accounting estimates of unit costs. Even when unit cost data are available, variations in program structure and mission, even within a single city or county, may make data from different programs incomparable. Variation across programs also makes the use of aggregate data impractical.

5.2.5 TIME AND PRODUCTIVITY

The total cost of mental illness and its treatment includes a variety of time costs incurred by patients, and in many cases, patients' relatives. As discussed in Chapter 4, time costs typically include the time patients and their relatives spend in treatment and traveling to treatment, the value of productive time lost by patients as a result of their illness, or time lost by relatives who forgo productive activity to care for ill individuals. Time costs are usually more difficult to estimate than more discretely defined treatment or service costs, and multiple considerations are involved in deciding how to characterize these costs, which costs to include in an analysis (as discussed in Chapter 4), and how to estimate those costs.

It has been traditional to distinguish between direct and indirect time costs. Typically, time spent in and traveling to treatment is considered a direct treatment cost, and lost productivity attributable to illness is considered an indirect cost. In practice, however, it is often difficult to distinguish direct and indirect costs. For example, it is not obvious whether the time a well relative spends in family treatment with an ill family member is a direct cost reflecting consumption of treatment resources or a loss of productive work time as a result of illness. The distinction between direct and indirect costs may vary with study context and is not a primary consideration in selecting methods for estimating time costs. It is essential, however, to avoid double-counting time costs as both direct and indirect costs. This kind of double-counting could easily occur if patient time spent in individual treatment contacts is included as a direct cost and the cost of lost productivity during the same period is counted as an indirect cost (Koopmanschap and van Ineveld, 1992).

Decisions about which time costs to include also will vary with the analytic perspective and the target group under study. It is appropriate to include the value of time spent in treatment and traveling to treatment when treatment participants give up work to take part. In studies of treatments for severe mental illness, however, many participants will be too disabled to engage in productive employment and are not giving up work hours to engage in treatment. Thus, it is inappropriate to use a wage-based estimate of the value of their time. One can take the perspective that these individuals are giving up leisure time, which has value, to participate in treatment. However, it is easy to imagine situations in which a disabled individual might well prefer certain treatment activities, such as participating in a socialization program with others in similar life circumstances, to his or her usual leisure activity of watching television alone. It is difficult to see how such a person has incurred a real time loss by participating in treatment. While all patients do not view treatment positively, it is likely that applying strict economic criteria to valuing time spent in treatment will overstate treatment costs for persons with disabling mental illness.

Standardized valuation of time spent in treatment poses other problems as well. Regardless of how time is valued, cost will increase with the duration of treatment. Thus, the most intensive treatments, such as inpatient hospitalization, will have the highest time cost. Since only the most severely ill persons are hospitalized, the value of such time is not obvious. Most severely impaired individuals would prefer not to be in the hospital, but it is doubtful that most could engage in productive work or enjoyable leisure activities were they not in treatment. Thus, including the value of time spent in intensive treatments could unreasonably overstate treatment costs.

Productivity

There is little question that the value of lost productivity is an important component of the societal cost of illness, and it should be included in societal cost analyses. The way lost productivity is included in an analysis may vary from study to study. In studies of treatments directed at target populations that typically have established a history of competitive employment, it is appropriate to use individual or aggregate wage rates to estimate the value of productivity lost as a result of illness. This approach may be less appropriate in studies of persons with chronic, disabling illnesses, such as schizophrenia, which often begin in adolescence or early adulthood before an individual has any significant record of labor force participation. As a result, prior wage rates for such individuals may yield unreliable estimates of their productivity. Aggregate, population-based wage rates are appropriate in cost-of-illness studies, which imply an illness-free comparison condition. In cost–outcome studies comparing specific patient samples, particularly persons with severe mental illness, aggregate wage rates are likely to overestimate true earning potential. For these reasons, many studies of treatments for the severely mentally ill have not included lost productivity as an indirect cost, but have collected data on actual earnings and included them in the analysis as outcomes (Murphy and Datel, 1976; Weisbrod, 1981; Hu and Jerrell, in press). This approach is desirable for several reasons. First, it avoids the inclusion of a large, unreliable cost component, which could obscure treatment differences. Second, it is based on actual patient data and avoids estimation using cumbersome external data sources. Third, it seems an appropriate perspective since many severely mentally ill persons are unemployed or underemployed, and improved vocational function is a specified goal of many treatment programs.

Patients' Time Costs

Time that patients spend in treatment, traveling to and from treatment, or time lost from productive activity as a result of illness can be valued in several ways. Regardless of the valuation method, it is crucial to keep in mind the caution against double-counting time costs as both a direct treatment cost and an indirect cost of lost productivity. If time spent in treatment is included as a cost, the time should not be valued at a wage rate unless the patient was actively engaged in the competitive job market, as evidenced by employment or substantive job seeking, or was clearly engaged in significant noncompensated activity, such as household work or child care.

Study-specific cost estimates can be calculated using actual wage rates in current or previous employment. This approach is both feasible and desirable in studies of patient groups in which employment is common. In such cases, actual wage rates will provide a more accurate estimate of time costs than aggregate wage rates. Current or prior wage rates may yield highly variable and unreliable estimates in severely disabled patient groups, which are characterized by limited work force participation, and aggregate data may be preferred. Even when actual individual wage rates are used for competitive employment, aggregate rates, as described below, are used to value nonmarket, household work.

Local administrative data sources rarely include information on wage rates for specific individuals. There may be some instances, however, in which obtaining wage data from study participants may be desirable. Calculating a study-specific average wage may be useful if external factors produce an unusual distribution of individual wage rates or if aggregate wage data are not available for the general population at a suitable level of detail.

Existing aggregate data on prevailing wage rates are used to estimate time costs in many studies. Earnings data can be aggregated in different ways to suit particular study goals. Rates specific to geographical areas (national, regional, local) or subgroups defined by gender, ethnicity, or occupation may be used. Average wage rates should be adjusted for level of work force participation in the population, since not all individuals would work even in the absence of illness. More specific estimates of work force participation rates will yield more accurate time cost estimates. For example, in their national study of the costs of alcohol and drug abuse and mental illness, Rice and her colleagues (1990) used data on average national income aggregated by age and gender and adjusted for the percentage income loss associated with each diagnosis. A variety of national and regional data on wages and labor force participation is available from the U.S. Department of Labor's Bureau of Labor Statistics (1992a).

Aggregate estimates typically are used to estimate the value of nonmarket work, such as housekeeping and childcare. These activities can be valued at the prevailing wage rate of domestic workers (Smith and Wright, 1994). Peskin (1983) presented a regression approach that values the time inputs involved in household work using the "specialist" cost of workers, such as cooks and cleaners, who perform similar tasks in the competitive market. For updated estimates using this approach, see Rice et al. (1990).

Family Members' Time Costs

Family members often provide extensive informal care to a severely disabled family member, and there are two approaches to estimating these costs that have different interpretations and are appropriate in different research contexts. The first method values time at the opportunity cost of the family member providing care. The second method values time at the substitution cost of the actual caregiving tasks performed (Zick and Bryant, 1990; Clark and Drake, 1994; Smith and Wright, 1994). The opportunity cost method is most appropriate from a societal, cost-of-illness perspective, since it reflects the value of the productivity loss society incurs when a family member gives up competitive employment to care for someone who is ill. This kind of estimate, however, may distort cost–outcome relationships in studies that focus on the relative cost-effectiveness of particular treatments. Consider, for example, two mothers who leave paid work to care for a schizophrenic child. One mother is an attorney earning $100,000 per year, and the other is a bank teller earning $25,000. If the opportunity cost method is applied using individual wage rates, the treatment of the attorney's child would appear to cost four times as much as the treatment of the bank teller's child. Unless there is reason to assume that the quality of the lawyer's caregiving is significantly superior, this valuation does not provide any meaningful information about treatment cost and its magnitude may have a noticeable impact on the overall cost–outcome relationship.

Thus, in many cases, it makes more sense to use either an aggregate wage rate as an estimate of opportunity cost or to use the substitution cost, calculated as the specialist cost of paid caregivers, such as home health workers or mental health workers. The substitution cost approach is particularly useful when the caregiving activities could be incorporated into a particular intervention. The relationship between opportunity cost estimates and substitution cost estimates may differ from study to study. In a study of family assistance provided to persons with both severe mental illness and substance use disorders in New Hampshire, Clark (1994) found that the opportunity cost method, applied using aggregate regional wage rates, yielded lower estimates than the substitution cost method. In a national study of informal care for the elderly, White-Means and Chollet (1996) found that the opportunity cost method, applied using individual wage data, yielded higher estimates than the substitution method. It is not clear whether this disparity is due to differences in study population or estimation method.

Study-specific cost estimates of the opportunity cost of family members' time inputs can be calculated using individuals' actual wage rates in their current or previous employment. A wage-based opportunity cost is only appropriate when there is evidence that a family member would have engaged in competitive employment had he or she not been caring for an ill relative. If there is no evidence that a family member would have engaged in productive employment, the substitution cost of informal care should be used to value his or her time. Study-specific estimates of substitution costs would only be appropriate in study samples in which formal care is substituted for informal care frequently enough that formal care costs are available.

As in the discussion of patient time costs above, local administrative data sources rarely include information on wage rates. There may be some instances, however, in which an average wage rate calculated for the group of family members in a particular study may be useful. Such an average rate may be desirable if external factors produce an unusual distribution of wage rates or if aggregate wage data are not available at a suitable level of detail.

Existing aggregate data on prevailing wage rates are a frequent source of opportunity cost estimates of family time costs and the most common source of substitution cost estimates. Opportunity cost estimates are calculated from aggregate earnings data using the same methods described above for valuing patients' time. Methods for calculating substitution cost estimates from aggregate wage data vary with the specificity and detail of utilization data on family time inputs. When detailed data are available on the nature and duration of actual tasks performed, the specialist cost method can be applied to value each separate task, such as cooking, transportation, or medication management. For example, Clark (1994) valued family time devoted to illness related tasks at the average reimbursement rate for mental health case managers and valued time devoted to housekeeping tasks at the local rate for home health care workers. If detailed data on task composition are not available, the reimbursement rate for home health care workers is usually the most practical substitution cost estimate.

5.2.6 OTHER FAMILY COSTS

As discussed in Chapter 4, families also often make direct cash contributions to the support of an ill family member (Franks, 1990; Carpentier et al., 1992; Clark and Drake, 1994). Many cash and in-kind contributions can be considered transfer payments from a societal perspective. From the family perspective these resources are costs, and from the ill person's perspective they are income. Information on cash contributions is valued at its reported amount. In-kind contributions are probably best converted to an estimated cash equivalent by the interview respondent at the time of the interview.

5.2.7 TRANSFERS AND OTHER INCOME

Traditionally, transfer payments are not considered costs from a societal perspective because they reflect only a transfer of existing resources rather than creation or consumption of resources. As a result, only the costs of administering transfer payments are costs from the societal perspective. However, transfer payments may be viewed differently from other perspectives. From the recipient perspective, transfer payments are clearly gains, not costs; from the governmental perspective, both benefits and administrative activities are costs. Even in societal cost studies of mental health treatments, transfer payments may be examined even if they are not treated as costs, since disability and welfare benefits tend to be extremely important to persons disabled by severe mental illness. Thus, it is typical to consider transfer payments and their administrative costs separately. Brent (1996) argues that transfer payments should not be excluded from cost outcome analyses because they are associated with real societal costs, particularly in programs for the severely mentally ill. Collecting complete data on transfer payments permits analysis of benefit and administrative costs as appropriate to different research questions.

In studies involving client or collateral interviews, study-specific cost estimates of transfer payments are commonly obtained by asking respondents about the type and amount of payments received.

Administrative costs of transfer payments must be estimated. In most cost–outcome studies it would be difficult to justify the effort necessary to estimate study-specific costs associated with administering transfer payments to a specific group of study clients. Obtaining access to entitlement program records or obtaining permission to observe program activities are major obstacles. Site specific costs may be equally difficult to obtain. Most estimates of the administrative costs of transfer payments are based on aggregate national data for nationally administered programs such as Supplemental Security Income (SSI).

The simplest and most common approach to estimating the administrative costs of transfer payments is to estimate administrative costs as a percentage of benefits paid using national aggregate data. Using this method to calculate 1985 costs of social welfare administration, Rice and her colleagues (1990) estimated that administrative costs ranged from a low of 1.2% of OASDI benefits to a high of 12.1% of unemployment insurance benefits; administrative costs for SSI were calculated as 8% of benefits. In light of this level of variation in administrative cost, it is advisable to calculate administrative costs separately for different entitlement programs in studies of populations that receive a high level of transfer payments.

The costs of different administrative activities also vary, and calculating administrative costs as a flat percentage of benefits may obscure true cost. For example, it is more expensive to evaluate and award a new claim than to maintain an awarded benefit (Schobel, 1981). Frisman and Rosenheck (1994, unpublished manuscript) used Social Security Administration data to calculate application and benefit maintenance costs separately. They found that the annual cost of a recipient with a new award would be at least $640, while annual maintenance costs for a previously awarded benefit could be as low as $55. Although costs for the subgroup of mentally ill beneficiaries could differ from these estimates, these results suggest that misestimation of the administrative costs of transfer payments could have an impact on the cost–outcome relationship in studies in which transfer payments are common.

Other sources of income, to the extent that they are relevant to the particular study, typically are gathered in monetary units so that no other value estimation is needed, except for the adjustments described below.

5.3 ADJUSTING COST ESTIMATES

It is often necessary to adjust cost estimates prior to analysis to ensure meaningful comparisons across treatments, locales, and time. These adjustments include adjusting costs for inflation occurring during or since the study period, adjusting costs for regional differences in prices, discounting costs to reflect the current value of future costs, and including or excluding personal maintenance costs, such as room and board costs, which may be part of some treatments but not of others.

5.3.1 INFLATION

Cost data often are collected over a period of years in longitudinal studies. Cost data collected in the last year of study are not directly comparable to data collected in the first year of the study, because inflation during the time interval has altered the value of the dollar and the meaning of cost estimates. Standard inflation or price indices typically are used to adjust costs in different years to the level established in an index year specified for the study. For example, in a 5-year cost study that started in 1990 and ended in 1995, investigators might make adjustments to present all cost data in 1995 dollars.

The Medical Care Price Index (MCPI), a subindex of the Bureau of Labor Statistics' Consumer Price Index (CPI) (1991, 1992b), is a standard source of inflation rates for cost adjustment. The CPI is designed to measure price changes experienced directly by consumers; the MCPI measures price changes in a particular "market basket" or set of medical services, such as physician and hospital services, and medical commodities, such as drugs and medical equipment. The MCPI is a consistent and reliable indicator of price changes in consumer transactions in the medical sector, although it may not provide an absolutely accurate measure of inflation in the medical care sector (Graboyes, 1994; Getzen, 1992).

One concern in mental health cost–outcome studies is that the inflation rate reflected by the MCPI may be inaccurate, because the set of services and commodities included in the MCPI may not correspond to the resources used in mental health treatment. In some situations, it may be desirable to look at lower level subdivisions of the MCPI, which reflect costs for specific services (e.g., physicians, hospital rooms, inpatient and outpatient care, nursing homes) and specific commodities (e.g., drugs, medical equipment). Specific indices also exist for hospital costs and nursing home costs, which may be appropriate in some studies (Graboyes, 1994).

It is also possible that MCPI calculations are based on a sample of consumers that is not representative of consumers of a particular mental health treatment. Specially focused CPI indices have been calculated for subgroups of consumers, such as retirees and self-employed individuals (Getzen, 1992), but it is not clear that specific groups of mental health consumers could be identified in CPI data. An alternative to adjusting for inflation is to use costs from a single "index" year to value utilization in all years; this approach provides a common, comparable cost metric for the full study period.

5.3.2 REGIONAL VARIATION

Regional variation is of concern in multisite studies because prevailing regional differences in costs of similar resources can obscure cost–outcome comparisons. CPI and MCPI data can be used to adjust for regional variation in cost because data are collected and tabulated for both large and small geographic regions.

5.3.3 DISCOUNTING

Discounting is the process of adjusting future costs to their present value. This adjustment is based on the economic principle that the present value of a dollar is always greater than the value of the same dollar in a future year, even in the absence of inflation, because the opportunity to use the dollar now is forgone, as is the opportunity to earn additional income by investing the dollar. Therefore, it is necessary to adjust the costs of interventions that continue for more than one year, so that costs in later years are expressed in terms of the present value. For example, at a 5% discount rate, the present value of a $100 cost to be incurred next year is $95.24, calculated as $100/(1 + .05)$.

The choice of an appropriate discount rate for cost–outcome analyses is a complex and controversial issue. There is apparent consensus in the applied literature in health economics on a range of discount rates between 2 and 10%, with a 5% rate most commonly employed (Krahn and Gafni, 1993). This prevailing standard, however, masks considerable theoretical disagreement among and between economists and philosophers about discount rates. This disagreement centers on which of two economic principles provides the best rationale for discounting the costs of health care and other social programs (Olsen, 1993a; Robinson, 1990). The first principle is that of time preference, according to which the appropriate discount rate reflects the rate at which individuals are willing to exchange present for future consumption. The second principle is that of opportunity cost, according to which the discount rate reflects the rate of return on an investment in an alternative program or activity (Krahn and Gafni, 1993). These principles may lead to equivalent discount rates, but the time preference approach usually results in higher rates than the opportunity cost approach. Controversy arises over whether consumers' revealed preferences for current consumption provide the appropriate standard for funding decisions that will effect those consumers and society at large in the future.

The discount rate used in any cost–outcome analysis can have a dramatic impact on results and conclusions; high rates favor programs with short-term therapeutic effects, while low rates favor programs with long-term preventive effects. It is difficult to justify the conventional rate of 5% to achieve comparability across studies, because different programs may have different values under different conditions. For example, different rates may be appropriate in considering or comparing public and private investments. Discount rates should be selected to be consistent with the perspective of the overall analysis. Thus, a societal discount rate would be appropriate in an evaluation of a government-funded program, but not in an evaluation of a privately funded program (Krahn and Gafni, 1993). At present, no optimal strategy exists for determining the ideal discount rate in any cost–outcome comparison. Therefore, it is important for investigators to document the discounting procedures used in any analysis and to conduct sensitivity analyses to determine whether variations in the discount rate substantively alter study findings. The discounting of outcomes is another important consideration, and it is discussed in Chapter 8.

5.3.4 JOINT COSTS

Joint costs are incurred when one facility or program provides two or more distinct services, such as day treatment and outpatient therapy, and the two services share resources such as space or staff. The cost of such shared resources must be allocated proportionately among the different services before the true cost of each service can be determined. Two general methods are used to allocate joint costs between services. One method is based on the amount of inputs used, such as amount of space or clinician time. The other method is based on the amount of outputs produced, such as number of clients treated.

5.3.5 MAINTENANCE COSTS

Personal maintenance costs represent resources required for subsistence whether or not an individual participates in mental health treatment, including food, shelter, and clothing. There is some debate about how to incorporate these costs into cost–outcome analyses of mental health treatment, and different approaches may be more suited to the study of some treatments than others. It is also possible to consider many maintenance costs as either public or private transfers and treat them similarly to transfer payments as discussed in Section 5.2.7 (Brent, 1996; unpublished).

Maintenance costs usually are incorporated into the administrative unit costs of inpatient and residential services. Questions arise, however, as to whether these costs should be part of the treatment cost, since every individual, whether healthy or ill, has some basic needs for food, clothing, and lodging, and only the added costs of meeting these needs in a special setting are truly treatment costs. In some studies, maintenance costs incurred in treatment settings have been considered treatment costs (Rice et al., 1992). In other studies, room and board costs have been subtracted from the unit cost of residential treatment. Dickey and associates (1986), for example, attributed one third of the cost of residential mental health programs to room and board. It is more common to separate maintenance costs from treatment costs for long-term residential than for short-term acute services, such as inpatient hospitalization, because inpatient care is temporary and patients are likely to continue to incur their usual lodging and other maintenance costs while they are in the hospital. It is less common for persons living in long-term facilities to maintain another residence.

Maintenance costs incurred by individuals living in houses or apartments alone or with family or friends typically are not included in cost analyses, because these are normal expenses not directly associated with mental illness. The costs of employing a caretaker to assist a patient with basic daily living activities, however, is an illness-related cost that should be included. Financial support from family members and friends may also be a cost of illness and could be included in cost analyses. It may be difficult, however, to determine the amount or nature of this assistance or to determine how much of the assistance provided to an ill individual exceeds that provided to other household members.

It may be more important to estimate maintenance costs in some studies than in others. For example, maintenance costs are likely to be more relevant in studies of treatments for severely mentally ill individuals who are likely to use a relative high level of residential and intensive treatments than in studies of other patient groups. Separating treatment from maintenance costs may be important in studies comparing a service that includes maintenance costs in its unit price to one that does not, such as a comparison of a residential program to a day treatment program. If maintenance costs were included in the unit cost for the residential program, it would spuriously appear more costly than the outpatient program. A valid comparison would require deducting maintenance costs from the unit cost of the residential program or calculating the maintenance costs incurred by patients in the day treatment program. It may not be necessary to separate maintenance costs for services that are not the focus of study and are used relatively equally by all treatment groups.

5.4 CHAPTER REVIEW

The accuracy and detail in estimating the value of the various resource units included in a study should match the relative importance of each type of unit. There are three general approaches to cost estimation that vary in accuracy, detail, and difficulty. The most detailed, specific, and difficult approach is direct estimation of actual costs incurred, which would be used for a few important costs most directly affected by the interventions under study. A simpler but less accurate approach used for resource units of intermediate importance is the analysis of local accounting data. The simplest but least accurate approach used for peripheral resource units is to use existing aggregate or survey data on the costs of resources similar to those under study.

Specific techniques and data sources used in valuing the types of resources introduced in Chapter 4 were discussed, including methods for estimating the costs of mental health treatments, physical health care, criminal justice activities, social services, time and productivity costs, family costs, and transfers and other income. The strengths and weaknesses of alternative methods were discussed in the context of different research goals.

The final section covered five kinds of adjustments to costs, some or all of which may be needed in particular studies. Both adjustment for inflation and discounting to present value are needed in studies that span more than one year. Multisite studies may require adjustment for local variation in costs. One may also need to deal with joint costs when more than one type of resource unit is delivered by the same accounting cost center. Finally, if cost data for some 24-hour services include personal subsistence or maintenance costs while others do not, one may need to estimate the fraction that represents maintenance costs.

6

MEASURING SERVICE PRACTICE

Investigators are conducting a four-site study comparing two styles of service practice for persons who have schizophrenia or bipolar disorder, who also have a persistent pattern of substance abuse, and who have experienced two or more hospitalizations in the past 3 years. One service style is each site's current array of services, including each site's practice of coordinating services through linkage case management. The investigators slightly modified this "usual care" style by training staff in a drug abuse treatment model. The second service style is assertive community treatment (ACT), in which most services are provided by a team of eight clinicians who have had training in the same drug abuse treatment model. Qualified clients who agree to participate are randomly assigned to usual care (all services except ACT services) or ACT (with the possibility of additional usual services except for linkage case management). At the end of the study the findings are similar in three of the sites, but different in the fourth. In three sites, ACT costs the same as usual care but produces better outcomes, as hypothesized. In the fourth site, the ACT model costs more but has no better outcomes. Because the investigators had not gathered adequate data on the clinical practices of ACT and usual care services in their four sites, they were unable to determine whether the pattern of findings reflected differences in clinical practice. For example, did the ACT team in the fourth site fail to practice the key aspects of assertive community treatment or the special drug abuse interventions as consistently as did staff in the first three sites? Or did the usual-service clinicians in the fourth site practice several key features of the style intended in the experimental program?

"Service practice" refers broadly to any procedure likely to influence client outcomes. It might be "treatment practices" such as psychotherapeutic or pharmacologic technique, or "program practices" like the frequency and type of client contacts, or "service system practices" like criteria for client eligibility, service capacities, and practice monitoring techniques using treatment guidelines.

6.1   WHY MEASURE SERVICE PRACTICES?

There are at least five reasons why an investigator might want to measure practices in mental health cost–outcome research. First, if an investigator is comparing outcomes for well-specified program models, he or she will want to measure practices to ensure that the intended models are properly implemented, as might have been done in the example above. This goal is a direct extension of the "fidelity check" in psychotherapy research.

Second, a researcher may hypothesize that measures of program practice will explain the effects of treatment assignment on outcome. In the case example above, the investigators might have hypothesized that high frequency of client contact sustained over time, faithful implementation of a multistage substance abuse intervention, and a vigorous supported employment intervention would additively account for the relative effectiveness of the assertive community treatment intervention and the variation in outcome from site to site.

Third, an investigator might want to specify the similarity of programs under study to "standard" service models. This might be of interest when the investigator has created a unique new intervention model and wants to characterize the degree to which it is similar to existing intervention models. For example, the NIMH Treatment Strategies in Schizophrenia study (Schooler et al., 1989; 1997) developed protocol-driven medication and family intervention clinics in each of the five study sites. Comparing their practices to samples of programs typical of three "standard" models, it was possible to show that the study clinics were intermediate in their "case management" intensity between the typical outpatient clinic and the typical case management or assertive community treatment (ACT) program, were similar to ACT programs in team functioning and other ACT innovations, and provided a structured family intervention more intensive and organized than seen in any program in the comparison sample, regardless of program model (Hargreaves et al., 1991).

Fourth, in studies of system changes, changes in program practices may themselves be the effect of primary interest. For example, an investigator might hypothesize that capitation contracting (in which the provider organization receives a fixed payment per member per month and is at risk for financial losses) typically induces provider organizations to adopt and vigorously monitor adherence to treatment guidelines, and different types of capitation contracting may induce more "restrictive" (cost–containment oriented) or "prescriptive" (prevention oriented) guidelines.

Finally, practices can also be dependent variables when an investigator wishes to study historical changes in practice, or wishes to examine equity issues, such as whether practices differ when the client is a member of an under-served minority.

There are cost–outcome studies in which the investigator correctly may choose not to measure service practice. In studies done quickly with little research funding in order to take advantage of a "natural experiment" it may be wise to focus on obtaining adequate measures of outcome, even though the nature of the service changes may be known only anecdotally. If large effects on outcome are observed, the primary importance of the study may be to stimulate further research using a more fully developed design. Similarly, an investigator may carry out a pilot study of a service innovation with the intervention remaining an unanalyzed "black box" until the preliminary evidence shows that the effects on outcome make a more fully developed study worthwhile. Even in fully developed cost–outcome experiments it may be possible to characterize the practices being compared relatively simply and inexpensively, as we shall see in this chapter.

6.2 MEASURING SERVICE PRACTICE: THE SPECIAL CHALLENGE OF COST–OUTCOME RESEARCH

In efficacy research, pharmacology and psychotherapy investigators have developed methods for measuring treatment practice under tightly controlled conditions. This measurement tradition guides the development of methods for measuring mental health service practices in cost–outcome studies.

In drug efficacy research, in which the focus is usually on the short-term physiological effect of a compound on symptoms and side effects, attention to treatment implementation typically has been quite narrow. Investigators usually measure the amount of medication each subject consumes or plasma levels of drug and active metabolites that are achieved. Complexities do arise when comparing two active compounds. Often the relative therapeutic potency of the two compounds is not known. Some even have an optimum therapeutic window such that higher doses are less potent. In either of these situations, it is difficult to design a comparative study in which the two drugs are given at an "equivalent" dosage. With antipsychotic drugs, there is also a question about whether onset of therapeutic effect is hastened by progressively increasing the dose until response or intolerable side effects, or by targeting a therapeutic range of dosage (or plasma level) and holding at that dosage. The psychosocial concomitants of medication administration rarely are examined unless drug and psychosocial interventions are being compared, as in the ground-breaking study by Elkin and co-workers (1985). In such studies the psychosocial aspects of drug (or placebo) management are important to specify, implement consistently, and verify, if results implying relative efficacy are to be interpretable (Fawcett et al., 1987).

In psychotherapy efficacy research, investigators have vigorously developed

methods for specifying and monitoring the implementation of different psychotherapy models (Waltz et al., 1993). This trend was greatly stimulated by the example of the NIMH Treatment of Depression Collaborative Research Program
(Elkin et al., 1985; 1989; Elkin, 1993). Investigators developed treatment manuals, trained experienced clinicians to a treatment performance criterion, and
monitored audiotaped treatment sessions throughout the study using detailed rating procedures (Waskow, 1984; Hill et al., 1992). Separate research groups were
responsible for the treatment design, training, and monitoring of each of the
three psychosocial modalities being compared: (1) interpersonal psychotherapy
(Weissman et al., 1982; Rounsaville et al., 1984; 1986; 1987; Chevron and
Rounsaville, 1983; Chevron et al., 1983), (2) cognitive therapy (Shaw, 1984;
Dobson et al., 1985; Vallis et al., 1986; Shaw and Dobson, 1988), and (3) antidepressant and placebo medication management strategies (Fawcett et al., 1987).
This example set a high standard for subsequent psychotherapy research, although a standard that is probably necessary if meaningful conclusions are to be
drawn.

Cost–outcome research has grown out of these psychopharmacology and psychotherapy research traditions, and it presents new challenges in monitoring
treatment practices. Some would say this is because health services investigators
have less experimental control over services than clinical treatment investigators. To some extent this is correct, driven by the emphasis on generalizability
and on examining interventions under conditions of usual service delivery. As
discussed in Chapter 1, the kinds of treatment management controls used in efficacy research sometimes may impair generalizability. On the other hand, health
services research needs to attempt a different level of control over experimental
services. An innovative treatment or service may require special management
practices in order to be delivered effectively. For example, health services researchers might examine the cost-effectiveness of incorporating structured diagnostic procedures as an aid to selecting appropriate treatments. A more general
issue for cost–outcome research is the specification of the operating nature of
whole service programs in their contacts with patients. One may wish to include
not only the specific treatments that are provided, but also the guidelines used to
select the sequence of treatments and other services that may need to be integrated with the treatment process, such as assistance in obtaining financial entitlements, adequate housing, and employment. The methods used to maintain
the continuity of services are also a central issue for some target populations.

6.3 TREATMENT THEORY: A GUIDE
TO MEASURING PRACTICES

Early efforts in mental health services research were often atheoretical. Studies were head-to-head trials of alternate service models, with no hypotheses
about what were the effective ingredients, and few if any measures of service

practice. In recent years mental health services researchers increasingly have called for theory-driven services trials, which have greater relevance, power, and precision than simple head-to-head "horse races" (Bickman, 1987; 1990; Chen, 1990; Finney and Moos, 1984; 1989; Lipsey, 1990; Lipsey and Pollard, 1989). By "theory" these researchers and theorists mean a specification of the hypothesized effective ingredients of the studied services, hypotheses about the relevant target population, and hypotheses about what different interventions are most useful depending on the specific stage of the disorder or the state of the person receiving the intervention.

6.3.1 LIMITATIONS OF "BLACK BOX" EXPERIMENTS

A policy maker distant from clinical practice may think of a service model as a "black box." The phrase is used in electronics to describe a complicated device that is packaged as a unit and whose internal mechanism is hidden and mysterious for the user. If the investigator thinks of service models in this way, studies are poorly designed, and findings can lead to crude or distorted conclusions. Theories of service effects not only help to improve research design, but they also enable the investigator to discover ways to improve cost-effectiveness and to guide practical application of research findings. A number of authors have discussed "small theories" of service effects (Bickman, 1987; 1990; Chen, 1989; 1990a; Lipsey, 1990). This section draws on a well-written paper by Lipsey (1990), which contains numerous thought-provoking examples that the reader may find helpful.

A "small" theory of treatment is based on common sense thinking about how programs produce benefit or harm (Chen, 1990b). One might identify an informative intervening variable that mediates the effect of treatment assignment on outcome, such as the extent of treatment participation. One might think of a pattern of intervening variables that could be organized into a causal diagram (Hargreaves, Catalano, Hu, and Cuffel, in press). For example, perhaps severity of disability, gender, and treatment assignment together influence the degree of treatment participation, which in turn influences social functioning and cost. Figure 6.1 represents these hypotheses as a simple causal diagram. The diagram reminds us, among other things, that we need reliable measures of baseline severity of disability and of treatment participation.

One might also think of a "stage-state" hypothesis that suggests how interventions should be adapted to the client's condition. For example, for severely mentally ill persons with comorbid substance abuse, one stage might be when they do not see substance abuse as a problem, and another stage when they see substance abuse as a problem and want to reduce substance use (McHugo et al., 1995). Confronting the patients with the number of times that substance abuse has led to their involuntary treatment or trouble with the law might be useful in the first stage by increasing the probability that they move to the second stage,

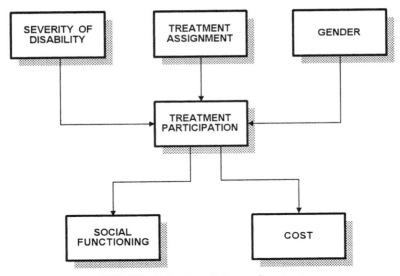

FIGURE 6.1   A small theory of treatment.

but it might not be useful during the second stage. Similarly, an intervention aimed at reducing substance use might only be effective in the second stage. Simple hypotheses of this sort suggest how interventions may need to be adapted to the user's current state. Such hypotheses suggest theoretically important measures of intervention practices. Incorporating measures from small theories of treatment improves the ability of a clinical trial to suggest mechanisms of effectiveness.

6.3.2 FOUR ASPECTS OF TREATMENT THEORY

Four aspects of treatment theory are emphasized by Lipsey (1990): (1) definition of the problem, (2) critical service ingredients, (3) stages in delivering the treatment, and (4) expected outcomes.

Problem Definition

Problem definition encompasses the illness or disability condition that represents the need for service and the particular subpopulations or circumstances for which the service is tailored. Is the service focused primarily on persons with schizophrenia, or on those with a variety of serious mental disorders, or on persons severely disabled by any mental disorder, or on a broad range of persons from the severely disabled to the mildly disabled? Is the service focused on persons who are in a particular service situation in the specialty mental health sector (e.g., presenting for psychiatric hospitalization or preparing to leave the hospital), persons identified in primary care as suffering from a psychiatric disorder, or persons with such disorders who have not been identified in any part of the medical care sector? Is the focus on how to optimize service for a particular problem or subgroup (service design), or on how to make an existing service accessible to the right recipients (service marketing)? A clear definition of the problem focuses one's attention on possible hypotheses about critical ingredients.

Critical Ingredients

Treatment theory hypothesizes which ingredients of service practice are crucial for effectiveness. Critical ingredients may extend beyond specific treatments, such as a blend of treatment and social services that may be cost-effective for persons who are severely disabled. We often think about factors that influence access to services, promote good working alliances between staff and users, and even program characteristics that enable users to shape a program to meet their particular needs. We also think about staff morale and leadership qualities that enable a program to function well or to implement a specific service model accurately. If specific elements are hypothesized to be crucial for an innovative service intervention, this will guide the choice of measures of program practice that can confirm that the innovative service actually embodies the crucial elements and usual care does not.

Stages in Delivering the Treatment

Some types of service are thought to bring patients along through a series of stages involving attitude and insight changes that must be matched by a sequence of distinct intervention strategies. Prochaska (Prochaska et al., 1992) articulated this for alcoholism treatment, and Drake and McHugo (Drake et al., 1993a; McHugo et al., 1995) for people with mixed mental and substance abuse disorders. If such stages of engagement and response are hypothesized to be important, then a measure of the stage of each subject and the timing of stage transitions may be important to understanding program effects. For example, in substance abuse treatment, people move ahead and fall back frequently and typically take years to reach stable abstinence. A cost-effective innovation can show advantage in the rate at which the distribution of stage occupancy moves forward compared to usual care, even if the number of subjects reaching ultimate outcomes is small when subjects are followed only two or three years (e.g., Drake et al., 1993b). Stages are a special case of how theory might suggest intermediate outcomes that would be useful to measure in understanding mechanisms of effect.

Expected Pattern of Outcomes

Finally, treatment theory implies the nature, range, and timing of treatment effects. It will identify side effects that may be a problem. It may suggest critical periods for accomplishing tasks such as establishing a therapeutic alliance, and it may even indicate how soon to expect short-term, intermediate, and ultimate outcomes. Stage-state treatment theories especially call for ongoing measurement of the relevant outcome stages or states that are expected to guide service interventions. Thus, theory allows investigators to plan the timing and content of outcome assessment to best portray the detailed structure of treatment effects on outcome, not just study which treatment "wins the horse race" at the ultimate follow-up measurement.

6.3.3 USING COLLABORATION AND CONSULTATION TO FORM SMALL PROGRAM THEORIES

Prior experience with services for the relevant target population is valuable in formulating small theories of service effect. Existing theories of service impact and evidence from prior studies are also relevant. Consultation and collaboration can be helpful to investigators who lack this kind of expertise. For example, program practitioners can describe how service interventions work, what user characteristics are important in matching users to services, and what are the common barriers to access, deleterious side effects, and timing of effects. One may hear multiple, conflicting hypotheses, but this is not a problem, since all viewpoints can stimulate thoughts about crucial variables to measure and service components to incorporate.

Drawing on theory and hypotheses, and on consultation and collaboration, an investigator's first task in measuring service practice is to identify the key ingredients. In the case example at the beginning of this chapter, investigators needed measures of key features of clinical practice in order to understand their findings. They could have turned to a considerable literature. Experienced leaders of ACT programs have offered their views about the key ingredients (Knoedler, unpublished; McFarlane and Stastny, 1987; McGrew et al., 1994; Test, 1992; Test and Stein, 1976). McGrew and Bond (1995) report the "judgements of experts" from a survey on the critical ingredients of ACT. Several investigators have suggested procedures for measuring key ACT practices (Brekke, 1987; 1988; Brekke and Test, 1987; 1992; McGrew et al., 1995). Conversations with other ACT investigators in 1996 would even have helped them locate an unpublished instrument then considered by many to be the current state of the art among measures of fidelity to the ACT model (Teague, written personal communication, 1996). When an investigator is studying a well-researched intervention model, there may be plenty of help available for identifying hypothesized or demonstrated key ingredients. The investigators could also have been spurred on by the large practice variations found by several investigators among intended replications of the ACT model (Bond et al., 1995; Deci et al., 1995; Rosenheck et al., 1995c; Teague et al., 1995).

In contrast to the case example, investigators are more often faced with the task of measuring a unique treatment or service model that has not been well studied. In this circumstance the investigator needs to develop an explicit specification of the service model, with its treatment theory, hypothesized key ingredients, and planned measures of these ingredients, all starting pretty much from scratch.

6.4 DEVELOPING A SERVICE MODEL SPECIFICATION

If a tested and recommended specification does not exist for a model to be studied, current service categories probably will be inadequate. Investigators will need to develop an operating manual, observe existing practice variations, and assemble or create relevant measures. In this way the measures of key ingredients can be understood in the context of the full treatment or service model.

6.4.1 LIMITATIONS OF CURRENT SERVICE TYPE DESIGNATIONS

We are used to thinking of the variety of services for persons with mental illness by the names of major program elements: inpatient, outpatient, day treatment, halfway house, and so forth (Leginski et al., 1989). Clinicians familiar with such programs will require only a moment's reflection to remind themselves that the practice variation within any of those program types can be huge, sometimes seeming greater that the typical differences between program types. Mental health services investigators seem to be in agreement that a program typology at this level is not specific enough for informative cost–effectiveness studies.

6.4.2 DEVELOPING AN OPERATING MANUAL

Often the first step in model specification is writing an operating manual. Sometimes published descriptions of model programs can serve this purpose, but when one attempts to operationalize measures of model components it becomes clear that greater clarity and specificity are needed. An example of a program manual is provided by McFarlane and Stastny (1987) for the assertive community treatment model. In some cases a program manual may need to incorporate within it established treatment guidelines for specific disorders and manuals for psychotherapies known to be efficacious.

6.4.3 OBSERVING PRACTICE VARIATION

The next stage of model specification often emerges from an expert consultant or site visit team that helps programs practice a model as originally intended. Examples of this are the dissemination of the Fairweather Lodge model (Fairweather, 1980), the dissemination of the assertive community treatment model (Test, 1992; Thompson et al., 1990), site visit activities of the International Center for Clubhouse Development (Propst, 1992) with regard to the Fountain House model, and the Boston University site visits of psychosocial rehabilitation programs (Anthony et al., 1982; Farkas et al., 1988). These consultants and site visitors see practice variations and sharpen their concepts of the key elements of the model.

6.4.4 ATTENTION TO COMPETING MODELS

The investigator needs measures of whether program practice is faithful to the intended program model. These measures should reflect the key features of the model being studied, but also the features of competing models that may or may not be incorporated into the practice of the program. When an innovative model is being compared to "usual services," adequate measures of usual service practices are also important. All of these purposes could be accomplished more easily if we had established psychometrically sound measures that encompass the range of key service elements across the entire spectrum of services for persons with mental disorders. At present only selected aspects of this methodology are available.

6.4.5 USUAL SERVICES: PROGRAM OR SYSTEM?

It is common to compare an innovative program model to "usual care." Often this means that experimental subjects will receive most services from the innovative program, while comparison subjects will receive services from many different programs. In one case, the investigator wants to measure the practice of a program, and in the other case the practice of a system of service programs. This is actually quite a general problem, since even subjects assigned to a specific program may drop out or receive additional services elsewhere. Therefore, measures of practice also must be measures of services received in a system, with some breadth of measures of sources of service along with more focused measures of the nature of services in the most commonly used service programs. In cost–outcome research, in which the investigator usually wants to measure total service cost, the effort of measuring utilization and measuring the nature of the services utilized sometimes can be coordinated.

Finally, the threats to practice stability mentioned in Chapter 2 also will need to be kept in mind as one develops a service model specification. Ideally one studies innovative and usual care practices that are well established with only modest staff turnover, changes in caseload ratio, or other threats to continued stable performance during the study period.

6.5 MEASUREMENT APPROACHES

Six sources of information on program practice commonly are used in mental health services research (Table 6.1). Key informant, staff survey, and user survey are the most feasible to use, if appropriate measures are available, although key informant is the most economical and user survey the most expensive. The

TABLE 6.1   Sources of Practice Data, Relative Cost, and Model Specificity

Source of data	Relative research cost	Model specificity
Key informant inventory	Low	General
Staff survey of practices	Low	Specific
User survey of practices	Low	Specific
Direct observation	High	General
Units of service records	Moderate	General
Staff time logs	Moderate	Specific

fourth source, direct observation, has taken two forms. One uses a rating instrument similar to the first three methods and a relatively brief site visit by an observer. The more usual form, however, is more intensive qualitative observation using ethnographic methods, although such observations can also form the basis for closed-end ratings with a predefined inventory. The final two sources—units of service records and staff time logs—while labor intensive and expensive, are usually necessary to estimate utilization and cost in controlled studies of cost-effectiveness. Units of service recording procedures and staff time logs are relatively well developed for nonresidential programs. Two more intensive approaches, work sampling and time-motion analysis, were discussed in Chapter 4.

6.5.1 KEY INFORMANT INVENTORY

A key informant is a program staff member, often the director, who is in a position to have a complete overview of a program. Program structure, policy, caseload, and staffing are objective features that usually can be recorded reliably by a key informant, although local records may need to be consulted by the informant. Within a given model or program type many of these characteristics are taken for granted by program staff and are not thought of as part of the program design, yet they necessarily provide context and influence the service process. Is the program reimbursed fee-for-service or does the program share financial risk? Are all physical spaces in the facility open to users or are parts reserved for staff only? Is public transportation available and the neighborhood safe? Do users typically come to a facility or is most user contact in the community? Is a residential facility locked or entirely open? Are necessary health and social services provided by the program, readily available, or relatively difficult to obtain?

Caseload and staffing also influence program practice, especially if the target group for the study is only a subset of the caseload. Important caseload features may include the age, gender, ethnicity, diagnosis, comorbidity, and level of functioning distributions of clients. Other caseload issues include the proportion who are involuntarily held, the proportion whose care is paid from income entitlement or various categories of health care reimbursement, length of stay distributions, and lifetime total time in hospital or other intensive 24-hour setting. Staffing is also crucial to type of service. Are there staff licensed to prescribe or dispense medication or give injections? Is staff focused on general nursing and medical care or are mental health skills well represented? Are mental health consumers or recovering substance abusers employed on the staff?

When a key informant item requires judgment, the reliability of a single respondent may be poor. The exact boundary between "objective" data and more judgmental data is best defined by empirical study of reliability and validity. Information on typical service practice, if it is not based on complete databases of units of service delivered, usually requires the judgment of multiple respondents, either staff or users (patients, clients, members, service seekers). Sometimes measures can be anchored with detailed criteria for each rating level, however, which may take more time to complete but may yield good reliability with a single rater. Key informant, staff, users, and outside observers may also bring different perspectives to some important judgments about practices. This echoes an issue raised in Chapter 4 about the value of "triangulated" measurement of utilization and anticipates a similar discussion in Chapter 7 about measuring outcomes.

6.5.2 STAFF SURVEY OF PRACTICES

When information cannot be reported reliably by a key informant, a sample of staff member respondents may provide more useful information. Staff surveys seem to attain adequate reliability and validity only if they focus on specific treatment and service practices rather than broad treatment philosophy. While a single key informant could complete such an inventory, the issues rated are not always easy to describe, and reliability (intraclass correlation) has been poor for single respondents, even in describing relatively concrete aspects of practice (Hargreaves et al., unpublished). About six respondents seem to be needed to attain adequate subscale intraclass correlations in distinguishing among programs. Items or subscale scores typically are averaged across respondents to maximize reliability. Where there are more potential raters than needed, good practice is to identify staff who have worked in the program at least a few months and are not students, volunteers, or clerical staff, and randomly sample among them.

6.5.3 USER SURVEY INSTRUMENTS

User survey instruments cannot only document the perceived availability of specific service technologies, they can also add information about the interpersonal style in which services are offered and experienced. This information may have an important impact on service accessibility, acceptability, and effectiveness. User survey instruments have been used in a number of studies, but no major instrument has yet been developed that could be applied widely. Some outcome instruments include questions about users' or family members' experience with mental health or substance abuse programs.

One limitation of user instruments is that the user may only know of services that he or she has been offered, not the whole scope of services in the program. Reliability and validity may also be reduced if one uses a binary (yes/no) response format. These problems may mean that larger samples will be needed to attain good reliability.

6.5.4 PARTICIPANT OBSERVER OR SITE VISITOR INVENTORY

A participant observer may be in a unique position to observe certain characteristics of a program, such as qualities of the interpersonal process between staff and users, among users, and among staff—processes that these participants may be unaware of or reluctant to report. Participant observation has been used in several ongoing cost–effectiveness studies of community programs for persons with severe mental illness, usually engaging a qualitatively trained anthropologist or sociologist for extensive participation in one or two programs. This type of qualitative observation and synthesis aims to identify unforeseen or unrecognized characteristics of service programs. However, participant observers (and site visitors with more structured and briefer program contact) also may complete a structured rating instrument.

The range of content that might be covered in staff and user response instruments is illustrated by the "sampler" in Table 6.2. Subscale titles for the expanded Community Program Philosophy Scale (CPPS), for the Residential Substance Abuse and Psychiatric Programs Inventory (RESPPI), and for the Program Environment Scale (PES) are grouped into empirical or conceptual subgroups. One can see that some concepts are quite general, while others are specific to particular program models.

6.5.5 UNITS OF SERVICE RECORDS AND OTHER ARCHIVAL DATA

Units of service information often are computerized and will be gathered at the individual user level for purposes of cost estimation, as discussed in Chapter 4. Service consumption also can provide useful information about program operating characteristics. Brekke and Test (1992) show an example of this in which the overall types of service units are similar across programs but the intensity and breadth of service drops off rapidly after entry in some programs and continues for months or years in other programs. Service units often are recorded with the amount of time involved, whether the contact was face-to-face, by telephone, or with a collateral, and whether the contact was in the office or the community. Other archival data needed in some studies may include medication prescription and dosage, problems with and treatment for medication side effects,

TABLE 6.2   Content of Selected Program Practice Measures[1]

CPPS[2]	RESPPI[3]	PES[4]
Innovation	Community accessibility	Program cares about me
Staff involvement in job	Physical amenities	Clarity
Clarity	Social-recreational aids	Energy level
Staff cohesion	Prosthetic aids	Free to be; accepted
Supervisory support	Safety features	Friendly and caring
Team model	Staff facilities	Openness
Out-of-office contact	Space availability	Optimism of staff regarding client
Housing	Resident social resources	Work within program
Link to entitlements	Client mental functioning	Support getting paid work
Emergency access	Client activity level	Emergency access
Referral advocacy	Activities in the community	Family and friends
Interagency orientation	Health and treatment services	Housing
Longitudinality of care	Daily living assistance	Link to entitlements
Psychotherapy	Social/recreational activities	Link to community activities
Family orientation	Involvement	Medications
Interest in SPMI clients	Support	Substance abuse
Clients exercising power	Spontaneity	Confidentiality
Cultural competence	Autonomy	Continuity of contact
Individualization	Practical orientation	Empowerment: program
Substance abuse orientation	Personal problem	Empowerment: treatment
Substance abuse versus SPMI[5]	Anger and aggression	Individualization of treatment
Substance abuse: 12 step	Order and organization	Place
Substance abuse: role play	Program clarity	Rules
Social skills training	Staff control	Client-client respect
Place and training rehabilitation	Physical attractiveness	Positive physical contact
Work in the program	Environmental diversity	Negative physical contact
Supported work	Resident functioning	Space
Job finding	Staff functioning	Staff-client respect
Employment models		Staff commitment

[1]Shading reflects factors or content domains from existing measures.
[2]CPPS = Community Program Philosophy Scale (expanded).
[3]RESPPI = Residential Substance Abuse and Psychiatric Programs Inventory.
[4]PES = Program Environment Scale.
[5]SPMI = severely and persistently mentally ill.

use of seclusion, physical restraint, and observation, restrictiveness of services, and referral for special services. Methods for gathering such data were discussed in Chapter 4.

6.5.6 STAFF TIME LOGS

Staff time logs are usually necessary to supplement and validate units of service data when detailed information on staff practices is required. Brekke (1988) used a log in studying community mental health programs. Dennis (Dennis et al., 1992) used a "client encounter checklist" for measuring substance abuse counseling. Required reporting of service units to payers often does not give sufficient detail and in many cases may be misleading. For example, some jurisdictions allow one program to bill psychotherapy units but not case management units, while for other programs the reverse is true, in an effort to force work patterns into cost centers for the purpose of cost accounting. When staff do both types of activities, they may all be recorded as psychotherapy in one program and case management in the other. Staff logs that record more specific details of the content and focus of patient contacts enable the investigator to further define the average meaning of service unit types in each program studied.

Staff logs are time consuming for staff and may distort the workload distribution slightly, but usually can be time sampled. For example, staff might be asked to keep logs for two-week periods two or three times per year. During this time it is advisable to audit the time logs against service units reported and resolve discrepancies immediately while staff can recall their activities.

Staff logs are used less often for inpatient and residential programs, since the unit of service is an inpatient/residential day. If the investigator plans to disaggregate the cost of a service day, however, staff logs or other time-and-motion sampling may be needed to determine how to disaggregate costs of different staff activities, as discussed in Chapter 4. When time-and-motion sampling is used to quantify the amount or cost of service received, such data may also help characterize qualitative differences among inpatient wards or residential programs.

6.6 EXISTING MEASURES

Existing measures are limited by a focus on specific treatment models, specific aspects of treatment, or the treatment of specific disorders. They provide a firm foundation, however, for developing more comprehensive and general measures. The most relevant of these measures are discussed below and are summarized in Table 6.3.

Rudolf Moos and his colleagues are responsible for an extensive body of work on measuring characteristics of psychiatric and substance abuse programs, including the Ward Atmosphere Scale (WAS; Price and Moos, 1975), the

TABLE 6.3 Existing Practice Measures, Model Coverage, and Respondent[1]

		Program Practice Measures[2]							
Model	WAS	COPES	MEAP	RESPPI	DAPTI	CPPS	PES	DCL	CCACTI
Acute inpatient (psychiatric)	S,C	C	K,S,C	K,R					
Acute inpatient (substance abuse)		S,C	K,S,C	K,R	K				
Skilled nursing (geriatric)			K,S,C						
Residential (psychiatric)		S,C,R	K,S,C	K,R					
Residential (substance abuse)		S,C	K,S,C	K,R	K				
Residential (geriatric)			K,S,C						
Supported housing (geriatric)			K,S,C						
Psychosocial		S,C					C	S	
Clubhouse		S,C					C	S	
Day treatment		S,C,R					C		
Assertive community team		S,C				S	C	S	R
Case management						S	C		
Vocational							C		
Outpatient clinic (psychiatric)						S			
Outpatient clinic (substance abuse)					K				
Methadone maintenance					K				

[1]Respondent types: K = key informants, S = staff, C = clients/users, R = research observers/raters.

[2]Rating scales: WAS = Ward Atmosphere Scale, COPES = Community-Oriented Programs Environment Scale, MEAP = Multiphasic Environmental Assessment Procedure, RESPPI = Residential Substance Abuse and Psychiatric Programs Inventory, DAPTI = Drug and Alcohol Program Treatment Inventory, CPPS = Community Program Philosophy Scale, PES = Program Environment Scale, DCL = Daily Contact Log, CCACTI = Critical Components of Assertive Community Treatment Interview.

Community-Oriented Programs Environment Scale (COPES; Moos and Otto, 1972), the Multiphasic Environmental Assessment Procedure (MEAP; Moos and Igra, 1980; Moos and Lemke, 1984), the Residential Substance Abuse and Psychiatric Programs Inventory (RESPPI; Timko, 1995), and the Drug and Alcohol Program Treatment Inventory (DAPTI; Swindle et al., 1995a, b). The MEAP, RESPPI, and DAPTI combine standardized measures of objective program characteristics with the kinds of subjective attitude scales used in the WAS and the COPES. Applications of these measures indicate that characteristics such as case mix, program size, and physical attributes of facilities can affect program implementation and client outcomes (Lemke and Moos, 1989; Timko, 1996). These investigators have set an excellent methodologic standard for developing, testing, and validating measures of program characteristics, although the specific measures are not broadly applicable to the full range of intervention programs and treatments in mental health.

The Community Program Philosophy Scale (CPPS), developed by Jerrell and Hargreaves (Jerrell and Hargreaves, 1991; Hargreaves et al., unpublished), is a staff response inventory designed to characterize a particular spectrum of nonresidential community programs from clinic-based outpatient models through linkage and clinical case management to the assertive community treatment (ACT) model, and successfully distinguishes these models (Brekke and Test, 1992; Rosenheck et al., 1993; Hargreaves et al., unpublished). The CPPS, however, focuses only on nonresidential treatment programs, measures only staff perspectives, and does not include objective information on programs.

The Program Environment Scale (PES), developed by Martha Burt and colleagues, measures consumer perceptions of nonresidential community support and rehabilitation programs such as day treatment, psychosocial rehabilitation, drop-in centers, and clubhouses of the Fountain House model. Like the CPPS, the PES applies to a limited range of programs and a single respondent group (Burt, written personal communication, 1997).

Brekke and colleagues have done substantive work in developing model-guided approaches for measuring implementation of ACT model programs and other community support programs using the Daily Contact Log (Brekke, 1987; Brekke and Wolkon, 1988; Brekke and Test, 1992). Although these methods are limited to a narrow range of nonresidential community programs, this work illustrates several crucial elements of meaningful implementation measurement. First, they advocate a theory driven approach to assessing the extent to which treatment is delivered in conformity with the stated design, which requires identification of the key elements of treatment models and specification of both intended and actual program practices. Their results also underscore the importance of multiple respondent perspectives in obtaining valid and reliable measures of program practices and the value of objective measures of program, client, and staff characteristics.

McGrew and co-workers (1994) also have developed a measure of implementation fidelity for the ACT model. Completed by research observers, the

Critical Components of Assertive Community Treatment Interview (CCACTI) consists of rating scale items based on the critical ingredients of the ACT model and accurately detects program evolution and drift across ACT programs. This work also illustrates an approach for identifying the crucial dimensions of a treatment model and the value of assessing ways in which broad program goals are implemented. Gregory Teague (written personal communication, 1996) and colleagues have developed a key informant instrument distinguishing ACT programs from linkage case management that is being used in several studies. It is currently the most detailed and sensitive measure of fidelity to the ACT model, as far as the authors are aware.

In summary, existing measures provide several usable approaches, and a conceptual and methodologic basis for further development and expansion. The experience with existing measures also reveals the particular strengths and weaknesses of various sources of data or types of respondents.

6.7 USING PRACTICE DATA
IN COST–OUTCOME RESEARCH

The most common use of practice data is to verify that the interventions under study took place as intended, as was needed in the case example at the beginning of this chapter. Analysis usually will benefit from a consideration of the importance of each of the features that are intended to distinguish the programs under study. One might construct a summary scale in which each component measure is weighted according to importance judgments made by an expert panel. Alternatively, one might have the expert panel directly judge the fidelity to the innovative model of each experimental and usual care condition, as Teague and his co-workers (1995) did in a seven-site (14 programs) randomized trial of services for persons who were severely mentally disabled and also engaged in substance use. They compared a modified assertive community treatment intervention (ACT) that included a stepwise substance abuse treatment intervention to a linkage case management condition (Drake et al., 1990). They found that in one of the seven sites the implementation of the innovative ACT team failed, and was not distinguished in its practices from the case management condition in that site. In the remaining six sites, the ACT teams scored significantly closer to the ACT model than did the case management programs, as expected. In one instance, however, the case management program received additional staff and progressively adopted many ACT practices (Teague, personal communication). This type of finding might lead one to examine treatment effects only in the sites with adequate differentiation among practice across treatment conditions.

Teague's findings (Teague et al., 1995) suggest an even more interesting potential use of practice data. There was variation in model adherence among sites, not just in the failed site. Such variation allows examination of whether the character of the practice in each condition in each site relates to individual differences in outcome. Analyses of this sort are sometimes referred to in economics as "production function" analyses (Yates and Newman, 1980; Knapp, 1979; 1993; 1995). Such analyses require multiple sites and large samples of subjects, but potentially allow a rich exploration of hypotheses about key ingredients in service models, including how they interact with baseline subject characteristics.

6.8 FUTURE DEVELOPMENTS

The measures reviewed in this chapter are promising and illustrate workable measurement approaches, although the measures reflect different perspectives and emphases that stem from the perspectives of each scale's authors and the specific research aims each scale was designed to accomplish. Experience with the more recently developed measures is still relatively limited; the newer measures probably have a number of limitations in subscale homogeneity, reliability, and ability to discriminate among programs. They certainly are not yet confirmed to provide the content coverage that is needed to assess all of the currently popular service models.

Intensive work on measurement methods is needed to develop a consistent and comprehensive set of measures with greater conceptual depth and psychometric quality. This psychometric work should capitalize on and be coordinated with development of instruments to aid in managing behavioral health care. Measures of service access may also provide valuable research information.

Treatment guidelines may play an increasingly important role in practice measurement. Managed care settings already are using treatment guidelines as a tool for managing care. Sometimes guidelines are primarily restrictive, specifying when a procedure should not be provided even when sought by the patient, and are criticized as managing costs rather than care. Other guidelines are more prescriptive, specifying when a procedure should be recommended proactively when the patient fails to seek it. Current guidelines usually are based on clinical opinion, and research validation of guidelines is an ongoing process. Treatment guidelines are important for practice measurement because they focus data collection attention on aspects of treatment process hypothesized (if not known) to be central to treatment quality and effectiveness. Use of treatment guidelines already is spurring the development of measures of guideline adherence and experiments on how to obtain optimal guideline adherence by clinicians. In the future, clinical triage and primary care as well as specialty care may be aided routinely by information support in the form of guideline retrieval and decision monitoring. Information systems that support decision monitoring will in turn become important sources of research data on clinical practice.

6.9 CHAPTER REVIEW

Practice measurement in cost–outcome research may serve as a check on the adequacy of delivering a standard service model, as an aid to explaining outcome variation among sites in multisite studies, as a way to calibrate the similarity of usual care programs across sites, as a measure of practice changes resulting from system-level interventions, and as a way to study natural variation in service practices. The overarching goal is to identify the key service or treatment practices that account for superior cost–outcome performance.

Studies are generally more informative if investigators articulate a treatment theory of the way an innovative service is expected to produce superior results. Such a theory would define the problem or target population, hypothesize the key ingredients of service practice thought to be necessary for cost-effectiveness, identify steps or stages in treatment when they are applicable, and specify the expected pattern and timing of outcomes. Such theory will suggest ways to make the study design more sensitive and focused, including ways to incorporate measures of hypothesized key ingredients and of the appropriateness of the staging or sequence of interventions.

Measures of practice, though not usually by that name, have become essential features of many kinds of efficacy research, and they are no less valuable in cost–outcome research.

If a tested and recommended specification does not exist for a service model to be studied, nor is there a consensus on relevant measures, the investigator may need to develop new practice measures, by developing an operating manual or treatment guideline, observing existing practice variation, and assembling or creating relevant practice measures. The innovative service may be provided by a single program, but a "usual services" comparison condition may involve many programs, indeed an entire service system, adding to the complexity of measurement. Practice drift during the study may also need to be measured, requiring multiple assessment occasions.

The six common sources of practice information (Table 6.1) include a key informant inventory, a staff survey of practices, a user survey instrument, a participant observer or site visitor inventory, analysis of existing program service records, and a staff time log created for the study. Each has its own advantages and limitations, and multiple measurement perspectives may be desirable.

Several measures of practice in mental health services already exist (Table 6.3) and more are being developed. In many studies it may be desirable to use one or more existing measures to allow comparison of intervention practices to broader norms, supplemented by one or more intervention-specific measures to tap hypothesized key ingredients not included in existing measures.

7

MEASURING MENTAL HEALTH OUTCOMES

The psychiatric services in Central City's jails have come under increasing scrutiny from the city council, the sheriff's office, the director of the Mental Health Department, and the Alliance for the Mentally Ill. Central City's jails are overcrowded and increasingly filled by persons with mental illnesses. The city council argues that jails expediently and appropriately deal with mentally ill persons who cause disruption for businesses, tourists, and neighborhoods and has pledged to crack down on the problems associated with mental illness in these areas. Others argue that housing mentally ill persons in jails is unethical, denies access to needed mental health services, and is counterproductive in reducing problems associated with mental illness in the community.

Central City's sheriff's office and the Department of Mental Health agree to fund a pilot project involving intensive case management of persons who are frequent users of the jail psychiatric service. The case manager meets clients in jail, arranges for postincarceration social services, and immediately engages the client in mental health treatment upon release to the community. Continued funding for these services is contingent on determining that the program is cost-effective. Everyone with a personal stake in the pilot project, however, has his or her own idea of what is a successful outcome. It has become clear to the investigators responsible for designing the cost–effectiveness study that whether or not the program is shown to be cost-effective depends on what outcomes are used to define effectiveness and on how these outcomes are measured.

Although much of this book is dedicated to estimating costs, measuring effectiveness is equally important. We have shown that perspectives on cost analysis vary from the narrowest to the broadest—from single payer costs to social cost.

Similarly, perspectives on effectiveness in mental health vary in breadth from a narrow focus on disorders and symptoms to a broad focus on health status, quality of life, and even public safety and societal welfare. This chapter examines issues unique to the measurement of mental health treatment effectiveness and describes measurement instruments in five outcome domains.

Any investigator new to effectiveness research in mental health might assume that a set of proven measures could be readily identified from a review of published measurement research in the field. This is not the case. The current status of the literature suggests that there is a large number of published outcome measures but very little accumulated knowledge about the principles, characteristics, and standards of good outcome measurement in effectiveness research. New outcome measures continue to be developed and published, replacing older measures that tend to drop from use without compelling evidence that newer measures are more reliable and valid. It appears that the saying about old generals applies equally to mental health outcome measures: "Old measures never die; they just fade away." Unfortunately, this has left the field with a large number of measures with different names and authorships, assessing similar constructs, using similar items, with nearly equivalent psychometric properties. We understand the sentiments of Endicott and Spitzer (1972) when they entitled their article, "What! Another Rating Scale?"

Rather than providing an exhaustive review of published outcome measures, we attempt to highlight emerging standards of measurement in the field. This chapter focuses on issues unique to the measurement of outcomes in effectiveness studies and focuses on measures for which there appears to be growing consensus on their use. For some domains, no clear consensus exists, and we attempt to provide a more comprehensive review of candidate measures within these areas.

The slow pace of methodological development in mental health outcome measurement assures that this state of affairs will continue and promises to limit the value of recommendations made about specific measures in this chapter. We encourage investigators to be aware of current research in the field. However, a body of useful research on outcome measures in mental health has been completed but never published. We encourage investigators not to rely entirely on published outcome measures, but to contact established investigators in the field to obtain state-of-the-art measures and recommendations about how to use these measures in various study populations.

7.1 MEASUREMENT CHALLENGES IN EFFECTIVENESS RESEARCH

Several issues challenge investigators seeking to mount an effectiveness study—issues that argue against adopting measurement protocols directly from efficacy trials of psychopharmacologic agents or psychotherapeutic interventions. As the case example at the beginning of the chapter illustrates, effectiveness research may be concerned with a broad range of policy-related outcome domains in heterogeneous samples and in a diversity of institutional, clinical, and community settings.

7.1.1 CHALLENGE 1: BROADER RANGE OF OUTCOMES

Effectiveness studies concern themselves with a broader range of policy questions, and thus outcome domains, than do efficacy studies. Efficacy studies, by contrast, ask a relatively simpler question, "Does the intervention affect specific outcomes for which the intervention is designed?" For example, does imipramine alleviate depressive symptoms? Or, does social skills training improve social skills? Effectiveness studies go beyond the initial efficacy question and ask whether other outcomes of interest to the consumer and to society are affected: "Does the intervention improve the specific symptoms for which it is designed *and* does it improve functioning, health status, and quality of life?"

Policy-relevant research questions often challenge investigators to obtain data on multiple outcomes and from multiple and imperfect sources, including consumers, family members, friends, mental health providers, and archival records. In the case example at the beginning of the chapter, medication adherence, symptom severity, substance use, violence, and social functioning are all outcomes that might be of interest and that cannot be validly measured from a single information source. On the other hand, collecting data on multiple outcomes from multiple sources adds to the expense of effectiveness research, raises concerns about the aggregation of discrepant information, and is problematic when sources of information other than the consumer are not available.

7.1.2 CHALLENGE 2: REPRESENTATIVE SAMPLES

Effectiveness research frequently is interested in the effects of an intervention in the full target population, not the narrow, homogeneous clinical populations represented in the typical efficacy study. Effectiveness research often examines interventions that do not target homogeneous clinical and diagnostic groups. Rehabilitative, preventive, organizational, and financing innovations serve populations with a variety of diagnoses and disabilities. The common practice in efficacy research of obtaining homogeneous samples defined by particular, age, gender, race, and diagnostic groups is not appropriate for effectiveness studies of interventions designed to affect a broad range of clinical populations. In Chapter 2, we explored how effectiveness studies are designed to examine the effects of mental health interventions in a representative sample of the intended target population. There may also be legitimate questions about whether some subgroups may respond differently to a particular intervention. In this case the investigator can still obtain a representative sample, but can oversample small subgroups in order to have adequate power to test hypotheses about differential response across subgroups.

Representative samples can be very heterogeneous. Outcome measures in a cost–effectiveness trial may need to perform adequately across heterogeneous subgroups. If the intervention studied is tested in multiple disorders, outcome measures designed for use with specific disorder groups may not be applicable. For example, measures emphasizing schizophrenic or manic symptomatology (e.g., the Brief Psychiatric Rating Scale or the Young Mania Rating Scale) may not be appropriate for use in heterogeneous samples that contain disorder groups in which psychosis is not prominent. Outcome measures need to be appropriate for all subgroups within the target population, have adequate psychometric properties, and measure the domains that may be most affected by the intervention within each subgroup. Pilot research on the characteristics of the target population in terms of demographics, primary diagnoses, comorbid conditions, and level of disability is valuable in selecting appropriate measures.

7.1.3 CHALLENGE 3: DIVERSITY OF CLINICAL SETTINGS AND COMMUNITY CONTEXTS

In contrast to efficacy research, effectiveness research is more likely to examine interventions in multiple settings and outcomes that manifest themselves in a variety of contexts. This places a heavy burden on outcome measurement in that the adequacy of measures may vary with context. Measures of symptoms, diagnosis, and functioning may be more reliable and valid when consumers are assessed in clinical settings than when they are assessed in community residences and public places. Similarly, measures of functioning and quality of life may perform quite differently for consumers assessed in rural, suburban, and inner-city settings.

Particularly troublesome is the possibility that differences in the performance of outcome measures across clinical and community settings confound control and experimental group comparisons and bias study findings. Sometimes this occurs when participants receiving the experimental intervention are seen more frequently in clinical settings than participants in comparison groups. Clinical settings may offer greater opportunity to observe and to talk with patients about their symptoms and functioning than other settings, and differences in the opportunity to observe symptoms and functioning may create biases in outcome measurement. Other potential sources of measurement bias occur if investigators attempt to use more than one source of information to assess an outcome domain. In general, using multiple sources is helpful in improving reliability and validity. If, however, the experimental intervention is associated with a greater number and more reliable information sources, then a measurement bias will be introduced into the design. In the study of case management for jail detainees, persons receiving the case management intervention will be more closely followed in the community, which will yield more information about potential negative outcomes such as violence, substance use problems, legal difficulties, and interpersonal conflicts.

7.1.4 CHALLENGE 4: LENGTHY
FOLLOW-UP INTERVALS

Cost–effectiveness studies are often challenged by the need for long-term follow-up data on study subjects. To date, policy makers and federal granting agencies have promoted studies that focus on the most costly users of the mental health system—what are sometimes referred to as the severely and persistently mentally ill. Effectiveness is observed over months or years, rather than weeks, because interventions must show evidence of sustained improvement in long-standing and relapsing disorders. Longer follow-up intervals allow investigators to capture improvements in outcome domains that occur months after the onset of treatment and to examine the long-term stability of recovery. Slow-response outcome domains further add to the length of cost–effectiveness studies. Typically, changes in functioning and quality of life will occur over longer periods than changes in disorder-specific symptoms. As a result, cost–effectiveness studies often investigate the mental health outcomes of individuals over periods of one to three years. This increases the risk of loss of cooperation with outcome interviews and increases the relative value of outcomes obtainable from unobtrusive sources such as arrest records, mortality data, and the like.

7.1.5 RESOLVING THE CHALLENGES
AND DEVELOPING A PROTOCOL

The practical steps in developing a strong outcome measurement protocol are summarized in Example 1.

The first step in designing an outcome measurement protocol to meet the above challenges is to identify outcomes that are of greatest policy relevance. Ideally, outcomes would be prioritized from several perspectives, including the investigator's theories and preconceptions, the consumers perspective, the payor's perspective, the provider's perspective, and other affected community stakeholders, such as informal caregivers, police, and community neighborhoods. Important questions include, Who is likely to be affected by the intervention? How will they be helped? In what ways might they be harmed, troubled, or inconvenienced?

Theory and the involvement of stakeholder perspectives in the design of measures will aid investigators in determining what is most important to measure

---

EXAMPLE 1. STEPS IN DEVELOPING STRONG
OUTCOME MEASUREMENT

Step 1:   Select measurement domains with a clear understanding of treatment theory, consumer, provider, and other stakeholder preferences.

Step 2:   Review the literature and contact other investigators in the field for measures of each selected domain.

Step 3:   Pilot test measures in the study setting.

Step 4:   Embed outcome measures in a strong research design.

---

and in assuring that the breadth of the intervention is matched by the breadth of the measurement protocol. In the example at the beginning of this chapter, a cost–effectiveness study that examined only the program's success at treating the mental health symptoms of released jail psychiatric service patients would not conceptualize effectiveness adequately. Instead, the development of the outcome measurement protocol needs to reflect the diversity of intervention goals and the diversity of stakeholder preferences. Chapter 8 will extend the discussions begun in this chapter by describing how to aggregate multiple outcome measures and take into account the various stakeholder preferences.

A second step in developing a measurement protocol is reviewing published measures and contacting experienced investigators in the field who have faced the measurement challenges in their own research. Investigators working in the field often will have unpublished improvements to published scales and psychometric data that can aid in the design of new cost–effectiveness studies. Methodological research in this area has been slow to develop and to appear in the published literature. Knowing the latest methodological developments in the field requires communication with investigators who are conducting cost–effectiveness research to avoid repeating mistakes or reinventing wheels. The complexity of cost–effectiveness research makes ongoing consultation with such colleagues especially valuable.

The third step is pilot research to determine the length, feasibility, and reliability of the planned outcome measurement protocol in the population and settings of the cost–effectiveness study. We encourage investigators to develop draft measurement protocols for administration to small samples prior to recruiting subjects for the cost–effectiveness study. These pilot studies should be designed to check interrater reliability of all or portions of the measurement protocol and can be used as a final check on the training of persons responsible for administering the measurement protocol. Such pilot experience should be integrated with testing of the sources of data for utilization, cost, and income, as discussed in Chapters 4 and 5.

The final step is to embed the outcome measurement protocol in a strong research design. The strongest designs involve comparisons between well-defined intervention models rather than between an intervention model and an ill-defined comparison group receiving usual care. Many outcome measurement biases are avoided in research designs when all study groups are engaged in treatment models that provide equal opportunity to observe outcomes. Such studies also benefit from clear intervention goals that allow a prioritization of potential outcome measures.

In the remainder of this chapter we present a conceptual framework of outcome measures that will aid investigators in selecting measurement methods for cost–effectiveness studies. We will also describe the major outcome measures used in mental health cost–effectiveness studies. The framework is designed to help the investigator think through the challenges of measurement in cost–effectiveness research.

7.2 CONCEPTUAL FRAMEWORK FOR OUTCOME MEASUREMENT

Outcome measurement protocols embody decisions about three questions:

1. What outcome domains will be assessed?
2. What sources of information will be used for each domain? and
3. How often and over what period will outcomes be assessed?

7.2.1 OUTCOME DOMAINS

There have been several attempts to conceptualize the broad range of mental health outcomes that are of policy relevance. Some theorists have characterized outcome domains in terms of dysfunction, disability, and handicap (Liberman, 1988). Some have characterized outcomes as clinical, rehabilitative, humanitarian, and public safety (Attkisson et al., 1992; Hargreaves and Shumway, 1989). Others have proposed clinical status, functional status, life satisfaction, and safety and welfare as mental health outcome domains (Rosenblatt and Attkisson, 1993). Taken together, the frameworks reflect the fact that the goals of mental health interventions go beyond the treatment of specific symptoms and mental disorders. Existing outcome typologies, however, do not lend themselves easily to the design of outcome measurement protocols, because they do not encompass critical outcome domains such as health status and quality of life.

Here, we modify existing typologies to aid investigators in the selection of outcome measures. First, we add health status as a domain encompassing measures of mental and physical health symptoms and functioning. There have been important advances in the definition and measurement of health status in the last decade, and this has been accompanied by increased recognition of the interdependence of mental and physical health symptoms and functioning. We describe these important measures in a section on general health status measures.

Second, we add quality of life as the broadest outcome domain of interest to cost–effectiveness studies. Existing typologies have not explicitly recognized quality of life as an independent outcome domain despite several adequate measures explicitly designed to measure the construct. Existing typologies place quality of life concepts in the clinical, functional, and life-satisfaction domains (Rosenblatt and Attkisson, 1993). It seems reasonable to propose that quality of life is the broadest outcome domain of concern to effectiveness research, subsuming narrower outcome domains such as symptoms, functioning, and health status (Ware, 1989).

The resulting typology of outcome measures (shown in Example 2) consists of five domains ranging from the most specific to the most broad: (1) measures of disorder and symptoms, (2) measures of functioning, (3) measures of general health status, (4) measures of quality of life, and (5) measures of public safety and societal welfare. Conceptualized in this way, outcome measures can be selected according to theoretical conceptions about the intended effects of the intervention. Certain outcome domains may be considered more proximal to the intervention and may be assessed more intensively. Other outcomes may be more distal from the intervention and may be assessed less intensively. For example, disorder specific symptoms may be a proximal outcome for a medication intervention but a distal outcome to a case management intervention. The hypothesized effects of the treatment will dictate the outcome domains that should be assessed most intensively.

EXAMPLE 2. DOMAINS OF OUTCOME MEASUREMENT

Domain 1:   Measures of specific symptoms and disorders.
Domain 2:   Measures of functioning.
Domain 3:   Measures of general health status.
Domain 4:   Measures of quality of life.
Domain 5:   Measures of public safety and societal welfare.

7.2.2 SOURCES OF INFORMATION

Recognition of the fallibility of mental health outcome measures has motivated the development of measurement protocols that incorporate multiple sources of information. Following a highly regarded measurement tradition in psychology, the multitrait-multimethod matrix (Campbell and Fiske, 1959), cost effectiveness researchers assess outcome domains using multiple methods and multiple sources of information. Use of multiple measurement methods allows the construct validity of any one measure to be verified and provides a test of the robustness of study findings to variation in measurement methods.

Measurement methods can vary with respondent type. Subjects may report on their own symptoms, behavior, functioning, and quality of life. In addition or alternatively, other respondents may be asked to report on the symptoms, behavior, functioning, and quality of life of the study subject. These respondents may be trained clinical raters, research observers, or collateral informants who are persons in the community, who have knowledge of the subject in community settings such as home, work, and school, and who have had an opportunity to observe the measured outcome constructs.

Measurement methods may also vary in the way that information is elicited from the respondent. Methods of eliciting information include direct behavioral observation, searches of medical and other archival records, biological assays, paper and pencil questionnaires, and structured and semistructured interviews.

7.2.3 MEASUREMENT WINDOWS
AND MEASUREMENT INTERVALS

A fundamental tenet of measuring effectiveness is that the measurement of change is estimated from repeated administration of cross-sectional measures rather than from any attempt to estimate change directly. Change is not "rated," but is "computed" on the basis of repeated administration of appropriate outcome measures at selected points in time.

Time considerations come into play in measuring outcomes in two important ways. First, cross-sectional measures inevitably have some retrospective window of time over which they assess the respondent's status at a particular point in time. The cross-sectional window may be a day, a week, or a month or longer, depending on the construct being observed and the reliability of the source for retrospective retrieval of information. Measures of relatively stable constructs (e.g., living arrangements, vocational activity) can be examined over longer cross-sectional windows than measures of highly variable constructs that cannot be characterized or reliably measured except in the very recent past (e.g., mood, daily functioning, and daily activities).

Second, we cannot talk about change without talking about change over a given time period. The interval between cross-sectional measures will vary depending on the research question, the nature of the intervention, and the population being studied. In a study having more than two measurement periods, the intervals between measurements may not be equal but varied in order to obtain different estimates of change at theoretically important points following the initiation and termination of the intervention. For example, measures may be obtained 1 month, 6 months, and 18 months following baseline assessment.

7.3 SPECIFIC OUTCOME INSTRUMENTS

We now take each of the domains of outcome and review candidate measures to illustrate the principles we have discussed, attempting to highlight emerging standards of measurement. We focus on measures for which there appears to be a growing consensus on their use. In domains in which no clear consensus exists, we provide a more comprehensive review of candidate measures.

7.3.1 OUTCOME DOMAIN 1: DISORDER AND SYMPTOMS

A cornerstone of efficacy trials is the assessment of disorder-specific symptomatic outcomes. Effectiveness studies may examine changes in morbidity (e.g., remission or relapse of major depression) and changes in disorder severity (e.g., increases or decreases in the frequency or severity of depressive symptoms) as they are affected by clinical, programmatic, and system-level interventions.

Disorder-specific measures tend to capture changes in outcomes that are unique to disorder groups, as well as subtle changes in clinical status that are not detectable using generic health status measures (Patrick and Deyo, 1989). They may be inappropriate, however, for assessing outcomes in diagnostically heterogenous samples and may not allow meaningful comparison of outcomes across diagnostic subgroups. When interventions are intended to have a broad impact on a very heterogenous clinical population, disease-specific measures may have lower priority than broader measures of functioning, health status, and quality of life. Study objectives and subject selection criteria will dictate the extent to which disease- specific measures should be included in any outcome measurement protocol.

Diagnostic Interviews for Adults

The Diagnostic Interview Schedule (DIS) is a highly structured interview developed by researchers at the National Institute of Mental Health (Robins et al., 1981). The DIS was used to collect data for the Epidemiological Catchment Area (ECA) program that surveyed five urban communities in the United States between 1980 and 1983 (Regier et al., 1993). The DIS was modeled after the Renard Diagnostic Interview, which operationalized the Feighner criteria for diagnosis (Helzer et al., 1985). The DIS also includes questions about service utilization over the past 12 months.

The Structured Clinical Interview for DSM-IV (SCID) is the gold standard of clinical diagnosis with adults (Spitzer et al., 1992; Williams et al., 1992). The SCID is a semistructured interview that guides a trained clinical interviewer through the differential diagnoses of the major mental disorders in the current Diagnostic and Statistical Manual (APA, 1994). Publication of DSM-III made previous structured clinical diagnostic interviews obsolete (e.g., Schedule for Affective Disorders and Schizophrenia and Present State Examination) and accelerated the emergence of the SCID as the most widely used clinician-administered diagnostic approach.

The SCID differs from fully structured interviews in that clinical, trained interviewers tailor the SCID to each subject and interview situation. The SCID encourages the clinical interviewer to complete a thorough clinical interview that can last from one to several hours depending on the morbidity and comorbidity of the respondent. Interviewers ask questions tailored to the experiences of subjects, ask elaborate questions, and use clinical judgment to determine whether the subjects articulation of their problems fit DSM-IV criteria. The SCID manual encourages the diagnostician to incorporate other sources of information such as family members, mental health providers, and medical records as needed.

The test-retest reliabilities of the SCID are adequate. Reliability coefficients for schizophrenia, mood, alcohol, and substance disorder diagnoses exceed .60 (Spitzer et al., 1992; Williams et al., 1992; Segal et al., 1994; Skre et al., 1991). Reliabilities for other categories vary by diagnosis. The costs of clinical diagnostic assessment with the SCID are high. The protocol is complex and requires a clinically trained interviewer who is knowledgeable about DSM-IV. In addition, the time required to complete the SCID may mean that other measures may have to be scheduled at a later time depending on the stamina of respondents. A version of the SCID for populations that are largely free of diagnosable psychotic conditions has been developed to streamline interview time in some situations. This version, known as the SCID with psychotic screen, largely eliminates sections that diagnose schizophrenia, schizoaffective disorder, and bipolar mood disorder. A version of the SCID, the SCID-II has been developed to assess personality disorders on Axis II (Fogelson et al., 1991; Segal et al., 1994). In addition, the SCID is designed to be modular, so that investigators interested in confirming the diagnosis of a particular disorder and who do not need identification of the full range of comorbid diagnoses can administer modules of the SCID that pertain to specific diagnoses (e.g., Psychotic Disorders, Alcohol and Substance Use Disorders, Posttraumatic Stress Disorder, and Anxiety Disorders).

An alternative to the SCID is the Comprehensive International Diagnostic Interview (CIDI). The CIDI is a structured interview that provides International Classification of Disease (ICD-10) diagnoses that are translatable into DSM-III and DSM-III-R codes. Several versions of the CIDI have been developed, beginning with the original version developed jointly by the World Health Organization and the Alcohol, Drug Abuse and Mental Health Administration (Robins et al., 1988; 1994). A modified version of the WHO CIDI was developed at the University of Michigan for use in the National Comorbidity Study (Kessler et al., 1994). Known as the UM CIDI, the layout, order of questions, and structure of stem questions are designed to improve the recall of mental-health-related symptoms and to reduce reporting biases as compared with the WHO version. A third adaptation of the CIDI has been developed for use in the Fresno study of "Mental Health Service Utilization among Rural Mexican Americans." The Fresno CIDI extends the UM CIDI to arrive at DSM-IV diagnoses and has refined language and expression to be more specific to that used by Mexican American and Mexican national populations (Aguilar-Gaxiola, et al., 1995).

The CIDI, like the DIS, is most appropriate for use in large sample studies in which diagnosis is of central importance and the cost of a clinical diagnostic interview using the SCID is prohibitive. Reliability of the CIDI and the DIS for assessing current psychiatric disorder has been well established in the literature (Robins and Regier, 1991; Helzer et al., 1985). The predictive validity of the instrument in estimating lifetime psychiatric diagnoses made by clinicians appears to be limited (Anthony et al., 1985; Wittchen et al., 1985). Because effectiveness studies are generally more concerned with current diagnoses, the lack of reliability in making lifetime diagnoses may be less problematic.

A third diagnostic instrument is the PRIME-MD, designed to be a rapid and accurate method to estimate DSM-IV diagnoses for the most common mental disorders seen in primary care settings (Spitzer et al., 1994). Diagnosis with the PRIME-MD proceeds in two stages. The first involves administering a one-page self-report questionnaire to the patient to screen for five major groups of mental disorders. This step commonly is done in the waiting room, administered by a receptionist or office nurse. The patient questionnaire screens for mood, anxiety, somatoform, alcohol, and eating disorders. The second stage involves administering a 12-page interview that guides a primary care clinician through the differential diagnosis of any disorder screening positive on the patient questionnaire. Clinician interview time is reported to be 5 to 11 minutes (Spitzer et al., 1994).

PRIME-MD diagnoses, made by primary care physicians, showed substantial agreement with diagnoses made by trained mental health professionals. In a sample of 431 primary care patients, face-to-face interviews by a primary care physician using the PRIME-MD were followed by telephone interviews by a trained mental health professional using the PRIME-MD and other questions taken from the SCID. Kappa coefficients for agreement between diagnostic methods were .71 for any psychiatric disorder, .61 for any mood disorder, .55 for any anxiety disorder, .71 for alcohol abuse or dependence, and .73 for any eating disorder. Agreements for the rarely observed somatoform disorder were not estimated. Agreement for specific diagnoses was lower in several instances such as minor depressive disorder, anxiety disorder not otherwise specified, and recurrent major depressive disorder. The pattern of disagreements suggested that a major source of diagnostic error in the PRIME-MD is low sensitivity. That is, for some diagnostic categories, the PRIME-MD is inadequate for detecting the presence of a mental disorder. Sensitivities for diagnostic categories ranged from .22 to .83. Alternatively, when the mental health professional did not find a diagnosable condition, it was very likely that no diagnosis was made by the PRIME-MD as well. Specificities were uniformly high, ranging from .88 to .98. That is, if the primary care physician identified a psychiatric disorder, the validation interviewer usually agreed.

The PRIME-MD appears to assess the most common mental disorders with a good degree of accuracy. It may be an appropriate diagnostic tool when obtaining full SCID or CIDI diagnoses, but it is not an appropriate investment of study resources in cases in which such disorders as schizophrenia, bipolar mood disorder, and substance use disorders other than alcohol are not anticipated. Its performance in settings other than the primary care settings in which it was developed and tested, however, is unknown. Investigators are advised to examine the psychometric properties of the PRIME-MD in their own populations and settings.

Finally, a fourth adult diagnostic aid is worth noting, the DSM Checklist. Psychometric work on the Diagnostic Interview Schedule led to the development of this diagnostic checklist suitable for use by clinicians in semistructured or unstructured interviews. The DSM-III-R Checklist (Hudziak et al., 1993), like the SCID, can also be used to organize data gathering from other sources such as family members, friends, and clinical records. The Checklist has been computerized by Przybeck et al. (1988) to increase administration and scoring efficiency. The feasibility, clinical utility, and interdiagnostician agreement have been examined in clinical and general population samples (Hudziak et al., 1993; Helzer et al., 1985; Helzer et al., 1987).

Diagnostic Interviews for Children

Clear advances in the diagnosis of child psychopathology have been made in the last 10 years, including the development of several structured and semistructured diagnostic interviews. A careful review of these instruments has been presented by Hodges (1993) and includes the Child Assessment Schedule (CAS), the Child and Adolescent Psychiatric Assessment (CAPA), and the Diagnostic Interview Schedule for Children-Revised (DISC-R), among others. Each has child and parent versions and is appropriate for samples with a range of psychiatric diagnoses. The DISC-R has been patterned after the Diagnostic Interview Schedule and is designed for epidemiologic investigations (Shaffer et al., 1993; Schwab-Stone et al., 1993; Piacentini et al., 1993). A revision of the DISC-R, the DISC-2, is in development, and some data on its reliability have been published (Fisher et al., 1993).

The CAS and the CAPA are semistructured instruments designed for use by clinicians to diagnose mental disorders in childhood. The CAPA has no published psychometric data. The CAS and other instruments mentioned by Hodges in her review shows psychometric properties equal to that of the DISC-R.

Measures of Symptom Severity

There is a vast array of self-administered and interview rating scales that assess a wide range of symptoms of psychosis, depression, and anxiety. Some are multidimensional in that they measure multiple symptom domains. Others focus on a single domain. We focus on the most widely used measures of four types: (1) multidimensional symptom measures, (2) depressive symptoms, (3) substance use measures, and (4) child measures.

Multidimensional Symptom Measures

The most widely used multidimensional symptom measures in the United States include the Brief Psychiatric Rating Scale (BPRS), the Scale for the Assessment of Positive Symptoms/Scale for the Assessment of Negative Symptoms (SAPS/SANS), the Positive and Negative Syndrome Scale (PANSS), and a family of self-report instruments centering around the Symptom Checklist-90-Revised (Derogatis, 1983). A wider variety of symptom measures is employed internationally (Manchanda et al., 1989).

The BPRS, SANS and SAPS, and PANSS are relatively similar in their administration and excel in assessing psychotic symptomatology. Trained clinical interviewers generally are required to conduct interviews lasting between 20 to 50 minutes depending on the comprehensibility and clarity of the respondent. Extensive training and ongoing monitoring of interviewer practices usually are required to assure that the BPRS is administered reliably across subjects and across interviewers.

The Brief Psychiatric Rating Scale (BPRS) was first published in 1962 and consisted of 16 symptom constructs rated on seven-point Likert scales during a clinical interview (Overall and Gorham, 1962). The scale has since been modified, and today the most commonly used form of the BPRS contains 18 items, is administered using a semistructured interview, and contains rating scales that are anchored by descriptors (Overall and Gorham, 1988; Woerner et al., 1988; Essock et al., 1996b).

The Positive and Negative Syndrome Scale (PANSS) expanded the BPRS and can be used to assess a variety of psychiatric symptoms with an emphasis on schizophrenia-related symptoms (Kay, 1987; 1988). The PANSS measures 30 symptom constructs using a semistructured interview format. The PANSS was constructed using the 18 items of the BPRS and 12 items from the Psychopathology Rating Scale (Kay et al., 1987). The items were derived rationally to assess positive symptoms, negative symptoms, and general psychopathology. With the PANSS, trained clinicians make ratings on operationally defined, seven-point scales that are patterned after those of the BPRS. These scales have shown good psychometric properties. In one study jointly comparing the PANSS and BPRS ratings, PANSS items showed greater interrater reliability than comparable items on the BPRS although items on both scales were quite acceptable (Bell et al., 1992). Strong correlation between comparable PANSS and BPRS items suggests that the BPRS is largely a subset of PANSS items and that research with the PANSS may be translatable to the vast body of research that has been completed using the BPRS.

Another choice for the assessment of psychiatric symptoms is the Scale for the Assessment of Negative Symptoms (SANS) and the Scale for the Assessment of Positive Symptoms (SAPS). Consisting of a total of 49 items, the SANS and SAPS were designed to provide a comprehensive assessment of symptoms characteristic of schizophrenia, although the symptom domains assessed by the SANS and SAPS are common to many other diagnostic categories (Andreason,

1982; Moscarelli, 1987; Andreason, 1986). The SANS facilitates detailed ratings of alogia, affective blunting, avolition-apathy, anhedonia-asociality, and attentional impairment. The SAPS facilitates detailed ratings of hallucinations, delusions, positive formal thought disorder, and bizarre behavior. Although assessing similar constructs with good internal consistency and interrater reliability, the SAPS and SANS are moderately correlated with the BPRS (Gur, 1991; Thiemann, 1987). It is likely that the SANS measures complementary aspects of negative symptoms that are not assessed by the BPRS.

Finally, the Symptom Checklist-90-Revised (SCL-90-R) provides a means of assessing a broad spectrum of mental health symptoms in a self-report, paper and pencil administered format (Derogatis, 1983). Derived from the Hopkins Symptom Checklist (Derogatis et al., 1974), the SCL-90-R contains nine items that form nine primary dimensions of psychopathology including somatic, obsessive compulsive, interpersonal sensitivity, depression, anxiety, hostility, phobic anxiety, paranoid ideation, and psychoticism. The SCL-90-R also yields three dimensions of global distress including a global severity index, a positive symptom distress index, and a positive symptom total.

The average time required to complete the SCL-90-R is between 12 and 15 minutes. Internal consistency and test-retest reliabilities are uniformly high and exceeded .77 for each dimension in one reliability study (Derogatis, 1983). A brief, 53-item version of the SCL-90-R is available (the Brief Symptom Inventory) in addition to clinician administered versions of the SCL-90-R (the Hopkins Psychiatric Rating Scale and the Brief Hopkins Psychiatric Rating Scale).

Depressive Symptoms

Turning to depressive symptoms, there are several widely used inventories for the assessment of depressive symptoms in adults. Three are brief self-report inventories that can be completed by subjects using paper and pencil or computerized administration formats: the Beck Depression Inventory (BDI), the Zung Self-Rating Depression Scale (SDS), and the Centers for Epidemiologic Studies Depression Scale (CES-D). The fourth is the Hamilton Rating Scale for Depression, a clinician administered rating scale that is considered the gold standard of depression severity rating measures.

The BDI contains 21 items measuring the cognitive, mood, and somatic symptoms commonly associated with depression (Beck et al., 1996). The psychometric properties of the BDI are well established and the measure has been widely used in efficacy trials of drug and psychotherapy interventions (Elkin et al., 1985; 1989). The BDI has been shown to discriminate depression from general negative affect and anxiety (Clark and Beck, 1995). The Zung Self-Rating Depression Scale (SDS) (Zung, 1965; 1967; Zung et al., 1965) has been widely used to assess depression severity in pharmacologic and psychotherapy efficacy trials, although problems with convergent and discriminant validity have long been known (Carroll et al., 1973). The CESD is a 20-item scale designed as a tool for screening for depression in the general population or in primary care populations (Burnam and Wells, 1990; Miranda et al., 1990).

The Hamilton Rating Scale for Depression facilitates ratings of depression severity during the course of an unstructured clinical interview (Hamilton, 1960). The Hamilton scale contains 23 items (although only 17 items contribute to the depression total score). Clinicians rate symptoms of depression on three- or five-point behaviorally anchored scales. Despite the lack of a standardized response format, the interrater reliability of the Hamilton rating scale has been shown to be quite good. O'Hara and Rehm (1983) showed that undergraduates given short training periods can administer the Hamilton scale with a high degree of interrater reliability and with excellent agreement with expert raters.

Although generally comparable in terms of ratings of internal consistency, interrater reliability, and concurrent validity, the BDI, Zung, CES-D, and Hamilton measures appear to differ in their sensitivity to change in outcome studies. Meta-analytic studies and studies comparing measures directly suggest that the Hamilton Rating Scale for Depression shows greater sensitivity to clinical change than do either the BDI or the Zung scales (Edwards et al., 1984; Lambert et al., 1986; Lambert et al., 1988; Senra, 1995). These studies suggest that the magnitude of effect sizes measured by the Hamilton Rating Scale are greater than that reported on the other measures when expressed in standardized units and that the Hamilton Rating Scale detects changes in depression earlier in treatment than either the BDI or Zung measures.

Substance Abuse Symptoms

Turning to substance disorder symptoms, one finds that although a considerable amount of published research has been directed toward the screening, detection, diagnosis, and classification of substance use disorders in a variety of clinical populations, little research has examined the extent to which any of these measures are appropriate for assessing the outcomes and effectiveness of substance abuse services. Historically, the most highly regarded indicator of effectiveness for substance disorder interventions was abstinence from alcohol and other problematic substances. As Babor et al. (1994) state in their review of outcome measures for alcohol treatment research, the proportion of days abstinent out of the total number of possible drinking days in a given period and the amount of substance consumed in a given period are hallmark indicators of treatment effectiveness.

It is not surprising then, that outcome measures for assessing the quantity, frequency, and intensity of alcohol and other substance use have received the most attention in the literature (Babor et al., 1994; Miller and Del Boca, 1994). The most common and direct methods involve some form of self-report on the part of the consumer with increasing evidence that self-report of alcohol and substance use by disordered individuals is not necessarily biased (Babor, 1994; Babor, 1987). There is growing consensus that self-report of substance use by disordered persons is consistent with other available sources of information (Hesselbrock et al., 1983; O'Hare et al., 1991). However, under certain conditions verbal reports are unreliable and inaccurate, affected by memory, desire to give socially desirable answers, poorly designed questions, and anxiety about confidentiality violations (Babor et al., 1994). The experienced investigator will recognize that each of these conditions is heavily influenced by how the outcomes are measured and is under the control of the researcher. The factors involved in obtaining unbiased assessment of the quantity and frequency of alcohol and other substance use include (1) use of structured assessments, (2) obtaining information from multiple sources, and (3) reassuring subject's of their confidentiality and their role as candid information providers (Babor et al., 1994).

The most rudimentary estimates of alcohol and other substance use consist of multiple-choice questions about how often subjects typically use and how much is consumed on each occasion of use (Miller and Del Boca, 1994). More systematic quantification of patterns of use is allowed by computing an average consumption grid as developed by Miller and Marlatt (1984) in the Comprehensive Drinker Profile. Respondents are asked to describe their morning, afternoon, and evening drinking patterns during a typical seven-day period. Exceptions to this pattern, either towards greater or less drinking, can be noted, and overall consumption patterns can be quantified by combining estimates of steady and the episodic drinking behavior. A third alternative is the time-line-follow-back method, in which a retrospective calendar is used to reconstruct the consumption of substances in each day of a given period. The interviewer helps the subject characterize his or her drinking or substance use for each day in terms of a Likert scale or in terms of the actual amount consumed. Self-monitoring extends the time-line-follow-back method by using a prospective calendar. A hybrid of the average grid and time-line-follow-back method has been developed by Miller and Del Boca (1994) and referred to as the Form-90. Each method appears to be applicable to subjects, collateral informants, and clinicians.

A variety of other outcome measures have been less widely used but may be applicable for certain studies. The most notable of these are global outcome ratings by clinicians that incorporate quantity and frequency of use, substance-related impairments and consequences, and mortality. (The scales are presented and summarized nicely by Babor et al., 1994.) Clinically meaningful criteria are established for scale points usually ranging from "abstinent" to "heavy drinking problems" or "mortality." Drake has used case-manager ratings of alcohol and substance use problems in persons with schizophrenia and has shown these estimates to have good interrater reliability (Drake et al., 1989; 1993).

In addition, substance abuse outcome measures attempt to assess negative consequences associated with substance use (Babor et al., 1994). These may be categorized as *intra*individual consequences, such as withdrawal, medical problems, and depression, or as *inter*individual consequences, such as fights, intoxication-related arrests, loss of employment, and failed relationships. These characteristics are quantified by a number of measures that have been used in the treatment of alcohol disorders literature and by diagnostic instruments such as the CIDI, the DIS, and the SCID. The alcohol and substance use disorder sections of these instruments generally have shown quite good reliability (Cottler et al., 1990). In their review, Babor et al. (1994) conclude that there is no standard or consensus on measurement of negative consequences associated with alcohol despite the importance and robustness of these outcome indicators.

Symptom Measures for Children

Turning to symptom measures used in studies of outcomes for children, the best known is the Child Behavior Checklist. Originally developed as a method for reviewing clinical records of children receiving mental health services, it yields ratings on 20 social competence items and more than 118 behavior problems (Achenbach and Edelbrock, 1978). Items were derived from reviews of the child psychopathology literature and reviews of 1,000 clinical records. The instrument was adapted for parents, teachers, clinicians, trained observers, children, and peers by wording items in simple language and asking respondents to rate whether a discrete behavior or social competence is "very or often true," "somewhat true," or "not true" of the subject. The Child Behavior Checklist is used extensively in epidemiologic studies of childhood behavior problems and in large scale effectiveness studies of mental health interventions for children. Interparent agreement, interinterviewer agreement, and one-week test-retest reliabilities were in excess of .90 for total behavior problems and total social competency in a large sample of children referred for outpatient mental health treatment (Achenbach and Edelbrock, 1981). Two broad-band subscales of problem behavior and social competencies have been developed using factor analysis (Achenbach and Edelbrock, 1978; 1979). Consistently identified across various age cohorts in children was an internalizing factor consisting of somatic problems, social withdrawal, uncommunicativeness, immaturity, anxiety, and depression. Also consistently found across various age cohorts was an externalizing factor consisting of hyperactivity, delinquent behavior, aggressiveness, and cruelty. One-week test-retest and interparent reliabilities on the subscales were generally high. In clinically treated samples, significant reductions in total problem behavior scores and increases in the majority of social competence scores suggest the CBCL is sensitive to clinical improvements (Achenbach and Edelbrock, 1979).

7.3.2 OUTCOME DOMAIN 2: FUNCTIONING

The goal of mental health intervention is not only the alleviation of symptoms but the restoration of functioning. Functioning is defined as the ability to engage in productive and socially valued activity and is demonstrated by the performance of expected self-care activities and in the fulfillment of social, occupational, and educational roles. Measures of two types are reviewed: (1) global ratings of functioning and (2) multidimensional ratings of functioning. Measures of functioning have been reviewed periodically since the early 1980s (Anthony and Farkas, 1982; Ciarlo and Windle, 1988; Goldman et al., 1992; Wallace, 1986; Weissman et al., 1981). We update these reviews with special attention to measures with broad-based applicability in effectiveness research. Many measures appear less applicable for effectiveness research because they are designed for use with special populations in restricted settings, such as residential or inpatient treatment facilities. To be included in this review, the measure must have reported the results of psychometric research on reliability and validity. Finding no clear superiority in the psychometric properties of any of these instruments, we do not detail the psychometrics of any. All appear adequate based on the published report of the test developers, and none are contraindicated based on published psychometric data. We suggest that choice of measure be based on ease of use, depth of assessment required, and whether global ratings of functioning are desired. Although all measures are English-language-based, some measures developed by European investigators may need to be adapted or modified for use in the United States due to idiomatic differences in language usage.

Global Functioning

We begin with global measures of functioning. In Chapter 8 we will describe methods of combining mental health outcome indicators to form an overall index of effectiveness. Clinical raters can also take into account multiple areas of functioning and make global judgments about the functioning of an individual. The most widely used indicator of functioning is the Global Assessment of Functioning Scale (APA, 1987; APA, 1994), the most recent version of which has been tested in the DSM-IV field trials (Patterson and Lee, 1995). The GAF was developed by modifying an earlier scale: the Global Assessment Scale (GAS) (Endicott et al., 1976). The GAF rates overall mental health functioning from the lowest to highest levels on a 100-point scale over a given interval. Within the 100 points, ten major levels of functioning are defined with behavioral anchors. The interrater reliability of the GAF was estimated in several independent samples and ranged from .61 to .91 with a standard error of measurement between 5 and 8 points (Endicott et al., 1976). Comparable reliabilities were found for trained psychiatrists, residents, and psychologists in a community mental health center (Dworkin et al., 1990).

The GAF can be used with adults and children alike, but there are two published modifications of the GAF specifically for children. The most widely used modification was developed by Shaffer and co-workers (Shaffer et al., 1983; Rey et al., 1995), and the second by Sorensen et al. (1982).

Variation in the GAF is not determined purely by the functioning of rated individuals, however, since symptoms are included in the GAF scale. This may be problematic for investigators who want independent ratings of symptoms and functioning. This concern led to the creation of the Social and Occupational Functioning Assessment Scale (SOFAS), which provides an overall rating of mental health functioning uncontaminated by symptom severity (Goldman et al., 1992). SOFAS is contained in Appendix B of DSM-IV (APA, 1994). Other clinical rating scales have been developed and reported in the literature but have been less widely adopted in research or clinical practice (Green and Gracely, 1987).

Multidomain Functioning

We turn now to multidomain functioning measures, often used when study objectives and research questions require detailed information about functioning. There is a wide variety of published outcome measures that allow quantification of functioning in specific areas of functioning such as social, work, school, and activities of daily living. We identify 14 measures that assess functioning in a broad variety of settings and have published psychometrics. A summary of each measure's areas of functioning and sources of information is found in Figure 7.1.

Functioning domains assessed by most measures include activities of daily living (ADLs); independent living skills (e.g., managing finances, housekeeping, shopping), sometimes referred to as instrumental activities of daily living (IADLs); general and leisure activity levels; social functioning; educational functioning; work functioning; legal problems; dangerousness towards self and others; legal problems and antisocial behavior; and symptoms and distress indicators. Some measures may also assess problems with alcohol and substances; manifestations of odd, bizarre, and problematic behavior in the community; and family burden. These domains are included less consistently across measures and appear to be less central to conceptions of functioning.

Measures vary in whether they elicit information from consumers, from collateral informants, or from both sources. The Katz Adjustment Scales, the Social Adjustment Scale, the Social Functioning Scale, and the Social Stress and Functioning Inventory for Psychotic Disorders all have parallel consumer and collateral versions (Katz and Lyerly, 1963; Weissman et al., 1981). Relatively few measures require significant interviewer judgments or ratings. The exceptions are the Katz Activities of Daily Living Scale (Katz and Lyerly, 1963), which is an observational rating scale, and the Psychiatric Status Schedule (Spitzer et al., 1970) and the Psychiatric Evaluation Form (Endicott and Spitzer, 1972), which requires some interviewer judgment in completing the measure. One measure solely obtains information from collateral informants: the Life Skills Profile (Rosen, 1989; Parker et al., 1991; Parker and Hadzi-Pavlovic, 1995). The remaining measures are based on patient or some other collateral source of information.

All measures in Figure 7.1 have at least adequate psychometric properties. No measure distinguishes itself, however, with uniformly higher reliability and validity coefficients. Instead, the measures are distinguishable in terms of areas covered and in how similar areas are conceptualized and operationalized. The most narrow are the Katz ADL and the Life Skills Profile, which focus on activities of daily living and independent living skills. These measures would be most appropriate for more disabled populations and for studies of interventions de-

SCALES	AREA OF FUNCTIONING										SOURCES			
	ADLS	IADLS	GENERAL ACTIVITY	SOCIAL	EDUCATION	WORK	LEGAL PROBLEMS	DANGER TO SELF	DANGER TO OTHERS	SYMPTOMS	PATIENT REPORT	INTERVIEWER RATING	COLLATERAL REPORT	STANDARD ADMIN
Community Adaptation Schedule (Burnes and Roen, 1967)														
Disability Assessment Schedule (De Jong et al., 1985)														
Denver Community Mental Health Questionnaire (Reihman et al., 1977)														
Endicott Work Productivity Scale (Endicott and Nee, 1997)														
Katz Adjustment Scales (Katz and Lyerly, 1963)														
Katz Activities of Daily Living (Katz and Lyerly, 1963)														
Life Skills Profile (Rosen, 1989; Parker et al., 1991; Parker and Hadzi-Pavlovic, 1995)														
Multnomah Community Ability Scale (Barker et al., 1994a, 1994b)														
Personal Adjustment and Role Skills Scale (Ellsworth et al., 1968)														
Psychiatric Evaluation Form (Endicott and Spitzer, 1972)														
Psychiatric Status Schedule (Spitzer et al., 1970)														
Social Adjustment Scale (Weissman and Paykel, 1974)														
Social Functioning Scale (Birchwood et al., 1990)														
Social Behavior Assessment Schedule (Platt et al., 1980)														
Social Stress and Functioning Inventory for Psychotic Disorders (Serban, 1978)														

FIGURE 7.1 Multidomain Functioning Scales: Coverage and sources of information.

signed to improve basic skills, such as feeding, grooming, maintaining a house, shopping, and managing personal finances.

Measures with the broadest areas of coverage included the Psychiatric Status Schedule, Family Evaluation Form, Psychiatric Evaluation Form, Katz Adjustment Scales, the Social Behavior Assessment Schedule, and the Multnomah Community Ability Scale. Each has well-developed administration and scoring procedures. The PSS and PEF have an audiocassette training tape that accompanies each measure. The KAS has been used frequently in published studies of mental health interventions, although it is among the oldest of the measures, first introduced in 1963 (Katz and Lyerly, 1963).

The list of measures identified in Figure 7.1 will assist the investigator in identifying functioning measures that are of particular relevance. Choice of functional outcomes in cost–effectiveness research is dictated by the research questions, the nature of the intervention, and the characteristics of the target population. Often, no single measure will offer exactly the right breadth and depth of assessment in all of the functioning domains of interest to a particular study. Assembly of a measurement protocol often entails assembling relevant functioning measures, and modifying, deleting, and adopting components that are most relevant to the particular study. This must be done with special regard to the conditions under which particular instruments were tested and validated. Modification of content or administration procedures render existing psychometric data inapplicable. Addition of measures and items may add to the interview burden and redundancy and may affect test performance. Deletion of items may subtly change the context of items and affect test performance. Significantly modified instruments should be pilot-tested to determine feasibility, reliability, and validity.

7.3.3 OUTCOME DOMAIN 3: HEALTH STATUS

Ultimately, our concerns in mental health care are holistic and broader than the alleviation of symptoms and the remediation of specific functional deficits. Mental health interventions seek to affect mental health conditions such that they improve individual's overall health status and well-being (Ware, 1989; 1996; Dickey and Wagenaar, 1996).

The importance of measuring holistic effects of mental health interventions is growing, and cost–effectiveness studies of mental health interventions usually benefit from inclusion of health status measures. The struggle to achieve parity in the funding of mental health interventions compared to other health interventions requires empirical evidence showing that mental health is a critical component of health status and that the cost-effectiveness of mental health interventions rivals that of other health care interventions. Health status measures quantify outcomes of diverse treatments and diverse target populations not specific to any one age, disorder, or treatment group (Patrick and Deyo, 1989). Some measures, such as the Quality of Well-Being Scale, yield an overall indicator of health status that weights multiple aspects of health related quality of life according to consumer preferences for various health states. We review two health status outcome measures, both of which have been used in a wide variety of settings and populations.

The Medical Outcomes Study Short Form 36 (SF-36) yields a profile of eight health status dimensions: physical functioning, role limitations due to physical problems, social functioning, bodily pain, general mental health, role limitations due to emotional problems, vitality, and general health perceptions using 36 self-report questions scored on Likert scales. The scale properties of the SF-36 have been well established in large and diverse samples (McHorney et al., 1994). The SF-36 is well suited for rapid assessment of large samples and can be incorporated easily into longer assessment batteries without adding significantly to the cost of data collection. The SF-36 appears appropriate for use in telephone interview and mail surveys (McHorney et al., 1994).

The second measure, the Quality of Well-Being Scale (QWB) yields an overall indicator of the health related component of quality of life that may be particularly useful in evaluating the cost-effectiveness of mental health interventions (Kaplan and Anderson, 1990). As in health care, mental health care policy makers are faced with difficult decisions about the investment of limited dollars in the delivery of care. Comparing alternative treatments or delivery modes may be analogous to comparing the value of apples and oranges unless outcomes are measured on a common scale (Kaplan, 1994a). Rational decision-making may be impossible if data on the cost-effectiveness of relevant alternatives is derived from different measures or the treatments appear to affect various outcome dimensions somewhat differently.

The Quality of Well-Being Scale addresses the apples-and-oranges problem by aggregating different attributes of health status into an overall indicator by weighting each aspect of health status by its usefulness to the individual. The degree of usefulness of any particular health state, such as physical mobility, is referred to as its utility. Methods for estimating health care utilities are described in Chapter 8.

The QWB health care utility index is expressed in terms of quality-adjusted life years, and incorporates mortality, morbidity (quality of life), and prognosis (duration in a disabled health state). The morbidity component is conceptualized as health related quality of life and is a function of mobility, physical activity, social activity, and health symptoms. Utility ratings for each combination of quality of life state show high stability over a one-year period and consistency across a variety of rater groups (Kaplan, 1994b; Kaplan et al., 1978). Among health utility measures, the QWB appears to have the highest correlation with health status measures such as the SF-36 (Revicki and Kaplan, 1993). In one study, QWB scores were regressed onto the health status dimensions of the SF-36. The regression model accounted for 56% of the variance in QWB scores (Fryback et al., 1992).

7.3.4 OUTCOME DOMAIN 4: QUALITY OF LIFE

The effectiveness of some mental health interventions, especially those for chronic and debilitating mental disorders, is measured in terms of quality of life. For chronic and debilitating disorders, etiologies are poorly understood, symptoms may recur over extended life periods, and available treatments manage but do not cure the disorder. Therefore, comprehensive mental health care for these disorders works to minimize the consequences of mental disorder on functioning and quality of life. The wide adoption of the stress-vulnerability model in the treatment of severe mental disorder has fostered the recognition that individuals' life circumstances dramatically affect stress and adaptation to mental disorder and thus affect the severity and course of these disorders.

Quality of life is the broadest of the four outcome constructs and includes mental health status, functioning, general health status, and subjective well-being. It is not surprising that the term "quality of life" often is used imprecisely and synonymously at times with functioning and general health status (Ware, 1989). Mental health status, functioning, and general health status are undoubtedly components of, but are not synonymous with, quality of life. Quality of life depends also on the adequacy and desirability of one's living arrangements, neighborhood, financial resources, and occupation. It is not surprising then, that quality of life measures often jointly assess attributes of symptoms, functioning, general health status, and life circumstances.

The majority of quality of life measures in psychiatry have been developed for adult populations with severe mental disorders (Lehman and Burns, 1990). Lehman and Burns (1990) in their review of quality of life measures conclude that measures of quality of life that have been developed for the general population are adequate for the study of nondisabling mental disorders. Among measures for severely disabled populations, two have achieved prominence based on their comprehensiveness and psychometric development: Quality of Life Interview and the Oregon Quality of Life Questionnaire.

The Quality of Life Interview (QOLI) (Lehman, 1983; 1988; 1996; Lehman et al., 1995) measures objective and subjective indicators of quality of life in several life domains including living situation, leisure activities, family relations, social relations, finances, work and school, legal and safety, and health. The health domain of the QOLI consists of the Medical Outcome Study Questionnaire as reviewed above in the section on general health status measures. As Lehman indicates in his introduction to the core version of the QOLI, the contents of the QOLI have been adapted to the purposes of various studies. Lehman has identified a set of items that constitute a "core version" that allows comparability across studies with varying research goals.

The QOLI is highly structured, permitting standardized administration and minimizing interviewer effects. The QOLI has an administration manual and easily can be given by trained nonclinical interviewers in about 45 minutes. The psychometric properties of the QOLI have been studied in several samples

(Lehman, 1988). On subjective satisfaction scales, internal consistencies ranged from .74 to .88 across several domains and several independent samples, indicating good to excellent reliability for the subjective scales (Lehman, 1988). One-week test-retest reliabilities ranged from .41 to .95 with 55% of the test-retest coefficients greater than .70, suggesting that the subjective scales of the QOLI show somewhat lower temporal stability. Objective life satisfaction scales show a similar level of internal consistency and test-retest reliability. Internal consistencies for the objective scales were comparable, ranging from .44 to .87 with 44% of the coefficients exceeding .70. One-week test-retest reliability coefficients for the objective scales ranged from .29 to .93 with 41% of the coefficients exceeding .70.

The Oregon Quality of Life Questionnaire (QLQ) (Bigelow et al., 1982) is a comprehensive measure that conceptualizes quality of life in terms of 15 domains including psychological distress, psychological well-being, tolerance of stress, total basic need satisfaction, independence, interpersonal interaction, role functioning as a spouse, social support, work at home, employability, work on the job, school, meaningful use of time, negative consequences of alcohol use, and negative consequences of drug abuse (Bigelow et al., 1982; 1991). Administration of the QLQ involves a standardized interview. Two different response formats of the QLQ can be used: interviewer rating and self-report. In the interviewer rating version, interviewers rate problems in each of the areas on four-point Likert scales. In the self-report version, interviewers ask respondents for their ratings of problems in each of the areas on four-point Likert scales.

Reliability and validity of the QLQ have been well-established in large samples. Internal consistencies ranged from .17 to .98 with 57% of the scale reliabilities exceeding .70 in a sample of 2,642 persons (Bigelow et al., 1991). In addition, construct validation of the QLQ indicates that it discriminates the quality of life of community mental health center clients in economically depressed communities from economically stable communities and discriminates community mental health program clients in expected ways (Bigelow et al., 1991). In addition, both the QLQ interviewer rating version and the self-report version discriminate clients receiving different intensities of community mental health services (Bigelow and Young, 1991; Bigelow, 1991).

7.3.5 OUTCOME DOMAIN 5: PUBLIC SAFETY AND WELFARE

Recognizing that the effects of mental disorder are experienced by more than the ill individual, typologies of outcome domains often include the safety and welfare of the public, including family members, friends, and the community at large (Hargreaves and Shumway, 1989; Attkisson et al., 1992). The narrowest conceptions define public welfare outcomes in terms of violence or the threat of violence towards self or others (La Fond and Durham, 1992). Mental disorder, however, affects others in many more ways than during occurrences of violent and self-harming behavior. At its broadest conception, measures of public welfare domain might encompass any way in which mental disorders affect others or the environment. In this section, we briefly review measures of violent behavior, disruptive behavior, and family burden.

Measures of public welfare constructs often use multiple sources of information about the behavior of mental health consumers. The use of multiple sources has been shown to increase the likelihood of accurately measuring problematic behaviors that affect public welfare by increasing the likelihood that a problem behavior is detected by at least one of the sources (Mulvey and Lidz, 1993).

Violence

Mulvey and Lidz (1993) have reviewed methods of measuring violence in persons with mental disorders. Information about the occurrence of violent behavior usually has been retrieved from archival sources such as police records, treatment records, consumer interviews, and collateral interviews. Mulvey and Lidz (1993) state that estimates of violence from any single source may significantly underestimate the actual level of violence and that, like measures of substance use, violent behavior is best assessed by combining information from multiple sources.

Several measures have been developed to assess violence, and they can be divided into those quantifying the frequency of violence on ratio scales (e.g., number of episodes of various violent behaviors) and on interval rating scales (e.g., clinician ratings of violence). An example of the former is the MacArthur Community Violence Scale (MCVS), which is being used in the MacArthur Foundation Study on violence in persons with severe mental illness (Steadman et al., 1994). The MCVS is suitable to interviews with consumers, collateral informants, and clinicians and assesses the number of occurrences of nine types of violent behaviors in the past 3 months. The Overt Aggression Scale (OAS) is an example of an interval rating scale of violence severity (Yudofsky et al., 1986; Kay et al., 1988). The OAS assesses verbal aggression, physical aggression against other people, physical aggression against objects, and physical aggression against self. Each area is rated on a four-point severity scale anchored by specific behavioral descriptors. Scales such as the OAS have been questioned as to whether severity ratings reflect an underlying interval scale (Mulvey and Lidz, 1993).

Disruptive Behavior

We would argue that behaviors that affect public welfare go beyond behavior that threatens bodily integrity of self or others. Broader measures of disruptive behavior are widely used in treatment outcome research for children (see the Child Behavior Checklist) and the demented elderly (Beck, et al., 1997; Cohen-Mansfield, 1988; Mungas et al., 1989). Measures such as the Disruptive Behavior Checklist (Beck et al., in press) and the Cohen-Mansfield Agitation Inventory (Cohen-Mansfield, 1988) produce valid assessments of problem behavior using reports of collateral informants. In addition, several of the functioning measures that we have already reviewed include measures of subviolent, disruptive behavior, especially the Katz Adjustment Scale, which contains a set of "social obstreperousness" items (Katz and Lyerly, 1963).

Caregiver Burden

Along with increasing awareness of the effects of mental illness on informal caregivers such as spouses, families, and friends, came increased attention to the development of methodologies for measuring family burden. The support systems in which consumers are embedded can have dramatic effects on the course of treatment, and attention to their outcomes in cost–effectiveness research is sometimes of particular interest to investigators. A comprehensive and systematically derived measure of family burden was developed by Richard Tessler using a sample of 305 family members associated with 175 severely mentally ill individuals in Ohio (Tessler and Gamache, 1995). The measure focuses on three dimensions of caregiver burden: (1) burden resulting from assisting with activities of daily living; (2) burden resulting from supervision and control of problem behavior; and (3) burden resulting from worry about the ill family member's safety, mental health treatment, social life, and living arrangements. Summary scales measuring total respondents showed adequate internal consistency and stability over a one-year period. The burden of assistance scale showed an internal consistency rating ranging from .70 to .78 across three assessments. The burden of supervision and control scale showed internal consistency less than .70 and the burden of worry scale showed internal consistencies ranging from .77 to .85.

7.4 FUTURE DIRECTIONS IN OUTCOME MEASUREMENT

Defining and measuring what we mean by "effectiveness" is critical to understanding the quality of the mental health treatments that we implement and in understanding how changes to existing systems affect consumers. Concerns about rising costs will continue to affect what mental health treatments are delivered and how they are delivered. It is critical that changes are not attempted without empirically sound knowledge regarding their effects on consumers. Just as the ideal in the measurement of cost is the societal cost perspective, the ideal in the measurement of effectiveness is a broad perspective that encompasses an individual's symptoms, functioning, general health status, and quality of life as well as social concerns, such as the safety and general welfare of the community.

The effectiveness of mental health care should be understood in terms of its effects on individuals and the communities within which they reside.

Outcome measures that encompass all relevant outcome domains are nonexistent, and we are a long way from the development and acceptance of such a broad measure. As a result, effectiveness studies in mental health care have been difficult to compare because outcomes are defined and operationalized in diverse ways across studies. When findings converge, diversity of outcome measures may lend more confidence in findings that are established across a range of outcome measures. Variability in outcome measurement standards across studies causes more problems when findings do not replicate, and the field is left to wonder whether the failure to replicate is attributable to differences in the content of items or their sensitivity to change.

The measures discussed in this chapter have achieved at least a moderate degree of use in the field and appear to show at least adequate psychometric properties. In the absence of consensus, it is hoped that this chapter is a guide to the more widely used and accepted measures in the field and will guide current research efforts in the selection of field-tested measures. The measures discussed in this chapter also define a benchmark against which newly developed measures can be evaluated. Within some outcome domains, the development of new measures has proceeded without regard to their additive advantage over existing measures. Methodological development of outcome measures should work to understand the core constructs within each domain and to critically evaluate the best means of assessing those constructs. Ideally, methodological work will help identify a core set of instruments within each domain that will form the basis for a well-accepted standard of outcomes measurement. Such a standard will go a long way toward defining what we mean by "quality" mental health care.

Finally, methodological work should also be directed toward the development of measures for newly conceived outcome domains. As theories of mental illness and treatment effectiveness evolve, new constructs will be defined and need to be measured in standard outcome measurement protocols. Recent work on therapeutic alliance, consumer empowerment, perceived access to care, and consumer engagement suggests future directions for the development of new effectiveness measures.

7.5 CHAPTER REVIEW

Effectiveness research raises new challenges for outcome measurement, as investigators move beyond the short-term symptomatic outcome focus of much of efficacy research. Effectiveness studies also ask whether the intervention improves specific symptoms, as well as functioning, health status, and quality of life over the long term.

In effectiveness research one often studies rehabilitative, preventive, organizational, and financing innovations intended to serve broad, heterogeneous populations. Outcome measures may need to be available in multiple languages, and cover outcomes such as comorbid substance abuse, legal difficulties, and interpersonal conflict. In diagnostically heterogeneous samples, symptom measures emphasizing disorder-specific symptoms may be insensitive to changes in other diagnostic groups.

The focus of effectiveness research on the full range of typical care settings and communities can also pose problems for outcome assessment. If one is using a usual-care comparison condition in which subjects vary considerably in the amount of services they receive, the settings and sources of outcome assessment must be planned carefully so as not to introduce a bias. If, for example, case workers are a source of outcome ratings, and they see the experimental subjects frequently but the control subjects rarely, some outcomes may be more visible in the experimental group, thereby introducing bias.

Effectiveness research often is focused within diagnostic groups on the subset that has a severe and relapsing course, so that the relevant time span is not weeks or months but one to three years or longer. This not only increases the expense of assessments and the difficulty of obtaining adequate research funding, but increases the risk of the bias introduced by loss to follow-up, and increases the value of unobtrusive sources of outcome data, such as hospitalization, arrest, and mortality records.

These challenges call for careful planning of assessment methods. The first step is to identify the outcomes of greatest policy relevance and give them the most attention. One then needs to review published measures and contact investigators currently working in the same area, since improvements in measures are slow to reach publication. The third step, during the training of assessment staff, is pilot administration of the assessment protocol to a small sample of the relevant populations and settings of the planned study. Pilot assessments provide a check on interviewer training, provide data on interrater reliability, and assure that outcome assessments are integrated appropriately with assessments of utilization and cost. Needless to say, the final step is to embed the outcome measures in a strong research design.

Outcome measures can be organized into five domains ranging from the most specific to the most broad: (1) measures of disorder and symptoms, (2) measures of functioning, (3) measures of general health status, (4) measures of quality of life, and (5) measures of public safety and societal welfare. Not all of these domains are relevant for every study. Even if all domains are relevant, those considered to be the most important and policy-relevant effects of the intervention will be the ones measured most carefully.

Source of information, measurement interval, and measurement window are choices that must be made in relation to the emphasis of the particular study. One usually seeks information from more than one source (self, clinician, informant, research interviewer/rater) on several important outcomes, allowing evaluation of construct validity in a multitrait-multimethod matrix. Change is not measured directly, but computed from repeated assessments of the same outcome measures. The intervals between assessments need not be equal, and should match the expected pattern of change (rapid following an illness exacerbation or during intense intervention, and slow over a longer period of growth or relapse prevention). The measurement window (How much ____ have you felt during the past week?) is constant at all measurement occasions, but may vary by content, since some outcomes are inherently variable, requiring a short window for adequate recall (e.g., mood or substance abuse), while others are very salient events that occur rarely and can be recalled over a longer interval (e.g., divorce, hospitalization, or arrest).

Specific instruments were reviewed in each of the five outcome domains. In domains in which a few instruments are dominant, only these were reviewed, while in less developed areas, a broader and more complete review was presented.

1. **Disorder and symptoms.** Diagnostic instruments include the SCID, CIDI, and PRIME-MD for adults, and the DISC-R (or DISC-2), CAS, and CAPA for children. There is a wide range of symptom instruments, including the BPRS, SAPS/SANS, PANSS, SCL-90-R for general symptoms; the HamD, BDI, SDS, and CESD for depression; several substance abuse measures; and the Achenbach CBCL for children.

2. **Functioning.** Global rating of function includes the GAF and SOFAS for adults and two modifications for children of the GAF. Fifteen multidimensional functioning measures, all with at least adequate psychometric properties, were also discussed (Figure 7.1).

3. **Health status.** The SF-36 and the QWB dominate this domain and facilitate comparisons with the results of a broad range of health services research.

4. **Quality of life.** These instruments include measures of subjective quality of life as well as scales covering mental health status, functioning, and general health status, and thus for some purposes may encompass the previous three domains as well. The most prominent instruments are Lehman's QOLI and the Oregon QLQ by Bigelow and colleagues.

5. **Public safety and welfare.** Measures of violence include the MCVS and the OAS, and a number of broader measures of disruptive behavior in both adults and children were mentioned. A comprehensive measure of family burden has been developed by Tessler and colleagues.

8

AGGREGATING OUTCOME
MEASURES

The investigators in the Schizophrenia Research Group felt a great sense of accomplishment as they put the final touches on the data set from their two-year cost–outcome study of antipsychotic medication in combination with an innovative group therapy. When they met to plan their data analyses, the economist quickly outlined her plan for computing the total costs associated with study treatments. The psychologist who had developed the comprehensive battery of outcome measures presented summary statistics showing that the instruments used had performed quite well, appearing both reliable and sensitive to change over the course of the study. This was a very satisfying finding, given the broad range of outcomes: client, clinician, and family assessments of symptoms and social functioning; a standard measure of health-related quality of life; psychiatrist ratings of short-term and long-term medication side effects; and client ratings of treatment satisfaction. Team members were impressed and relieved to learn that they had meaningful measures of all the important treatment outcomes. Then the economist inquired, "How are we going to add those up to get a total outcome measure to go with total cost?" The psychologist replied, "You can't just add them up. They all use different scales." Other investigators asked, "Can't you just standardize them to a common scale and add them up?" "Can you analyze each outcome separately?" "Is there one measure that is complete and comprehensive?" "Can we just use the one outcome that's most important?" "What if all the outcomes aren't equally important?" "What if clients, clinicians, and family members disagree about how important the outcomes are?" Members of the group began to wonder if they had wasted time and effort measuring all those outcomes, and they agreed to discuss the problem at their next meeting.

Given the diverse array of mental health outcome measures described in Chapter 7, it is easy to see why many investigators face the challenge of aggregating multiple measures into a single, comprehensive outcome indicator. Mental health researchers and practitioners have devoted extensive effort to the development of valid and reliable measures of the many objective and subjective outcomes of mental health treatment, and most treatment researchers use a variety of measures to assess treatment impact. As the investigators in our case study realized however, the wealth of information these multiple measures offer is not easily reduced to the kind of comprehensive outcome indicator that is compatible with total cost. Some analysts avoid the problems of aggregating multiple outcomes by conducting a separate cost–outcome analysis for each outcome measure or outcome domain and by allowing each decision maker to weigh the evidence and decide which treatment is superior (Drummond et al., 1987). While it may be useful to provide decision makers with data at this level of detail, this approach yields rather incomplete results because it does not identify a single superior treatment. There is also potential for considerable confusion as different decision makers assign different values to outcomes and reach different conclusions about the overall results of a study (Read et al., 1987). Thus, some form of aggregation is necessary to meaningfully compare the costs and outcomes of alternative treatments. In this chapter, we present several approaches to aggregating outcomes and discuss two kinds of adjustments made to aggregate outcome indicators: converting outcomes to quality-adjusted life years to permit cross-study comparison, and discounting to account for time preference for outcomes.

8.1 APPROACHES TO OUTCOME AGGREGATION

We begin with brief discussions of approaches to aggregation that are generally not suitable in mental health cost–outcome studies—using a single outcome, using comprehensive health-related quality of life scales, averaging the scores obtained from multiple measures, and monetizing outcomes. The majority of the chapter is devoted to methods for obtaining numeric preference or utility weights that reflect the importance of different outcomes. These numeric values can then be used to compute preference-weighted aggregate outcome indicators for cost–utility analysis, as described in Chapter 3.

8.1.1 CHOOSING ONE OF MULTIPLE OUTCOMES

One way to avoid the complexities of aggregating multiple outcomes is to conduct a cost–outcome analysis using only a single important outcome. In some medical contexts, it makes sense to use simple outcome indicators, such as mortality. For example, it is reasonable to assume that the most important outcome of trauma surgery is whether the patient's life is saved. Even life-saving emergency treatments, however, have risks or side effects that would be of interest in comparing competing treatment alternatives. Mortality is rarely an appropriate outcome indicator in evaluations of mental health treatments, and it is usually not possible to identify one outcome that truly dominates all other outcomes. This is particularly true of treatments for chronic illnesses, such as the schizophrenia treatments mentioned in the case study, because side effects are more significant in ongoing, maintenance treatments than they are in brief treatments for acute disorders.

8.1.2 USING A COMPREHENSIVE HEALTH-RELATED QUALITY OF LIFE MEASURE

An alternative to choosing just one of several outcome measures is to use a single comprehensive measure. As discussed in Chapter 7, health-related quality of life (HRQL) instruments provide global measures of the impact of illness and its treatment by integrating multiple outcomes, including patients' perceptions and traditional clinical indicators of treatment effectiveness. Health-related quality of life is typically conceptualized as having four domains: physical and occupational functioning, psychological state, social interaction, and somatic sensation (Schipper et al., 1990). There are two broad categories of health-related quality of life measures. Generic measures assess general concepts that apply across all illnesses and health states. Specific measures assess particular diagnostic groups or patient populations. These measures are useful in cost–outcome analyses, but cannot typically replace all other outcome measures in comparative analyses of mental health treatments. Following is an overview of the characteristics, strengths, and limitations of generic and specific HRQL measures. All of these measures are described in greater detail elsewhere. (See Spilker, 1990, and Patrick and Erickson, 1993, for detailed reviews.)

Generic HRQL Measures

There are a number of generic HRQL instruments, such as the Quality of Well-Being Scale (QWB), described in Chapter 7, which are designed to provide summary assessments of the complex effects of illness on life quality across the full spectrum of health states and disease entities. Other popular instruments include the Sickness Impact Profile (Bergner et al., 1981), the SF-36 (Stewart et al., 1989), and the EuroQol (Williams, 1990). General measures have been proven valid and reliable in studies of mental illness (Dickey et al., 1996a; Wells et al., 1989).

These measures are appealing for cost–outcome analysis both for their comprehensiveness and their generalizability, which facilitate comparisons across a wide range of illness and interventions. Unfortunately, the very breadth of coverage that permits comparison across varied treatments and health conditions tends to limit their sensitivity to more subtle differences that distinguish competing treatments for the same disorder. For example, a generic HRQL measure would be better suited for comparing a treatment for schizophrenia to a treatment for asthma than for comparing two treatments for schizophrenia. As a result, global HRQL measures are usually most appropriate in epidemiological studies designed to characterize and compare population groups. Most cost–outcome studies require more specific measures tailored to examine the key features of interventions under study. For example, in a comparison of two medication treatments, a generic HRQL measure might not reveal important distinctions between disease symptoms and medication side effects. Because of this important limitation, it is rarely possible to use a generic HRQL measure as the sole outcome measure in cost–outcome studies comparing mental health interventions. A generic HRQL measure may be a valuable adjunct to other more specific measures, because it would permit comparisons to other studies of other types of interventions.

Specific HRQL Measures

Specific HRQL measures are used to assess specific diagnostic or patient groups. The Lehman Quality of Life Interview (QOLI; Lehman et al., 1983), described in Chapter 7, is designed to measure health-related quality of life in persons with severe and persistent mental illness. These specific measures focus on the signs and symptoms associated with a particular diagnostic group or type of treatment. Many specific measures, such as the QOLI, have proven to be valid and reliable. However, study-specific measures may be necessary to detect subtle differences between alternative treatments for the same disorder, although investigators may sacrifice validity and reliability when they develop a new measure for their study. One of the generally desirable features of HRQL measures also limits their use as the sole outcome measure in a cost–outcome study. The HRQL perspective puts patient perception center stage. Patient perceptions are essential to evaluation, but they may not be sufficient because patients may not be able to accurately distinguish between health changes that occur as a result of treatment and changes that are part of the natural disease course. As a result, more objective clinical measures are typically needed in treatment comparisons. Thus, quality of life becomes one of the multiple outcomes that investigators must combine into a single outcome indicator.

8.1.3 AVERAGING ACROSS OUTCOME MEASURES

An intuitive approach to combining outcome measures is to average or sum their scores. An initial obstacle to combining values obtained with multiple outcome measures is that different measures have different scales and metrics. For example, one instrument may have 10 items, all scored as either 0 or 1, producing a range of possible scores from 0 to 10. Another instrument may have 40 items, each rated on a 7-point scale, producing scores that range from 1 to 280. If the raw scores were combined, the second instrument, which can yield much higher scores, will have more effect on the combined score than the first instrument, which has a much smaller range of possible scores. The obvious way to solve this problem is to standardize the scores to a common metric, so that all measures have the same range. When all scores have the same range, each of the outcome domains contributes equally to the combined score, solving the problem encountered with the raw scores, in which the relative contribution of a particular outcome measure depends on the range of its scores. Treating all outcomes as equal, however, is not appropriate if the outcomes are not equally important. In our case study, for example, the different outcomes of schizophrenia treatment may be valued differently. Reducing psychotic symptoms may be more important than reducing medication side effects, but it may be less important than improving social functioning. Simple averaging across outcome measures cannot reflect these differences in the value of the multiple outcomes.

8.1.4 MONETIZING OUTCOMES

A common metric that reflects the relative value of the different outcomes would be an improvement over the simple averaging methods described in the last section. This is one of the strengths of cost–benefit analysis. As noted in the discussion of analytic approaches in Chapter 3, cost–benefit analysis converts all outcomes into monetary terms. Using dollar values provides a common metric that reflects the relative value of the outcomes and makes it very easy to sum across multiple outcomes to compute an aggregate outcome indicator. Unfortunately, it is very difficult to assign meaningful dollar values to most mental health outcomes, and resulting monetary valuations may not reflect the true societal value of different outcomes. Furthermore, dollar values may not reflect different valuations made by different stakeholder groups. In the context of schizophrenia treatment, for example, clinicians may think symptom reduction is more important than eliminating medication side effects, whereas patients may place a higher value on eliminating side effects. Thus, the ideal approach to outcome integration would reflect the relative importance of different outcomes and allow examination of differences in valuations across various stakeholder groups.

8.1.5 USING PREFERENCE AND UTILITY WEIGHTS

Aggregation methods that employ preference or utility weights allow us to compute summary outcome indicators that reflect the relative importance of different outcomes. These methods involve measuring individual preferences, utilities, or values for health states or health outcomes to obtain numeric importance weights for different outcomes. The resulting importance weights can then be multiplied by the scores obtained on different outcome measures and used to compute a single outcome indicator. These methods facilitate examination of trade-offs between outcomes, such as between symptoms and side effects, as well as comparison of the value of outcomes across different subgroups, including stakeholder groups such as patients, clinicians, and the general public.

Preference and utility measurement approaches are designed to order health states in terms of their desirability. The terms "preference" and "utility" are commonly used interchangeably, although there are technical distinctions between them. "Preferences" are associated with riskless decisions, or judgments made with certainty. "Utilities" are associated with risky decisions, or judgments made with uncertainty (Gold et al., 1996; Patrick and Erickson, 1993). Thus, a person asked simply to choose the more desirable of two hypothetical health states is expressing a preference. A person asked to choose between two health states, one of which occurs with probability of .3 and the other with probability of .7, is expressing a utility, because the probabilities reflect a specified level of risk. These distinctions are usually not as clear or important in practice as they are in theory. First, most people recognize that virtually nothing is certain; thus, they assume some level of risk even when the level is not clearly specified. Second, the artificial nature of most judgment tasks tends to alter individuals' attitudes toward risk and obscure subtle distinctions between risky and riskless choices (Von Winterfeldt and Edwards, 1986). Here, we use the terms "preference" and "utility" interchangeably, but emphasize the use of "preference," because it conveys a little more intuitive meaning to most people who are not experts in decision theory. The next sections describe applied methods for measuring preferences.

8.2 METHODS FOR MEASURING PREFERENCES

Medical decision analysts have developed strategies for measuring preferences and utilities for health outcomes by synthesizing methods from psychology, economics, business, and other disciplines (Froberg and Kane,1989a–d). Health-state preferences have been evaluated in a broad range of contexts. Group preferences have been determined to guide resource allocation and individual preferences determined to aid patients' actual treatment choices (Torrance, 1982). Preferences have been measured for the complete range of health states and for the limited outcomes of treatments for specific diseases (Patrick et al., 1989).

In this chapter, we focus on preference assessment methods that are most useful in cost–outcome studies. With these methods, individual respondents make ratings of specific health states. The next section describes approaches to developing and presenting descriptions of health states, and the subsequent section describes approaches to obtaining respondents' preference ratings of health states.

8.2.1 HEALTH STATE DESCRIPTIONS

Most preference assessment methods use narrative vignettes to elicit ratings. The vignettes describe a particular health state in terms of a fixed number of outcome domains chosen to match a study's research goals and outcome measures. The validity of preference ratings rests on the validity of the health-state vignettes (Smith and Dobson, 1993). Thus, investigators must develop their vignettes with great care so that all respondents can understand them. The next paragraphs describe various aspects of health-state vignettes and factors that guide decisions about health-state construction, including vignette content, presentation format, and analytic framework.

Content

Heath-state vignettes should include descriptions of outcomes relevant to the interventions being evaluated, and the range of outcome domains presented should be linked to study outcome measures. For example, vignettes developed for use in the project described in our case example would describe health states associated with schizophrenia in terms of the outcomes measured in the study, including symptoms, social functioning, and medication side effects. The levels of outcome described for each domain should be appropriate to the population under study. For example, investigators studying schizophrenia treatment would probably include a more restricted range of social functioning than investigators studying psychoanalytic treatment.

In selecting outcome domains for inclusion in health-state descriptions, it is important to acknowledge that human information processing capacities are limited. Evidence suggests that most people have difficulty considering more than seven domains simultaneously (Miller, 1956). Persons experiencing cognitive deficits as a result of mental illness may well have more limited capacities. Since many studies may assess more than seven different outcome domains, investigators may need to consider the study goals, as well as the quality of the data available, to select the outcome domains that are most important and most sensitive to change over the course of treatment.

There are some outcome domains that can typically be excluded from health-state descriptions. Subjective domains, such as treatment satisfaction and quality of life, are important indicators of treatment effectiveness, but may unduly influence ratings if they are included in vignettes. Measures of these outcomes imply a particular valuation of other outcomes. For example, if a vignette includes a statement that the hypothetical person in a health state is very happy or very unhappy, respondents are likely to base their preference ratings on the level of satisfaction built into the vignette rather than carefully evaluating all other aspects of the health state.

Duration and prognosis are also crucial elements of any health-state description (Torrance, 1982; Sackett and Torrance, 1978). Typically, descriptions of temporary conditions include durations based on clinical evidence, while chronic conditions are assumed to persist until death. These standards are difficult to apply to many mental illnesses, which may be chronic, but are characterized by episodes of relapse and recovery of unpredictable duration. Since it is unreasonable to assume that most health states associated with major mental disorders will remain unchanged until death, a shorter period, such as one year or five years, may be specified to reflect the persistent nature of the illness as well as the possibility for changes in disease course and outcome.

The descriptions of the outcome domains that comprise the health-state vignettes are usually based on clinical literature; they can also be derived from the outcome measures to which they are linked. Regardless of their basis, it is a challenge to develop health-state descriptions that convey the same meaning to all respondents. There is great potential for confusion because health-state descriptions are commonly designed to present a wide range of complex information about symptoms, side effects, and treatment outcomes in a condensed format.

Concerns about comprehension are heightened when health-state preferences are compared across multiple stakeholder groups, such as patients, patients' relatives, clinicians, or members of the general public. Clearly, these groups differ in their familiarity with the health states associated with any specific illness. Patients and, to a lesser extent, their relatives know an illness intimately through their own experience, but they may not know how others experience the same illness. Clinicians, through their education and experience, are likely to have a much more comprehensive and technical understanding of an illness, but they may lack the personal perspective of patients and family members. Members of the general public have a stake in public health policy, but they may be unfamiliar with a specific illness and the health states associated with it. It is easy to imagine that these varied perspectives would lead to varied interpretations of health-state descriptions. Comprehension problems may be particularly likely in studies of mental illness, in which ill persons may suffer from cognitive impairments that affect their participation in preference assessment tasks and their ability to accurately express preferences judgments. In addition, the subjective nature of many psychiatric symptoms may make them difficult to describe accurately to persons who have not experienced them.

Researchers developing health-state descriptions may want to conduct pilot studies to assess comprehension across stakeholder groups. A range of structured, systematic methods developed in survey research and related disciplines permits evaluation of respondent comprehension (Willis et al., 1991). These techniques range in complexity from asking respondents to paraphrase descriptions (Goodman and Greene, 1989) through asking a fixed set of open- and closed-ended questions (Groves et al., 1991) to complex interview techniques, which involve detailed, multifaceted probing of respondents' understanding of each element of a sentence or question and exploration of the process by which respondents arrive at their answers (Belson, 1985).

Presentation Format

Health-state vignettes are usually presented in one of two formats, a brief list format or a more complex paragraph format. Empirical comparisons of the two formats do not show either format to be universally superior. Some evidence indicates that complex narratives may be confusing or distracting compared to simple lists (Llewellyn-Thomas et al., 1984). Other evidence, however, suggests that the presentation of multiple domains in an explicit list format may encourage subjects to simplify the judgment task by averaging across domains, thus invalidating the preference assessment task by weighting the domains equally (Barron, 1979; Ebbesen and Konecni, 1980).

The individual, personal attributes associated with health states can affect ratings. Studies of health-state descriptions and other vignettes frequently demonstrate that the demographic characteristics of hypothetical persons (e.g., gender, age, and race) can bias ratings of vignettes (Ciampi et al., 1982; Alexander and Becker, 1978). Therefore, reliability and validity may be increased by excluding potentially biasing demographic information from health-state vignettes. Other evidence indicates that individuals' own perceptions and values strongly influence estimates of others' judgments, such as when physicians are asked to estimate patients' preferences (Danis et al., 1988). Thus, some respondents may ignore personal characteristics described in vignettes in favor of their own perspective. Since some respondents tend to impose their own perspective, reliability may be enhanced by encouraging all respondents to evaluate health states from their own perspective. This can be done by presenting descriptions in a first-person format, using "I," or a in second-person format, using "you," and asking respondents to imagine themselves in the health states described.

Some research suggests that the order in which domains are presented within descriptions and the order in which descriptions are presented can affect responses (Perrault, 1976). For example, persons who have difficulty evaluating multiple domains may focus just on those presented first (Krosnick and Alwin, 1987). To avoid order effects, the order in which the domains are presented in descriptions and the order in which descriptions are presented to subjects can be randomly varied.

Analytic Framework and Design

A study's design and data analysis plan are major considerations in the construction of health-state descriptions. The types of inferences investigators want to draw from preference ratings dictate the strategy for assembling descriptions of different outcomes into health-state vignettes. There are three common frameworks for vignette construction and presentation that meet different analytic goals. These three approaches—holistic, explicit decomposition, and statistically inferred decomposition—are described below.

Holistic Presentation

Holistic presentations are used when investigators wish to obtain preference ratings for specific health states. For example, in a short-term study of two competing drugs, researchers might wish to focus on a finite number of health states thought to differentiate the two drugs. In such a study, vignettes would be designed that described the multiple attributes of these specific health states. The resulting set of vignettes would not necessarily encompass the full range of health states associated with the illness under study and might present some outcome domains in greater detail than others. In a study comparing drugs that have similar efficacy in controlling symptoms, but have contrasting side effect profiles, different vignettes would portray a number of different types and levels of side effects, while portraying only a limited range of symptoms.

The holistic approach to vignette construction is extremely common. It yields a manageable number of vignettes by focusing on specific health states relevant to a particular study. This approach is limited, however, because it yields preference scores only for the health states described. It does not allow investigators to determine how individual outcome domains contribute to the preference ratings of a health state or to examine trade-offs and interactions among the outcome domains. This last limitation is particularly problematic in evaluating treatments for chronic mental illnesses because trade-offs between desirable effects and undesirable side effects are extremely important in long-term treatments.

Explicitly Decomposed Presentation

Explicitly decomposed presentations allow subjects to rate the multiple attributes, or outcome domains, of a health state one at a time. This approach simplifies the rating task, but typically requires respondents to make many more ratings than methods that present the multiple attributes in vignettes. While each judgment is simpler, subjects may become confused or fatigued when they have to make many different ratings. Explicitly decomposed presentations are also limited because they make the assumption that the multiple outcome domains are independent of one another. This assumption is probably inappropriate in most mental health contexts, in which preferences for one outcome are likely to depend on other outcomes. In our schizophrenia research example, preferences for medication side effects would likely vary with positive symptom level. Persons with high levels of psychotic symptoms might tolerate more side effects to alleviate the psychotic symptoms than would persons with lower levels of psychotic symptoms.

Statistically Inferred Decomposed Presentation

Statistically inferred decomposed presentations represent a powerful hybrid of the holistic and decomposed models. Subjects rate multiattribute descriptions like those used with holistic presentations, but the descriptions are constructed using a factorial framework that yields importance weights for each outcome domain and statistical tests of relationships between domains using standard analysis of variance and regression procedures (Anderson, 1981; Veit and Ware, 1982; Louviere, 1988). The levels of the various outcome domains relevant to a particular study are identified and a factorial design chosen to allow examination of the main effects of each outcome domain as well as interactive effects among the domains. A wide variety of factorial designs can be used to test different hypotheses and are described in research design books such as Cochran and Cox (1957).

Statistically inferred decomposition is particularly well suited to studies in which trade-offs between outcome domains are of central interest, and this approach has been recommended to remedy the deficiencies of the holistic and explicitly decomposed strategies (Barron, 1979; Froberg and Kane, 1989a; Veit and Ware, 1982). Despite its appeal, statistically inferred decomposition has been applied rarely in health-state preference assessment, primarily because a full factorial design incorporating multiple attributes at multiple levels requires an unwieldy number of descriptions. Fractional factorial designs, however, involve only a subset of theoretically relevant interactions, and reduce the number of descriptions required. Fractional factorial designs have been suggested by Barron (1979), demonstrated by Cadman and Goldsmith (1986), and examples suited to different hypotheses can be found in Dey (1985) and Montgomery (1976). These more focused designs allow investigators to use statistically inferred decomposition to obtain importance weights for individual outcome domains and statistical tests of the relationships between domains using a manageable number of health-state vignettes. Methods are being developed that use cluster analytic approaches to devise descriptions that reflect the range of health states occurring in real life (Sugar et al., 1996). These methods promise to improve both the accuracy and efficiency of measuring preferences for health states associated with a particular illness or treatment.

8.2.2 OBTAINING PREFERENCE RATINGS

The previous section describes a variety of approaches to presenting health states for preference assessment. This section describes an even wider variety of approaches for quantifying respondents' preferences for such health states. Some of these approaches arise from decision theory, others have roots in economics, while others are adapted from psychology and psychophysics. We first discuss the three most commonly used response modes, including standard gamble, time trade-off, and category rating, followed by less common modes, including paired comparison, magnitude estimation, and person trade-off. Any of these response modes can be used with any of the presentation formats previously mentioned. There is no empirical evidence suggesting that any one response mode is clearly superior to the others. There is evidence that most methods are generally comparable, yet the degree of comparability varies from study to study (Froberg and Kane, 1989b; Nord, 1992). As the following notes, however, some methods may be preferable in certain contexts.

Standard Gamble

The standard gamble approach is based on the axioms of classical decision theory (von Neumann and Morgenstern, 1944) and is frequently considered the "gold standard" for preference assessment. It applies to risky decisions, or choices made without certainty. Subjects are offered a choice between two alternatives: living in one health state with certainty, or taking a gamble on a treatment that leads to a specified health improvement with probability p, or death with probability $1-p$. The probabilities are varied until the subject is indifferent and does not prefer either alternative. Although theoretically appealing, the standard gamble technique is often difficult to implement because many people have difficulty thinking probabilistically (Kahneman and Tversky, 1982; Schoemaker, 1982). In addition, the emphasis on the risk of death may confuse subjects rating health conditions that are not typically life threatening.

Time Trade-Off

To remedy some of the problems encountered with the standard gamble, Torrance and colleagues (1976) developed the time trade-off approach. The time trade-off technique reframes the standard gamble probabilities in terms of time spent in different health states and does not directly incorporate risk. Subjects are asked to compare years in an optimal health state to spending the rest of their life in a specific health state. Using visual aids representing different time periods, subjects evaluate these periods sequentially until they come to a period of years in perfect health that is equivalent to spending the rest of their life in the ill state. This method is quite widely used, though it lacks the firm theoretical foundation of the standard gamble and may be confusing to subjects rating health states unlikely to persist for long periods of time.

Category Rating

Category rating procedures require respondents to rate the desirability of a health state using rating scales anchored by the best and worst possible states. It is often considered the most tractable preference assessment method because of its similarity to familiar questionnaire formats (Froberg and Kane, 1989b; Nord, 1992). Although it has been criticized for producing nonlinear scales because subjects allegedly attempt to use all scale categories equally, category rating has been shown to produce consistent, interval-scaled responses when endpoints are clearly anchored and respondents are reminded that intervals between scale points are equal (Kaplan et al., 1979; Kaplan and Ernst, 1983).

Paired Comparison

Paired comparison procedures, based on Thurstone's law of comparative judgment (1927), offer a simpler and potentially more realistic approach to quantifying preferences. Other common preference assessment methods ask subjects to explicitly express the strength of their preferences in numeric terms. Daily life rarely demands such definitive judgments; most decisions reflect only relative preferences, such as "I would rather eat an orange than an apple." Hadorn et al. (1992) recently demonstrated that the Thurstonian paired comparisons method may provide a more natural and intuitive approach to preference assessment. The main limitation of the paired comparison approach is that compared to other preference assessment methods, each paired comparison yields less information about preferences, but requires the respondent to process more information. As the number of outcome domains increases, the number of health-state pairs needed grows quite large. Thus, the reduction in cognitive burden attained by simplifying each rating may well be offset by the increase in the number of ratings each subject must make.

Magnitude Estimation

Magnitude estimation procedures are based on techniques used in psychophysical experiments measuring perceptions of the brightness of lights or the loudness of sounds. Subjects provide ratio judgments of the relative desirability or undesirability of two health states, as in "State A is 7 times as desirable as State B" (Kaplan et al., 1979; Patrick et al., 1973). These procedures are somewhat more intuitive than standard gamble procedures, but the mathematical operations required are still perplexing to some respondents. Some subjects also become confused because the response scale has no upper bound.

Person Trade-Off

Person trade-off, or equivalence, procedures ask respondents to decide how many persons in one health state are equivalent to a given number of persons in a second health state (Patrick et al., 1973; Nord et al., 1993). This task is technically quite similar to the time trade-off, but even the hypothetical trading of ill individuals may be disturbing to some respondents (Froberg and Kane, 1989b).

Administration Format

Regardless of which approach to preference assessment an investigator chooses, the mode of administration is an important consideration. Most health-status preference assessment is done in individual interviews with specially trained interviewers, who may use various visual aids in obtaining ratings. Although some investigators have used paper-and-pencil questionnaires (Nord, 1993), the complexity of the rating tasks makes individual interviews desirable because subjects can ask questions and interviewers can monitor comprehension throughout the rating process. The flexibility of the interview process has the potential, however, to induce interviewer bias if interviewers provide different information or assistance to subjects. Computer-based assessments are becoming increasingly popular, particularly as technology for multimedia presentations becomes more widely available. Computerized multimedia interviews can use audio and video to present more realistic, personalized, and detailed depictions of health states. This approach also standardizes interview procedures and is less dependent on literacy level than standard procedures. Early studies suggest that computerized, multimedia interviews can improve the quality of preference ratings (Goldstein et al., 1994; Lenert et al., 1995). It remains to be seen, however, whether all subject groups are capable of interacting successfully with computers.

8.2.3 CHOOSING PREFERENCE ASSESSMENT METHODS FOR MENTAL HEALTH RESEARCH

At present, there is little definitive data demonstrating that any one method is superior for measuring health-state preferences. There is some indication in the published literature that although the more economic and decision analytic methods, such as the standard gamble and the time trade-off, are often favored on theoretical grounds, their complexity may confuse respondents and produce less valid preferences ratings than more psychological methods, such as rating scales (Kaplan et al., 1993).

The relative paucity of studies of preferences for health states associated with mental illnesses makes it even more difficult to identify a superior strategy for mental health research. Most standard methods—category rating, paired comparison, and standard gamble—have been used with some success in early studies of preferences associated with major mental illnesses (Morss et al., 1994; Revicki et al., 1995; 1996; Chouinard et al., in press). Initial studies of the feasibility and comparability of these methods, however, suggest that they may be less feasible and/or comparable for measuring preferences for health states associated with schizophrenia than for other types of health states (Lenert et al., 1995; Shumway and Battle, 1995). Clearly, additional methodological work is needed to identify the most valid and reliable preference assessment methods.

8.3 QUALITY-ADJUSTED LIFE YEARS

A comprehensive outcome indicator calculated as a preference-weighted sum or average of the outcome measures used in a single study facilitates cost–outcome comparisons among treatments provided in that study and to other treatments assessed using the same outcome measures. In their original form, however, such indicators cannot be readily compared across different studies that assess different outcomes. The quality-adjusted life year (QALY) approach provides a standard metric for comparing the outcomes of treatments for similar disorders assessed with different instruments, as well as treatments for very different health problems (Gold et al., 1996). The generalizability that QALYs offer is extremely desirable for informing policy choices, but they have a number of limitations, some of which are particularly relevant to studies of mental health interventions.

The traditional QALY approach yields a single summary measure of treatment effectiveness that encompasses both quality and quantity of life. In its most basic form, a QALY is calculated by standardizing the preference-weighted outcome indicator for a particular health state to a 0-to-1 scale, where 0 is typically equivalent to immediate death and 1 is equivalent to a full lifetime of optimal health. This standardized value is then multiplied by the time spent in that health state to obtain the QALY value. This value can then be combined with cost to obtain the cost per QALY, which can be compared to values from diverse cost–outcome studies. Varied methods have been developed to calculate QALYs at the individual and aggregate level and to account for different health states experienced over the life course (Patrick and Erickson, 1993; Gold et al., 1996).

Despite the appeal of the QALY method, there has been considerable debate about its validity. A major concern is that QALYs may seem more generalizable and comparable than they actually are. Because different preference assessment methods often yield different preference ratings, these differences will be carried forward to the calculation of QALYs, and QALYs based on different preference assessment methods will not be truly comparable (Gafni and Birch, 1995). A second concern is that traditional QALY methods are appropriate only in the evaluation of chronic health states that remain unchanged and not in the evaluation of health states that change over the life course (Loomes and McKenzie, 1989). Gafni and colleagues (Mehrez and Gafni, 1991; Gafni et al., 1993) have developed an alternative method, the Healthy-Years Equivalent (HYE) to deal with this problem. Others, however, argue that the QALY and HYE approaches are not equivalent (Culyer and Wagstaff, 1993).

This latter concern about the variability of health status over the life course is particularly relevant to the study of mental illnesses, many of which are episodic. The HYE approach, which involves assessing preferences for varying health states of different durations across the life span, is a desirable solution. Assessing preferences for many different health states of varying durations is nevertheless difficult and time consuming. One alternative is to measure preferences for individual states as if they lasted a lifetime and compute a composite preference rating for the more realistic series of changing states (Gold et al., 1996). This may not be a valid approach if the individual states cannot reasonably be assumed to last a lifetime.

The standard QALY reference range, from immediate death to a lifetime of optimal health, may also pose a problem in studies of mental health interventions. While many mental disorders are associated with increased mortality, death is not commonly a direct treatment outcome. As a result, preference assessment in mental health studies may focus on a narrow range of health states that capture the anticipated outcomes of study treatments and do not necessarily include death or perfect health. Preference ratings obtained using a restricted range of health states cannot be used to compute standard QALYs comparable to those obtained in other studies. It is, however, possible to include specific health states that provide a link to the death-perfect health continuum while focusing assessment on a targeted range of health states.

In weighing the strengths and weaknesses of the QALY approach, it is difficult to see QALYs as the ideal metric for comparing competing mental health programs. Mapping preferences for health states associated with similar treatments onto the broad death to perfect health scale is likely to obscure the differences between them (Donaldson et al., 1988). In spite of the variability associated with different preference assessment methods, QALYs do provide a useful tool in making policy choices among different kinds of health interventions. They are not, however, sufficiently accurate to determine such choices.

8.4 DISCOUNTING OUTCOMES

Regardless of the aggregation method chosen, investigators must carefully consider the discounting of outcomes for time preference, just as they considered discounting of costs. The preference for dollars spent now over dollars spent in the future has long been explicitly acknowledged and reflected in cost–outcome analyses of health care programs, but some are reluctant to explicitly assume that society values lives saved or improved in the present over lives saved or improved in the future (Parsonage and Neuberger, 1992). Both empirical and theoretical evidence, however, demonstrates the need to discount outcomes as well as costs.

Recent surveys of individuals (Olsen, 1993b; Redelmeier et al., 1993; Cairns, 1994; Cropper et al., 1994) and analyses of labor market data (Moore and Viscusi, 1990) show that individuals do discount health outcomes and show strong preferences for health improvements in the near term over those occurring in the future. Keeler and Cretin (1983) showed mathematically that failing to discount outcomes at a rate at least equal to that used for costs leads to strange and uninterpretable results by making programs appear more desirable if their implementation is delayed. Olsen (1993a) states that this finding is consistent with a broad range of economic theories of discounting and argues that it is essential to discount outcomes at the same rate as costs.

Agreement on a common discount rate for costs and outcomes does not provide a final solution, but merely returns us to the discount rate controversies discussed in Chapter 5. If anything, the empirical literature on time preferences for health outcomes raises even more questions about appropriate discount rates. Empirical studies of individual time preferences reveal that individuals discount health outcomes at much higher rates than the investment linked rates recommended for costs. While discount rates typically used for costs range between 2 and 10%, studies that ask individuals to value specific health outcomes at different time intervals yield average discount rates of 16.8% (Cropper et al., 1994), 15% (Olsen, 1993b), and 25% (Cairns et al., 1994) for health outcomes delayed 5 years. In contrast to these studies of individuals, analysis of labor market data reflecting wage differentials paid for risky jobs, yields discount rates from 1 to 14%, which are similar to discount rates typically applied to costs (Moore and Viscusi, 1990). Both survey and database studies, however, suggest that individuals discount health outcomes and monetary gains at similar rates. The differences in rates may well be associated with the research methods used, since individuals asked to evaluate hypothetical health states are likely to express their own individual preferences whether the task is framed as an individual or societal choice. As a result, their responses are likely to reflect personal concerns about current health instead of societal concerns about the future health of others.

Results of several of these studies, however, are additionally troubling because they also indicate that individuals do not discount health outcomes consistently over time, nor do they value health outcomes equally for persons in different age groups (Olsen, 1993b; Redelmeier et al., 1993; Cropper et al., 1994). Even experts in the field have yet to reach consensus about how these findings should be applied in conducting cost–outcome analyses, offering the recommendation that investigators conduct sensitivity analyses comparing the impact of different discount rates (Olsen, 1993a; Krahn and Gafni, 1993).

8.5 CHAPTER REVIEW

The multiple measures investigators use to assess the many subjective and objective outcomes of mental health care make it difficult to obtain a single aggregate outcome indicator that is comparable to total cost. Simple indicators such as mortality or global health-status life measures rarely capture the detail required to meaningfully compare mental health interventions. Usually the best approach in cost–outcome studies is to use information about preferences for alternative outcomes and outcome trade-offs to weight the different outcomes. The weighted outcome measures can then be summed to obtain a single, comprehensive outcome indicator that reflects the relative importance of different outcomes.

A key step in measuring preferences is to construct health-state descriptions. Narrative health-state vignettes describe a particular health state in terms of a fixed number of outcome domains chosen to match a study's research goals and outcome measures. Vignette content should match specific outcome measures used in the study, such as symptoms, functioning, and medication side effects. The levels of symptoms in vignettes should reflect the actual range of outcomes observed. Typical human information processing capacity suggests that no more than seven outcome domains should be included. It may be wise to employ even fewer than seven outcome domains if subjects are suffering cognitive deficits as a result of mental illness. The time span for the duration of the health state should be included in the instructions; a period of 1 to 5 years may be appropriate for disorders that are relatively persistent but relapsing.

Health-state descriptions should be pilot-tested for clarity. Techniques range from asking respondents to paraphrase descriptions to more complex questioning and interview procedures to identify words that carry ambiguous meanings.

A variety of research suggests that perceptions of health-state descriptions can be biased in a variety of ways by presentation format. Presentation in a brief list or in a more complex paragraph format each has its difficulties and neither is clearly better in all situations. The order in which domains are presented in descriptions and the order in which descriptions are presented to respondents should be varied randomly.

Inferences the investigator wants to draw from preference ratings also may influence the combinations of outcome domains that are presented. The simplest is a holistic presentation of several vignettes covering the range of outcome configurations that are either theoretically important in relation to the treatments being compared or are derived from the set of outcomes actually observed in a study. A holistic presentation, however, does not allow the investigator to determine the relative importance of the outcome domains. Information about the relative importance of the outcome domains and interactions among different domains can be obtained by using factorial design frameworks.

A variety of methods are used to elicit preference ratings. The most common methods are the standard gamble, time trade-off, and category rating methods. Any rating technique can be used with any mode of presenting health-state descriptions. There is no empirical evidence of the superiority of any of the available rating methods. The three most common methods have all been used in some mental health studies. It is plausible to mix the methods to obtain both ease of use and theoretical relevance. Further methodological work is needed to identify the most valid and reliable preference assessment methods, and the most applicable methods for mental health services research.

The quality-adjusted life year (QALY) approach provides a standard metric for comparing the outcomes of treatments for similar disorders assessed with different instruments, as well as treatments for very different health problems. Calculating the cost per QALY for different treatments allows decision makers to compare their relative effectiveness. Despite the appeal of the standard QALY metric, concerns remain about the calculation and interpretation of QALY values.

Regardless of the aggregation method chosen, investigators should usually discount outcomes for time preference in the same way that they discount costs. The discount rate used for outcomes should be at least as high as that used for costs, though it is advisable to conduct sensitivity analyses to determine the effects of different discount rates.

9

ANALYZING COST-EFFECTIVENESS

Capitation, a fixed prepayment to a provider for each member in a program, is being used as a new financing method for containing health care costs. One issue regarding capitation is its effect on the outcome of health care services. One state has carried out a capitation experiment in which severely mentally ill clients were randomized to capitated funding or usual care services in selected communities. After a three-year study, the director of the Department of Mental Health was very pleased to announce the findings to a mental health services advocacy committee. The study had found that participants in the experimental group were employed more often and increased their earnings as compared to clients in the control group. This was welcome news to the advocacy committee, and it recommended that the state implement the capitation program in every county.

A mental health services researcher was asked by a state senate committee to review the recommendation. The researcher pointed out that while the outcomes for the group under capitation were favorable, the cost per client under capitation was about $10,000 higher than in usual care. Furthermore, the direct comparison of outcomes between clients in experimental group versus clients in control group might have been influenced by a nonrandom attrition rate, such that clients remaining in the experimental group could be a biased subgroup that was more satisfied with the outcome of their services. These issues raised a question as to whether capitation was unequivocally better than usual care. Therefore, this researcher suggested the legislature look more deeply at the findings of the capitation study before concluding that capitation should be implemented in all counties.

9.1 MAKING COST–EFFECTIVENESS
COMPARISONS: BASIC CONCEPTS

In traditional cost–benefit analysis, in which both benefits and costs are measured in monetary terms, the two most common comparison criteria are the benefit–cost ratio and net benefit (benefits minus cost). As long as we can measure both costs and benefits in monetary terms, the cost–benefit comparison is straightforward. Most mental health outcomes, however, are measured in non-monetary terms, such as level of functioning, quality of life, life satisfaction, and social interaction. Cost–effectiveness analysis is more appropriate with these numerical but nonmonetary outcome measures. In such cases, a cost–effectiveness ratio can be calculated for program comparison, but it is not possible to calculate net benefit. Although it may be possible and desirable to construct utility indices from various effectiveness measurements so that cost–utility analysis may be used, the statistical analysis issues are similar. Since most studies in mental health services research examine cost–effectiveness, for simplicity we will use the term cost–effectiveness analysis in this chapter.

In this chapter we also assume the reader is familiar with multiple regression analysis and its variations: logit, probit, and tobit analysis, all of which are extensively used in economics. For readers who have a more limited knowledge of statistics or would appreciate a refresher, the following five paragraphs review briefly the statistical concepts used in this chapter. Readers should refer to these paragraphs when the subsequent equations seem unfamiliar. In spite of the difficulty of plunging into unfamiliar mathematical territory, we encourage the reader to gain an understanding of the motivation and concept of each data analysis approach described. The chapter is not intended to enable readers to undertake these analyses without consultation.

Multiple regression analysis is a method for constructing a weighted sum of several variables (the "independent variables") in order to estimate another variable (the "dependent variable"). Regression analyses are presented in this chapter as regression equations of the form

$$C = b_0 + b_1 T + b_2 x + u \tag{1}$$

where C is the dependent variable (such as treatment cost per client), T is the treatment "dummy variable" (a dummy variable is a way to code category membership using the values 1 or 0, such as experimental group = 1, comparison group = 0), x is another variable (e.g., a baseline client sociodemographic characteristic), and u is the error term. In multiple regression analysis, the data from a set of subjects would contain measures of C, T, and x. The primary interest is in the "regression coefficients," the terms b_0, b_1, and b_2 (there may be more) that are estimated from the C, T, and x variables by the regression analysis computations. Regression analysis programs also perform statistical tests to determine whether the population value of each regression coefficient can be concluded to be different from 0, and estimate a standard error for each coefficient, to enable the user to construct a confidence interval estimate of the population value of the coefficient. In Equation (1) it can be seen that if the regression coefficient b_1 is 0, the estimate of C is the same no matter what the value of the variable T (treatment assignment). Thus if b_1 is not statistically different from 0, one has no evidence that treatment assignment is associated with cost. If the data are from a randomized trial, then there is no evidence that treatment has a causal effect on cost.

In Equation (1), b_0 is the "intercept." The reason for this is also clear from the equation, since b_0 is the estimated value of C (except for the random error u) whenever the independent variables (in this case T and x) are all 0. Thus if T is a dummy variable and x is a standard score representing some quantitative variable, b_0 is the mean cost in the control group (when T = 0) for subjects with mean values of x (when x = 0). The coefficient b_1 shows the average difference in C between the treatment and the control group, when other variables (x, in this case) are held constant. Similarly, the coefficient b_2 shows how much the estimate of C is increased with one additional unit of x, if treatment is held constant.

A moment's thought will make it obvious that the scale of measurement of the variables will affect the size of the coefficients. Regression analysis computer programs usually produce two sets of coefficients, one for the raw scores as they were entered, the other for standardized scores. In this chapter we always discuss coefficients of raw scores, since this allows us to interpret the coefficients in terms of the scale of measurement of the dependent variable, as in the previous paragraph. However, when independent variables are not dummy variables (like T), but are quantitative measures (like x), we will often assume that they have been converted to standard scores prior to analysis, so that their mean is always 0. In interpreting the meaning of regression coefficients in practice, the investigator needs to pay attention to the scale of measurement of each variable and whether the output coefficients are raw score coefficients or standardized coefficients.

Regression equations are very flexible. Suppose one were estimating total cost, C, as a function of treatment assignment (T), severity of illness (a quantitative variable, higher score means more severe illness), and site (Chicago = 1, San Francisco = 0). One might also want to estimate the size of the interaction between severity of illness and treatment—the degree to which the difference in cost between the experimental treatment and the comparison treatment depends on the patient's baseline severity of illness. A sequence of two regression models would be required:

$$C = b_0 + b_1 T + b_2 \text{site} + b_3 (\text{severity of illness}) + u \qquad (2)$$

$$C = b_0 + b_1 T + b_2 \text{site} + b_3 \text{severity} + b_4 T \cdot \text{severity} + u \qquad (3)$$

where in Equation (2), b_0 and b_1 have the same meaning as before, b_2 indicates how much higher costs are in Chicago relative to San Francisco, and b_3 shows how much higher costs are for each unit of severity. Equation (3) is identical except for an additional term. Coefficient b_4 in Equation (3) shows how much the effect of treatment varies depending on the patient's severity of illness (or, equivalently, how much the effect of severity varies depending on the treatment to which the patient was assigned). Notice that the test of the interaction is accomplished by including a term that is the product of the treatment assignment dummy variable and the severity score. A side effect of adding the interaction term is to render coefficients b_0 through b_3 in Equation (3) uninterpretable under certain conditions, so interactions are evaluated using a sequence of regression models like these, which are often called "hierarchical" models. Equation (2) provides the correct values of the coefficients b_0 to b_3, while Equation (3) provides the correct value of coefficient b_4.

What we have been discussing so far is "ordinary least squares" (OLS) regression. OLS regression works well when the dependent variable (C in this case) is a continuous variable with a normal distribution. Sometimes an investigator wishes to analyze a dichotomous dependent variable (one that takes only two values), as when examining whether baseline variables predict that certain kinds of patients will drop out of the study (i.e., dropout, yes or no, is the dependent variable). With dichotomous dependent variables, the estimates of the regression coefficients can be inaccurate under certain conditions, and usually either logit or probit analysis is used. The reader may be familiar with the term logistic regression, which is another name for logit analysis, the most commonly used of the two methods. Both logit and probit analyses use a transformation of the dichotomous dependent variable to make it mathematically more tractable, and also use a different mathematical approach for estimating the regression coefficients, a maximum-likelihood procedure instead of a least squares procedure. These modifications in the analysis produce accurate regression coefficients, which can be interpreted in the same way, except for their scaling. Finally, neither OLS regression nor logit or probit analysis works properly when the dependent variable has many 0 values and many discrete non-0 scale values. Tobit analysis, also computed with a maximum-likelihood method, is used when one wishes to predict the value of such a variable from a set of other variables. An example of the use of tobit analysis is mentioned later in the chapter.

9.1.1 THE COST–EFFECTIVENESS RATIO

If statistical analyses of cost and outcome data yield significant differences that allow the investigator to conclude that the cost of an innovative treatment is less than usual care but the outcome of the innovation is better than usual care, one can immediately conclude that the innovative treatment is preferable. In decision analysis one would say that the innovation is the "dominant choice" (i.e., that it is unambiguously better than any other choice being considered). Similarly, usual care is the dominant choice when it is cheaper but more effective. Such findings provide the strongest type of evidence that one intervention is more cost-effective than another. If, on the other hand, the investigator concludes that both the cost and the outcome of two interventions are equivalent (see "equivalence testing" in Chapter 2), then either is acceptable. If only cost is equivalent, then the more effective intervention is preferable, and if only outcome is equivalent, then the cheaper intervention is preferable. Only when the evidence shows that one of the two interventions is both more costly and more effective is there no unambiguous conclusion. In this case one must judge whether the additional cost is worth the greater effectiveness. To aid in this judgment, the investigator usually estimates the population value of what is called an incremental cost–effectiveness ratio:

$$R = \frac{C_T - C_C}{E_T - E_C} \tag{4}$$

where C_T is the cost in the population of the experimental intervention, C_C is the cost of the control or comparison intervention, E_T is the effectiveness of the experimental intervention, and E_C is the effectiveness of the control intervention. This ratio is positive when one of the two interventions both costs more and produces a superior outcome. The ratio is negative in one of two circumstances, both of which, as we previously noted, have obvious policy implications: (1) cost savings, when the innovative intervention costs less but has superior outcomes, and (2) a bad investment, when the innovation costs more but produces worse outcomes. The ratio is not informative when either the numerator or the denominator is 0, although policy implications are still clear in these circumstances. In any circumstance, policy interpretation of an incremental cost–effectiveness ratio depends on the validity of the evidence about the population value, and this evidence is never perfect.

An investigator estimates an incremental cost–effectiveness ratio by measuring the difference in average cost between two interventions, by measuring the difference in average outcome between two interventions, and by computing a sample cost–effectiveness ratio with the estimated incremental cost in the numerator and the estimated incremental effectiveness in the denominator.

As an example, consider an intensive community treatment program that is associated with a $5000 average cost per participant in their first year, and in which the average program participant shows an improvement from 35 to 45 on the Global Assessment Scale in their first year. In comparison, comparable people receiving usual care incur costs of only $2000 in their first year and show an average improvement from 35 to 37. We compute the cost–effectiveness ratio as the difference in cost over the difference in outcome:

$$\frac{C_T - C_C}{E_T - E_C} = \frac{\$5000 - \$2000}{10 - 2} = \frac{\$3000}{8} = \$375 \tag{5}$$

This observed cost–effectiveness ratio estimates the increased average cost necessary to gain an average of 1 point of improvement per year, as rated by the

Global Assessment Scale. Equivalently, one could estimate that the innovative program produced an average gain of 8 points improvement over usual care, at an added cost of $3000.

The effectiveness–cost ratio is an alternative to using the cost–effectiveness ratio. This subtle change implies the increment in effectiveness produced per dollar. One advantage of using the effectiveness–cost ratio is that it is commonly reported in cost–outcome research and therefore makes it easier to compare findings across studies.

In the previous example, in which an additional 8 points of improvement measured with the Global Assessment Scale was attained by a program that incurred an additional $3000 in cost, one could divide 8 by $3000 to obtain the outcome gain of .00267 per additional dollar. One could report this by saying that each $1000 invested seems to produce an outcome gain of 2.67 GAS points on average. Whichever ratio is used, it is sensible to report the result in terms that are similar to the actual range of cost and outcome differences observed, since an investigator is usually on shaky ground to extrapolate much outside the ranges observed.

As we discussed in Chapter 8, abstract outcome scales can be hard for a policy maker to interpret, and preference-weighted outcome scores or utilities can sometimes improve the meaningfulness of outcome measures. Furthermore, no practical study can directly measure the value of the intervention over participants' subsequent lifetime. Modeling techniques described in Chapter 10 can show the policy maker what the lifetime cost-effectiveness of an intervention would be under various assumptions about the long-term trajectory of costs and effectiveness.

Raw-score outcomes are most meaningful when they inherently summarize the important effects. For example, in a cost–effectiveness study of drug regimens in the treatment of duodenal ulcers carried out in Finland by Sintoen and Alander (1990), effectiveness was measured in expected number of healthy days gained, and costs were expressed as total treatment costs. The experimental drug omeprazole produced a cost–effectiveness ratio of 6.5, and an effectiveness–cost ratio of 0.155. A ratio of 6.5 implies that the expected cost to produce one more healthy day is 6.5 Finnish marks, or for a cost of 100 Finnish marks, one can expect 15.5 more healthy days by choosing omeprazole treatment. One can imagine vocational rehabilitation cost–outcome findings reported as cost per work days gained, or suicide–prevention findings reported as cost per life saved.

The foregoing examples of cost–effectiveness comparisons are typically designed to assist policy makers or program managers in deciding whether to allocate additional resources to providing additional units of the innovative service. The findings do not directly apply to this question, because they are based on the particular levels of funding and volume in the programs studied. Therefore they suggest what would be the cost–outcome result were new programs of the size studied initiated as a substitute for usual care for the type of clients studied. In situations in which it is feasible to add the innovative procedure to usual care without creating entire new organizations (e.g., using a new drug in place of an old one), it would be ideal to determine the additional, or "marginal," cost a program must incur to achieve additional (marginal) units of effectiveness. To accomplish this one must be able to estimate marginal cost and marginal effectiveness, so as to compute a marginal cost–effectiveness ratio. Marginal cost means an additional cost incurred to the program as a result of providing an additional unit of service or serving one additional client. Marginal effectiveness means additional effectiveness units realized as a result of providing each additional unit of service or serving each additional client. In some cases (e.g., substituting a new drug for an old one) the additional cost (e.g., higher price of the drug, initial cost of training physicians in use of the new drug) may reasonably be assumed to have a linear relation to the additional effect. That is, treating 10 more patients or 100 more patients with a new drug is likely to yield the same increased effectiveness per patient treated. In other cases, in which using the innovative intervention with additional patients means forming new organizational units, the policy generalization is more complex, since start-up costs and the availability of appropriately trained clinicians may make it easy to get the observed cost-effectiveness with a small increase in patients served but harder when the increased number of patients to be served is very large.

An example of marginal cost is provided by a cost–effectiveness analysis of hepatitis B vaccine in predialysis patients (Oddone et al., 1993a). In a 2×2 design, marginal cost–effectiveness ratios were estimated under two scenarios: (1) predialysis vaccine versus no vaccine and (2) vaccine during dialysis versus no vaccine. The results (Table 9.1) indicate that if patients are vaccinated prior to dialysis, the additional costs of preventing hepatitis B infection is about $31,000 per infection avoided (marginal cost divided by marginal effectiveness). This means that $31,000 additional dollars would be spent on vaccinating patients for every case of hepatitis B infection prevented. The cost of vaccinating a patient during dialysis is lower, so even though each vaccination is slightly less likely to prevent a new infection, the cost per infection prevented is only about $25,000 when vaccination is performed during dialysis. Each of these can be interpreted as a marginal cost per infection prevented so long as there is no reason to expect that under either scenario the preventive effect of an additional person vaccinated would differ depending on how many are vaccinated. The policy choice between

TABLE 9.1   Marginal Cost–Effectiveness Ratios Comparing Vaccination Strategies

Strategies	Marginal cost to vaccinate one person	Marginal effect from vaccinating one person (N of cases prevented)	Marginal cost / marginal effect (cost per case prevented)
Predialysis vaccine versus no vaccine	$140	0.0045	$31,111
Dialysis vaccine versus no vaccine	$81	0.0032	$25,313

Source: Oddone et al. (1993a).

the two scenarios (predialysis versus dialysis vaccination) involves a further value trade-off between total vaccination expenditure and prevention efficiency on the one hand (which favors dialysis vaccination) and a distributional effect (i.e., that fewer total people would suffer infection under the predialysis method).

There are several reasons why researchers have avoided using marginal cost and marginal effectiveness. One is that marginal costs are difficult to estimate from routine accounting data, since one needs data on the cost of a program at various levels of volume of service, together with a statistical cost model to estimate marginal costs. The magnitude of marginal costs is often influenced by program size. Therefore observed variation in marginal cost may not generalize to programs of different size. For simplicity, researchers assume that when a program is operating at a constant cost, the cost of each additional unit produced is the same, so that marginal cost is equal to average cost. While this is a practical compromise in the design of research, it does leave an additional logical gap between study findings and policy application, a gap that is often overlooked.

Finally the reader should keep in mind that all references to effectiveness assume that improvements seen are the result of consumption of the intervention and not the natural course of recovery. Also implied is that no improvement means no benefit from the intervention, rather than the benefit of preventing expected deterioration or relapse. Usually, either random assignment to interventions or other suitable comparison conditions are necessary to make such interpretations. It is arithmetically simple, however, to compute a cost–effectiveness ratio for a program any time one has an estimate of the average cost per client and the average client outcome. Such a ratio has virtually no meaning, since there is no way to conclude that each increment in cost is producing an increment in outcome. An expensive program can be totally ineffective with a group of clients, and they may improve anyway due to maturation or other factors. In spite of this logical problem, it is not hard to find published nonexperimental comparisons of cost–effectiveness ratios between two different interventions, when in fact there is no basis for their meaningful interpretation. Two interventions that are compared in a randomized cost–outcome experiment may not have meaningful cost–effectiveness ratios when considered as individual programs, but when comparability of clients is assured by randomization (in large samples before attrition, not necessarily in every study), and other explanations for differential outcomes are examined and can reasonably be ruled out, then *differences* in cost and *differences* in outcome between programs can be interpreted as causally related.

9.1.2 DISCOUNTING COST–EFFECTIVENESS RATIOS

The concept of discounting costs was discussed in Chapter 5, and discounting effectiveness was discussed in Chapter 8. It is understood that costs should be discounted if measured for more than one year. The question is whether effectiveness should also be discounted before the estimation of a cost–effectiveness ratio. If one follows the same logic of time consideration used for discounting costs, one could argue that consumers would have similar time preference for better program outcomes. That is, participants place a higher value on getting treated and getting better sooner. If a program takes a relatively long time to achieve effectiveness, its effectiveness is less desirable than if it achieved effectiveness quickly. Therefore, one should calculate the present value of effectiveness using the same discounting procedure employed for costs, using the discount rate as an adjusted weight, such that:

$$PV_E = \sum_{t=1}^{n} \frac{E_t}{(1+i)^{t-1}} \qquad (6)$$

where PV_E is the present value of effectiveness, t is the year, E is the effectiveness measurement, i is the discount rate, and n is the number of years for which effectiveness data are available. While the authors recommend that investigators discount effectiveness when studying outcomes beyond one year, this issue continues to be debated in the literature (Viscusi, 1995).

A Swedish cost–effectiveness study of group living versus home living for dementia care (Wimo et al., 1995) illustrates the effects of discounting effectiveness. The eight-year cost of care, without discounting, was $172,852 (U.S. dollars) for group living and $215,022 for home living. At the same time, effectiveness was measured in quality-adjusted life years (QALYs) using the Index of Well-Being. The average QALY gained was 3.267 for group living and 2.985 for home living. With a 10% discount rate over the eight-year study period, the cost for group living was $144,760 and $176,278 for home living. The discounted QALY for group living was 2.76 versus 2.54 for home living. In other words, the cost per QALY gained before discounting was $52,908 for group living and $72,034 for home living. With a 10% discount, the cost per QALY gained was $52,449 for group living and $69,400 for home living. This example shows that without discounting, the difference between two care programs was $19,126, whereas after the discounting the difference was $16,951. While the conclusion is the same, the difference becomes smaller, because the time course of costs and well-being were different in the two conditions.

9.1.3 COMPARING MULTIPLE EFFECTIVENESS MEASUREMENTS TO A SINGLE COST ESTIMATE

As discussed in Chapter 8, mental health treatments have multiple outcomes, such as change in symptoms, social functioning, and life satisfaction, and may have an impact on the utilization of services. In cost–effectiveness comparisons, a common approach is to compare each individual outcome or effectiveness measure to one estimate of total cost. This approach assumes that each of these alternative outcomes can be produced with an incremental increase of $1.

For example, consider a community case management program with three outcome measures. For the average client, psychosocial functioning improved 5%, role functioning improved 8%, and life satisfaction improved 10%. Inpatient costs were reduced by $8000 at an average per client case management cost of $2000. In this case, there are four possible comparisons:

$$\frac{\$2000}{5\% \, ps \, adjustment}, \frac{\$2000}{8\% \, role \, function}, \frac{\$2000}{10\% \, satisfaction}, or \frac{\$2000}{\$8000}.$$

These ratios imply that a 1% improvement in psychosocial adjustment would cost $400, a 1% improvement in role functioning would cost $250, a 1% improvement in life satisfaction would cost $200, and it would take a $1 investment in case management to generate a $4 savings in inpatient costs. While these multiple cost–effectiveness ratios are useful in evaluating the different aspects of programs, two essential pieces of information are missing. First, these comparisons do not reflect the relative importance of the multiple outcomes. It leaves policy makers and program managers to weigh these outcomes. There is no global measurement of program effectiveness, which makes it difficult to make interprogram comparisons. That is why some researchers are engaging in cost–utility comparisons so that a preference-based summary score can be used for effectiveness–cost comparison, as discussed in Chapter 8.

The second problem with multiple cost–effectiveness comparisons with one single cost estimate is that information is lost regarding the relative efficiency of using a certain amount of resources to achieve a given outcome. It is just like a fixed cost for a five-course dinner. Although one enjoyed the main course and the dessert, it would be difficult to know how much cost is needed to produce a good main course or a dessert. To begin thinking about this issue it is often useful to work with program clinical staff to understand the processes of providing treatment services, and whether some services are seen as specific to certain outcomes. While this may not enable the investigator to break down costs and outcomes into different meaningful cost–effectiveness ratios in the current study, it can identify hypotheses about how to differentiate services for particular clients so as to improve cost-effectiveness for clients with particular problems or goals. It will usually require subsequent experiments with more specific client selection, intervention packages, and control conditions to evaluate these cost–outcome hypotheses. Even better, it would be valuable to develop these hypotheses in advance of an initial experiment, in order to accomplish these research objectives more efficiently, as described in Chapter 6.

9.2 PROCEDURES FOR COMPUTING COST–EFFECTIVENESS RATIOS

9.2.1 ADJUSTING FOR DIFFERENCES IN CLIENT CHARACTERISTICS IN COST ANALYSIS

The goal of cost analyses is to compute the average cost per client in experimental and comparison programs so that costs can be compared with effectiveness measures. This direct cost comparison is appropriate if client characteristics such as severity of illness, age, gender, and ethnicity are similar in the two programs. There is no guarantee, however, that client characteristics will be similar across groups even when clients are randomly assigned. The possibility of chance group differences in client characteristics as well as a group difference in attrition or dropout during treatment may introduce spurious sources of variation in costs. Even when study groups are equivalent, within-group cost variance may be associated with client variables. If a client variable explains more than 25% of within-group cost variance, covarying that client characteristics will usually reduce the error term enough to increase the statistical power of the test of the treatment group effect.

In order to compare costs in two different programs, it is best to form a regression model in which the total cost incurred by each client is a dependent variable, and the independent variables include not only the dummy variable indicating treatment group assignment but also client characteristics such as severity of illness, age, and gender. In a simple two-group comparison, in which the experimental treatment is coded 1 and the control treatment is coded 0, the coefficient of the treatment dummy variable is the cost difference between the average experimental client and the average control client, holding other characteristics constant. This approach is appropriate for estimating an adjusted cost difference between two programs.

The investigator uses the cost regression equation to estimate the adjusted cost of each program, holding other variables constant. For instance:

$$C = b_0 + b_1T + b_2x + u \qquad (7)$$

where C is the treatment cost per client, T is the dummy variable (experimental group $= 1$, comparison group $= 0$), x is another baseline client sociodemographic variable expressed as a standard score, and u is the error term. The coefficient b_1 is the cost difference between the treatment group and the control group ($C_T - C_C$), after taking into account the x variable, or covariate. When the covariate x is at its mean ($x = 0$), the estimated adjusted cost for the average experimental client is $b_0 + b_1$, while the adjusted cost for a comparison client is b_0.

An example of an estimated cost function for a case management program as compared to a usual care program might be as follows:

$$C = 645 + 67T - 12AGE \qquad (8)$$

where C is the individual total treatment cost, $T = 1$ for experimental clients and 0 for control clients, and AGE is a standardized score representing age at baseline. The equation indicates that the average cost of the case management program is $67 more than the usual care program, controlling for baseline age. Thus $C_T - C_C = \$67$, adjusting for age. The average adjusted cost of the case management program for a person at the mean age at baseline is $712 ($645 + $67), while the adjusted cost for such a person in the control program is $645. Younger clients in both groups cost more, and a client who is one standard deviation below the mean age at baseline (score of -1.0) costs $12 more on average. Since the equation contains no interaction term, it assumes that the relative cost of case management compared to control is not affected by the client's age.

9.2.2 ADJUSTING FOR DIFFERENCES IN CLIENT CHARACTERISTICS IN EFFECTIVENESS ANALYSIS

Treatment outcomes, like costs, are often influenced by factors such as client severity of illness, age, and gender. A regression model can be formulated to estimate the effects of the difference in treatments while examining such covariates. An appropriate measure of effectiveness is change in outcome status (e.g., role functioning, social adjustment, life satisfaction) between the baseline and follow-up measurements, which is represented here by the symbol ΔE. In practice, more than two measurement occasions are common, as are variations in the actual timing of measurement from subject to subject and unavoidable missing data for some of the measurement occasions. More advanced hierarchical models or random regression approaches may be superior in these situations (Laird and Ware, 1982; Gibbons et al., 1989; 1993; Gibbons and Hedeker, 1994). In this case E might represent a change slope or growth curve coefficient.

The explanatory variables in the regression model include the treatment variable and other variables depicting differences in client characteristics. The coefficient of the treatment variable is an estimate of the net effect of treatment on the outcome variable. It reflects not only the direction of the effect but also its magnitude. We can also compute a confidence interval on the estimate and test its statistical significance. The relative effectiveness of the treatment program, the coefficient of the treatment variable, is an adjusted effectiveness estimate, adjusted for the covariates.

The effectiveness regression model can be estimated as follows:

$$\Delta E = a_0 + a_1 T + a_2 x + u \tag{9}$$

where ΔE is the change in the effectiveness measure between baseline and follow-up measurements and u is the error term. The coefficient a_1 is the difference between the treatment group and the control group in change in effectiveness ($\Delta E_T - \Delta E_C$), while the constant a_0 is the average change in effectiveness for the control group (ΔE_C), after taking the other explanatory variables into account.

$$\Delta E = 20 + 2.20T + 1.4SEV \tag{10}$$

In Equation (10) the coefficient 2.20 might indicate the average difference in improvement of life satisfaction between the experimental group and the control group, controlling for baseline severity (SEV). Thus, the average improvement for a client of average baseline severity in the experimental group is 22.20 (20 + 2.20), and the average improvement for a similar client in the control group is 20. Clients with greater baseline severity show greater improvement. If the treatment groups differ on baseline severity, the adjusted coefficient of T will be different from the raw average difference in improvement in the two treatment groups. If the experimental group had more clients with high baseline severity, the mathematics of the regression analysis will lower the coefficient of T compared to the raw difference in mean change scores between groups.

The interaction with treatment assignment of a covariate like baseline severity may also reveal important facts about how the two treatments are working. This applies to both cost and effectiveness equations. In the above effectiveness example, adding a term for the interaction of baseline severity with treatment assignment might reveal a statistically significant effect. To understand this effect, it is helpful to draw a graph of the relationship of baseline severity to estimated change. Compute points on the graph using the coefficients from the equation that includes the interaction. Set T to one and estimate improvement with high baseline severity and low baseline severity (e.g., standard scores of 2.0 and −2.0), and plot that line for the experimental group. Repeat the process with T set to 0 and plot that line for the control group. This might reveal, for example, that clients with high baseline severity show more improvement in the experimental treatment than in the control condition, but clients with low baseline severity do not. This would suggest that applying the experimental treatment to clients with high baseline severity would maximize the effectiveness of the experimental treatment compared to control. A similar analysis of the cost equation would reveal how such a treatment assignment policy could be expected to affect costs.

9.2.3 USING REGRESSION COEFFICIENTS TO COMPUTE COST–EFFECTIVENESS RATIOS

The use of average incremental cost and average incremental effectiveness to construct cost–effectiveness ratios assumes that participants in both experimental and control groups have similar sociodemographic characteristics and other attributes. As we discussed earlier, it is likely that individuals will vary within and across groups. Therefore, it is often best to calculate cost–effectiveness ratios using treatment–effect regression coefficients, one obtained from a regression equation for cost and the other obtained from a regression equation for effectiveness. Both regression equations should include the same subject characteristics as independent variables. In such equations, the treatment regression coefficient then reflects the net effect of the experimental treatment on cost and effectiveness, holding other factors constant.

Assuming that both cost and effectiveness are significantly related to treatment, the investigator uses b_1 from Equation (7), the cost equation, and a_1 from Equation (9), the effectiveness equation, to form a cost–effectiveness ratio comparing two programs:

$$\frac{b_1}{a_1} = \frac{C_T - C_C}{\Delta E_T - \Delta E_C} \qquad (11)$$

Continuing the examples in previous sections, \$67 ($C_T - C_C$) is the average per-patient additional cost for the experimental group, and 2.20 ($\Delta E_T - E_C$) is the increased improvement in average life-satisfaction score for the experimental group. Thus,

$$\frac{C_T - C_C}{\Delta E_T - \Delta E_C} = \frac{67}{2.20} = 30.45 \qquad (12)$$

which implies that on average assignment to the experimental program consumes \$30.45 per patient more than the control program in order to attain each point of superior improvement in life-satisfaction score.

9.2.4   ESTIMATING INDIVIDUAL COST–EFFECTIVENESS RATIOS

Siegel, Laska, and Meisner (1996) discuss an approach in which an effectiveness–cost ratio is formed for each individual, and these ratios are used as the dependent variable in a regression model:

$$\frac{E}{C} = b_0 + b_1T + b_2x + u \qquad (13)$$

where E, C, T, and x have the same meaning as in earlier equations. Equation (13) is a simplified version of the Siegel model. The coefficient b_1 reflects the amount of difference in the effectiveness–cost ratio between the experimental group and the control group. For instance, if b_1 is equal to 0.50, then the average E/C ratio for experimental clients is 0.50 higher than the average E/C ratio for control clients. In other words, for every dollar in cost, there will be a half unit increase in effectiveness. The coefficients for the sociodemographic variables (x) provide additional information about how these factors influence the variation in effectiveness–cost ratios. If one is interested in examining whether the relative effect of two treatments depends on some other factor x, such as gender, ethnicity, or baseline severity of illness, an interaction term such as the product of T and x can be introduced into the equation.

9.3   STATISTICAL INFERENCE IN COST–EFFECTIVENESS COMPARISON

9.3.1   IDENTIFYING DOMINANT AND ADMISSIBLE ALTERNATIVES

We noted that if an investigator can conclude that an intervention was less costly and more effective than other alternatives, one would usually say that this intervention "dominated" the alternatives. Siegel et al. (1996) suggest a complementary concept, the "admissible" intervention, an intervention that can be considered because no other intervention had been shown to be both less costly and more effective (i.e., it is not dominated by any other intervention). This initial step in interpreting findings (ruling out inadmissible or dominated alternatives) has been elaborated and formalized with an explicit statistical testing procedure by Siegel et al. (1996, p. 399), to which the reader is referred.

9.3.2 JOINT TESTS OF SIGNIFICANCE ON COST AND EFFECTIVENESS

Individually testing the significance of a treatment comparison effect on cost and on effectiveness has been a common approach in cost–effectiveness studies, even though the study conclusion depends on the conclusion about both effects. One can test the joint effect of an intervention difference on cost and effectiveness using multivariate analysis of variance (MANOVA), using both cost and effectiveness as dependent variables, yielding a single test of significance. Most MANOVA programs output the traditional individual regression results as well. Note that if the MANOVA finds the population means of cost and effectiveness are different for two interventions, it does not provide any information about the size of the incremental cost–effectiveness ratio, or indeed even whether it is positive or negative. To understand the probable size of the cost–effectiveness ratio the investigator will go on to construct a confidence interval estimate.

9.3.3 CONSTRUCTING CONFIDENCE INTERVALS

No matter how cost–effectiveness ratios are estimated, the values estimated are point estimates subject to error, and it is desirable to portray the precision of the estimate by constructing a confidence interval. This is not possible in economic modeling studies in which one starts with aggregate mean values for cost and effectiveness. Economists have tended to use sensitivity analysis, based on upper and lower values of plausible but arguable assumptions in their proposed model, as a heuristic substitute for confidence intervals. Even as recently as 1994, O'Brien and colleagues (1994) felt it necessary to argue for collection of individual subject data on both cost and outcome so that the variance of cost, effectiveness, and its ratio could be estimated.

Among cost–outcome statistics, the net benefit (when both cost and outcome are measured in the same units, such as dollars) allows the simplest method for estimating its 95% confidence interval. If net benefit = NB is the sample mean of patient-level net benefit, then the confidence interval for net benefit is given by

$$\text{NB} \pm \frac{t_{N-1}s(\text{NB})}{\sqrt{N}} \tag{14}$$

where N is the number of subjects, t_{N-1} is the 97.5th percentile of a T distribution with N-1 degrees of freedom, and s(NB) is the sample standard deviation of NB. As with all confidence intervals, if the 95% confidence interval does not include 0, this is equivalent to finding that the statistic is significantly different from 0 at the 5% level.

Estimating confidence intervals for cost–effectiveness ratios is more complex, because normal distribution theory fails. The theoretical distribution of the ratio of two normally distributed random variables has undefined variance. Alternative approaches to constructing confidence intervals are coming into common use, but this area of statistical estimation continues to develop and in this chapter we do not provide specific estimation procedures. The reader is encouraged to review the citations below and possibly seek consultation from a biostatistician.

Two approaches to constructing confidence intervals are in use (Drummond et al., 1997). The first uses approximate methods for estimating the variance of the cost–effectiveness ratio, an approach taken by O'Brien et al. (1994) and refined by Siegel et al. (1996), Willan and O'Brien (1996), and Chaudhary and Stearns (1996). The second approach uses bootstrap resampling methods (Efron and Tibshirani, 1993; Pollack et al., 1994). The advantage of bootstrap approaches is that there is no issue of whether the sample statistic conforms to a particular theoretical sampling distribution. The bootstrap process forms an empirical probability distribution similar to the one observed in the sample. Bootstrapping can be used with any test statistic. While it requires programming and computing effort, it is practical on current desktop microcomputers.

Chaudhary and Stearns (1996) compare five methods applied to an incremental cost–effectiveness ratio in a data sample with a highly skewed distribution. Only three of the five methods they tested produced reasonable results, but those three were reasonably comparable. All of the acceptable methods were methods that produce asymmetrical confidence intervals in the presence of skewed distributions. One was a method similar to the ones suggested by Siegel et al. (1996) and Willan and O'Brien (1996). The other two were percentile-based bootstrap methods. Subsequent investigation of these methods under various conditions will reveal whether one is uniformly preferable.

9.3.4 STATISTICAL ADJUSTMENT DUE TO BIAS IN SELF-SELECTION AND ATTRITION

Attrition and selection bias also pose threats to the analysis of treatment costs and outcomes. The concern is that characteristics of the treatment or the comparison group are associated with the receipt of the treatment and its outcome. Attrition and selection biases pose special threats to the analysis of treatment effects because they often result from factors that are difficult to anticipate prior to treatment implementation or result from unknown and unobserved factors that operate during that selection of subjects or during implementation of treatment.

The statistical method for detecting and adjusting for treatment biases due to observed or unobserved factors that bias subject selection and attrition is called the "instrumental variable" technique, a way to reduce bias in estimates of treatment effects (Hu, 1982; Pindyck and Rubinfeld, 1993). The instrumental variable technique is widely used in economics.

The instrumental variable technique is based on the fact that selection factors and attrition can be thought of as a problem in the *measurement* of who has and has not received treatment (Maddala and Lee, 1976). In this approach, error in the dummy-coded treatment variable (T) occurs when an individual does not receive treatment because of selection or attrition. If no systematic selection or attrition factor were operating, then a completely representative sample of persons for whom the treatment is intended would be coded "1 = Received treatment" and an equally representative sample coded "0 = Did not receive treatment." If a systematic selection factor is operating, then the dummy coding of T is in error to the extent that a nonrepresentative sample of subjects is coded as 1 or 0.

If we specify the outcome equation as we did in Equation (8), and there is measurement error in the treatment variable (T), the error term u will be correlated with T, which will lead to a biased estimate of the coefficients. To adjust for the selection bias or attrition bias, the proper procedure is first to regress T as a function of variables that influence selection, such as age, gender, or prior health status, but are not correlated with u. Because these variables can be assumed not to be correlated with u, the value of T predicted from these variables also will not be correlated with u; thus, the estimated coefficient will not be biased. An estimated value of T, $\hat{T}$ (pronounced "T hat"), is therefore constructed using a logit or probit regression model of the following form:

$$T = b_0 + b_1 \text{age} + b_2 \text{severity} + \ldots + u \qquad (15)$$

While each subject's value of T is used in this logistic regression, one also obtains the estimated values of T, or $\hat{T}$, from the output for use in the second step in the analysis.

The second step is to express ΔE as a function of $\hat{T}$ instead of T:

$$\Delta E = a_0 + a_1 \hat{T} + a_2 x + u \qquad (16)$$

The resulting coefficient a_1 for $\hat{T}$ will be an unbiased estimate of the effect of the treatment on ΔE.

Heckman (1979) developed an alternative technique, assuming that important variables that explain the selection of subjects or attrition from the study may not have been measured and cannot be used in analyses about treatment participation directly. It may not be clear, for example, why some subjects choose to drop out of the study and others choose to complete the study. Thus, the outcome equation may have omitted some important variable. The statistical presentation of this extension, which involves the "inverse Mills ratio," is beyond the scope of this book, but interested readers may consult Heckman (1979) or

Mullahy and Manning (1994). Foster and McLanahan (1996) illustrate the use of instrumental variables in a study predicting school dropout.

9.4 ADDITIONAL ISSUES IN COST–EFFECTIVENESS ANALYSIS

9.4.1 ANALYSIS OF COST-EFFECTIVENESS IN MULTIPLE SITES

Many clinical trials of mental health services are implemented in more than one site. Multiple-site trials are attractive because they can improve the ability to generalize findings across diverse treatment settings. Multiple-site trials also provide larger sample sizes to improve the power of inferences. In cost–effectiveness analysis, questions arise about whether to combine data on costs and effectiveness measures from all sites or to analyze data from each site separately. The answer depends on the comparability of the sites. Whenever possible, it is better to combine data from all sites to estimate overall cost-effectiveness. To do this, one needs to adjust across sites for possible differences in cost-of-living, such as between urban and rural, or between East Coast, Midwest, and West Coast. The Department of Labor, Bureau of Labor Statistics, publishes cost-of-living statistics regularly for major cities in the United States. There is no need to adjust effectiveness measures that are not measured in monetary terms. Possible site-related effects on program implementation and efficiency can be examined by introducing dummy variables identifying the different sites. By using these site dummy variables, one can explore possible variations in costs and effectiveness, in addition to calculating the overall cost–effectiveness ratio.

If sites have distinctly different philosophies and program implementation styles, it may not be very meaningful to combine data across sites to estimate a single cost–effectiveness ratio. An experiment on treating severely mentally ill patients in two counties—one in urban Long Beach, California, and one in rural Stanislaus County in Central California—illustrates this concern (Chandler et al., 1996; 1997). The Long Beach site emphasized work rehabilitation much more than the Stanislaus site, and so it was more appropriate to conduct separate analyses for each site.

9.4.2 ANALYSIS OF COST-EFFECTIVENESS IN MULTIPLE PERIODS

Many mental health treatments last more than one year, and it may be appropriate to evaluate the costs and outcomes over a two- or three-year period. For two- or three-year follow-up studies, costs and outcomes are typically measured at four to six evenly spaced time intervals. Thus, it is essential to estimate cost-effectiveness with repeated measures. Several alternative approaches are available. One is to use a simple time-trend regression model to estimate growth rate as a summary of the multiple measures for each individual subject. One then uses the individual growth rate as the dependent variable in a regression model that includes a treatment dummy variable and other sociodemographic variables. This method is recommended by Rogosa and Willett (1985) and has been applied in a pilot study of the cost-effectiveness of case management programs (Jerrell and Hu, 1989). While a linear growth rate measure is a convenient approach to summarizing multiple measures over time, it sacrifices detailed information about the patterns of change over time, such as how long it took the treatment to become effective and the durability of effectiveness over time.

Another simple analytical model can be used with repeated measurements. A series of regressions can be estimated using the change scores between each follow-up assessment and the baseline as the dependent variables (Jerrell et al., 1994). The coefficients for the treatment dummy variable in each regression equation can be used to interpret the magnitude and statistical significance of the effectiveness of the treatment program in each period. It is possible that the coefficient is not significant in the initial period, becomes significant two or more periods later, and is not statistically significant in the final period, suggesting that the treatment effect is delayed and diminished over time, or that the experimental treatment produces early benefits but that subjects in the control condition eventually catch up.

Another approach is to pool all the effectiveness measures and estimate a pooled time-series and cross-section regression model. In this pooled model, dummy variables for time and a term representing the interaction between treatment group and time are included as explanatory variables, along with other sociodemographic variables (Hu and Jerrell, 1993). To obtain appropriate tests of significance, this model is structured as a repeated-measures analysis of variance. This kind of model is not appropriate when there is autocorrelation among the repeated observations or other violations of the assumed "sphericity" or "compound symmetry" characteristics of the covariance matrix over time, when multivariate analysis of variance (MANOVA) is required. These methods do not handle missing data, or efficiently model commonly seen autocorrelational patterns in repeated measures. For this purpose random-effects models are more appropriate (Laird and Ware, 1982; Gibbons et al., 1989; 1993). Random effects methods accommodate error due to time series, error due to cross-section, and random error. The estimation method first finds the variance and covariance of the time series, cross-section and random error, and then forms a covariance matrix to be used as additional input in the regression model to account for these variations in the repeated observations. These calculations can be accomplished in SAS PROC MIXED or using the MIXREG and MIXOR programs developed by Hedeker (1993a, b).

9.4.3 DISTRIBUTIONAL IMPACT
OF COST-EFFECTIVENESS

The purpose of studying the cost-effectiveness of a treatment program is not only to determine a program's overall effectiveness and cost, but also to determine who received more benefit and who received less benefit. It is very important to learn which groups benefit more from a program so that future implementation of the program can be improved or more specifically targeted to client groups. To study distributional impact in a cost–effectiveness comparison, one can conduct various subsample analyses, such as comparing males to females, various ethnic groups, low functioning subjects to high functioning subjects, or severely ill clients to less severely ill clients. Once separate costs and outcomes are estimated from each subsample, the same methodology for cost–effectiveness comparison can be used for each subpopulation. In order to have statistically reliable inferences, it is necessary to have a sufficient sample size for each subpopulation. In many studies, subgroups of interest are too small to yield meaningful results. An alternative approach to subsample analysis is to use interaction terms (i.e., treatment dummy variable multiplied by a given sociodemographic characteristic) as an additional variable in the regression equation, so that the limitations of small subsample size are partly overcome by using the entire study sample to estimate the error variance.

In a randomized clinical trial comparing three different drug regimens for asthma patients (Molken et al., 1994), the authors used a regression model to examine the impact of different patient attributes (e.g., smoking, hypertension) on longitudinal cost data by using product terms representing the interaction of treatment and smoking and the interaction of treatment and hypertension. In the entire group of subjects, treatment A led to lower costs than either treatments B or C. For smokers, however, treatment A led to higher costs than did the other treatments. Without examining the interaction of smoking and treatment, this important finding would have gone undetected.

Similarly, in mental health treatment research, it is possible for a treatment program to be more effective for males than for females, or more effective for severely mentally ill patients than for less severely ill patients. Effects of a novel intervention on cost may vary greatly with the subject's recent history of service utilization. These potentially important questions require some kind of subsample or interaction analysis.

9.4.4 SENSITIVITY ANALYSIS
IN COST–EFFECTIVENESS COMPARISON

In performing cost–effectiveness analysis, investigators must make a number of assumptions, beginning with principles of cost estimation (e.g., depreciation, discounting, value of time) and principles of outcome measurement (e.g., quality of life, discounting outcome, life satisfaction). It is important to know whether a change in these assumptions alters the results so much that they lead to different conclusions. To determine this, investigators carry out sensitivity analyses to determine how robust findings are to changes in the underlying assumptions and uncertainties in estimation procedures. The original analysis is often called the "base case" and the sensitivity analyses produce alternative cases to be compared to the base case.

The most common form of sensitivity analysis involves repeating an analysis using different values of a key variable selected from the plausible range of that variable. For instance, a well-known cost–benefit analysis in mental health services was carried out by Weisbrod (1983; Weisbrod et al., 1980) of the training in community living model developed by Stein and Test (1980). The cost per patient in the experimental program was $8093, while the cost per patient in the control group was $7296. Thus, on average, the experimental group cost $797 more per patient. The effectiveness of the program was measured in terms of employment earnings (benefits per patient), which amounted to $2364 for the experimental program versus $1168 for the control program. The patients in the experimental program had earned $1196 more than those in the control program. Thus, the experimental program showed a $399 greater net benefit than the control group. The study also used nonmonetary measures of effectiveness, including symptomatology, social relationships, and satisfaction with life. Researchers found that these effectiveness measures favored the experimental group over the control group.

One of the key cost elements in this analysis was the capital cost of treatment facilities. When capital costs were estimated as 8% of capital there was a $399 cost savings associated with the experimental treatment. McGuire (1991) used this example, however, to show that if the investigator had assumed a 4% cost of capital, the training in community living costs would be $1268 higher than the control program. Furthermore, if one did not consider capital cost at all, the experimental program would become more costly by $542. Thus, the choice of assumptions affects the conclusions. The key to sensitivity analysis is to define what is a reasonable range for a key variable and to examine cost-effectiveness at different values across this range.

Sensitivity analysis can be carried out by multiple methods. For example, an investigator may assume a discount rate of 3% but then explore the impact of using 0% or 10% discount rates. By applying these different rates, one may find whether the results are sensitive to changes in discount rate. One could also examine the estimate of the cost of home care services, ranging from $6 per hour to $10 per hour. Briggs, Schulpher, and Buxton (1994) review alternative approaches to sensitivity analysis in cost–effectiveness evaluation. It is always useful to provide alternative scenarios so that policy makers and program managers can appreciate the limitations of cost–effectiveness findings. While sensitivity analysis is no substitute for statistically derived confidence intervals on intervention effects, sensitivity analysis is helpful whenever the investigator makes parametric assumptions that cannot be empirically verified.

9.5 CHAPTER REVIEW

The purpose of estimating cost-effectiveness is to obtain information to guide future program planning and resource allocation so that resources can be used in the most beneficial way. In cost–effectiveness comparisons, one can calculate cost–effectiveness ratios or effectiveness–cost ratios. There may be multiple ratios to consider when a treatment program produces multiple outcomes. Cost–effectiveness ratios can be calculated using average value or marginal values. They can be calculated from group means, from coefficients from regression equations that adjust for relevant subject characteristics, or calculated for each subject. A variety of regression methods have been used in health services research in recent years. Regression models can yield more meaningful cost–effectiveness ratios for complete study samples and in specific subgroups. It is important to remember that these ratios are only point estimates, and it is useful to evaluate them in the context of variance estimates or confidence intervals to get a clearer picture of results.

In spite of the importance of cost–effectiveness comparisons, relatively few studies in mental health services research have provided actual cost–effectiveness ratios. This may be due to the fact that mental health outcome measures are frequently more complex and subjective than outcomes measured in medical care. For instance, the number of healthy days or quality-adjusted life years may be seen as more concrete measures than the percentage improvement in psychosocial functioning. Furthermore, in many cost–effectiveness studies for the severely mentally ill, psychosocial functioning has not differed significantly between the experimental and control groups (Hu and Hausman, 1994). It is not particularly meaningful to estimate cost–effectiveness ratios when there is little variation in effectiveness. Nonsignificant findings may be partly due to problems with program implementation, small sample size, a lack of sensitivity of measurement instruments, or the true equivalence of different treatments. Mental health services researchers need to find ways to better solve these problems in cost–effectiveness analysis.

Numerous assumptions are made in the process of estimating cost–effectiveness ratios. It is important to keep these assumptions in mind when interpreting cost–effectiveness ratios. Sensitivity analyses will show whether changing the assumptions changes the conclusions of a cost–effectiveness comparison.

The finding that cost or effectiveness does not differ between two interventions is often an important finding from a policy perspective. Because the failure to find evidence of difference is not the same as finding evidence of equivalence, such findings should be carefully examined, using confidence intervals in order to put an upper and lower bound on the estimated difference between two intervention strategies.

Given the complexity of estimating cost–effectiveness ratios, the degree of uncertainty in drawing inferences from estimated cost–effectiveness ratios, and the fact that many studies cannot provide conclusive findings, why is there still increasing demand to carry out cost–effectiveness analysis? The answer lies in the fact that it is a rational approach that leads researchers and policy makers through the logic of decision-making about allocating resources among competing alternatives, given budget constraints.

10

USING COST–OUTCOME DATA
TO GUIDE POLICY AND
PRACTICE

Research on assertive community treatment (ACT) for persons with severe mental illness (Test, 1992) is the strongest and most coherent body of cost–effectiveness investigation in mental health. ACT services are designed for people with serious mental disorders with psychotic components, including schizophrenia, bipolar disorder, and major depression with psychotic features, who are also frequent users of hospitals and emergency services and are unable to function well in the community between crises. As late as 1990, ACT was the only full-service intervention for this group that had been tested in multiple randomized clinical trials. From 1965 to 1980 a group of innovative clinicians experimented with new ways to help such persons minimize hospital time and maximize living and working in the community. In a series of seminal papers, the group described the evolution of the ACT clinical model and reported two experiments testing preliminary forms of the model (Marx et al., 1973; Stein et al., 1975; Test and Stein, 1976; 1978; 1980; Stein and Test, 1978; 1979; 1980; 1982; 1985; Test, 1979; 1992; Knoedler, 1979; 1989; Weisbrod et al., 1980; Weisbrod, 1981; 1983; Estroff, 1981; Diamond, 1979; 1984; Stein and Diamond, 1985).

The second of these two experiments, published in 1980, was a well-designed cost–benefit study (Test and Stein, 1980; Stein and Test, 1980; Weisbrod et al., 1980; 1981; Weisbrod, 1983). In this study the experimental treatment was applied for 14 months with a 14-month follow-up period during which all subjects received usual care. Subjects in the experimental program had less time in the hospital, more time in independent living situations, better employment records, increased life satisfaction, decreased symptoms, and improved treatment adherence. Family and community burden did not appear to increase. Societal cost was found to be slightly lower in the experimental treatment when wages earned were considered monetary benefits and income support was considered a cost.

These positive results were tempered by other findings. After the innovative treatment was withdrawn, outcomes in the experimental group gradually decayed to the level of those in usual care, indicating that the new treatment might need to be continued indefinitely. Furthermore, for a subgroup with personality disorders, the experimental treatment was much more expensive than usual care, suggesting that the intervention was most cost-effective for those with schizophrenia or severely disabling affective disorder. Finally, while costs were slightly lower in the experimental treatment, in the financing environment of the time (in Madison, Wisconsin) the experimental treatment was likely to distribute the payer burden differently, shifting the burden away from the state and onto the local tax base (Stein and Test, 1980; Test and Stein, 1980; Weisbrod et al., 1980; Weisbrod, 1983; Frank, 1993).

These findings stimulated great research interest in the U.S. and other English-speaking countries. By 1996 reports on more than a dozen further experiments had appeared (Mulder, 1985; Hoult, 1986; Hoult et al., 1981; 1983; 1984; Jerrell and Hu, 1989; Hu and Jerrell, 1991; Bond et al., 1988; 1990; 1991a; Test, 1992; Muijen et al., 1992; Morse et al., 1992; McFarlane et al., 1992; Merson et al., 1992; Lehman et al., 1993; Marks et al., 1994; Audini et al., 1996; Rosenheck et al., 1995a; Essock and Kontos, 1995; Chandler et al., 1996a, b; 1997; in press). These studies focused on persons with schizophrenia and affective disorders who were at high risk for repeated hospitalization. Some studied special subgroups, such as the homeless. In all studies, the model tested was one of indefinitely continued support in the community, though few studies followed participants for more than 2 years of treatment. A notable exception was a 12-year study by Test (Test et al., 1985). At least 11 ACT studies were published from 1986 to 1995 (Hargreaves and Shumway, 1989; Olfson, 1990; Chamberlain and Rapp, 1991; Rubin, 1992; Solomon, 1992; Test, 1992; McGrew et al., 1994; Bond et al., 1995; Burns and Santos, 1995; Santos et al., 1995; Scott and Dixon, 1995), and in 1995 numerous other studies were in progress (Randolph, 1992; Burns and Santos, 1995). The studies in progress utilize stronger usual care conditions, reflecting the widespread adoption of linkage case management in the U.S.

Across the nation, adoption of ACT has been slow, and a meta-analysis of nine studies suggests that as programs depart from the full ACT model they lose cost-effectiveness (Bond et al., 1995; Essock and Kontos, 1995). A 1992 survey of state mental health directors identified about 350 ACT programs in the U.S., of which only one third were estimated by the survey group to be sufficiently faithful replications of the ACT model to be cost-effective (Deci et al., 1995). The location of ACT programs was uneven. Wisconsin and Michigan accounted for 44% of the identified programs. Forty states had fewer than ten reported programs, including the two largest states—California with three and New York with none.

Has research on the effectiveness and cost of assertive community treatment had an appropriate impact on policy? Advocates claim the research evidence for the cost-effectiveness of ACT is the strongest we have on any method of service organization for the severely mentally ill, which is certainly correct. They also assert that the findings clearly support a policy of widespread adoption. This latter conclusion is somewhat less obvious. Burns and Santos (1995) noted that recent ACT research had provided "further evidence of the positive effects of [ACT] in reducing hospital use and increasing patient and family satisfaction; by testing [ACT] in a wider range of populations . . . ; and by studying the integration of . . . family psychoeducation" (p. 674). They noted the limited effects found on client-level outcomes, and suggested that "the brief duration of most studies, enriched control interventions, and problems in . . . establishing the [ACT] condition, retaining subjects, and measuring outcomes" may account for these findings (p. 674). They suggested future studies use "longer duration, better monitoring of implementation, and increased targeting of interventions [toward] substance abuse . . . and employment" (p. 674). They noted that research thus far has not informed the issue of the role of ACT in systems of care: whether to reserve it for highly noncompliant patients, use it for all the severely mentally ill, or reserve it for special subgroups; whether and when to transfer clients to a lower level of community care; whether ACT adapted for rural areas can be cost-effective; and how its key elements can be maintained while streamlining its cost. They note that many of these issues may be examined without expensive new studies by using meta-analytic techniques.

This extended case example, a brief history of ACT research, illustrates difficulties that can arise when mental health decision makers try to use cost–effectiveness data to guide policy and practice. In this particular case, the question of whether ACT research has had an appropriate impact on policy is too simplistic. The research clearly had an impact on initial adoption of the ACT model. Further research and more incisive integration of existing research findings are needed to address important remaining policy issues. The history of these studies illustrates how strengthening the generalizability of findings improves policy relevance. More important, this history illustrates the fact that a collection of individual studies is not sufficient without methods for reviewing and integrating findings and arguing for their policy implications.

A primary reason to undertake cost–outcome research is to make mental health care more effective and economical. This can happen only if research findings affect policy and practice. Research has an uneven record of success in affecting policy. Decrying this fact, however, is less useful than attending systematically to the steps needed to enable research findings to have their optimal impact. In this chapter we begin with a discussion of the concept of policy itself, and the ways research can aid policy formation. Then we consider four techniques for reviewing and synthesizing research findings to facilitate choice among policy alternatives: qualitative reviews, meta-analysis, clinical decision analysis and modeling, and cross-design synthesis.

10.1 WHEN IS MENTAL HEALTH POLICY NEEDED?

A policy is a definite course of action selected among alternatives to guide present and future decisions. Two types of policy are relevant to mental health cost–outcome research. The first is an overall plan adopted by government or a large organization about how to allocate health care resources. The second is a clinical policy in the form of guidelines for choosing among alternative interventions in caring for specific health problems. In this chapter we address both types of mental health policy.

In Chapter 3 we observed that in health care, and especially in publicly funded mental health care, there is not a classical "free market" in which providers make informed decisions about how much service to produce and how much they should charge and in which consumers make informed decisions about how much service to buy and what price they should be willing to pay. There are three factors that may prevent market forces from doing an adequate job of regulating the amount of service provided and the prices charged and paid. These three factors are asymmetric information, externalities, and distributional inequity (Wolf, 1988).

10.1.1 ASYMMETRIC INFORMATION

Asymmetric information means either the buyer or the seller lacks essential information to judge the value of a mental health service. It is often hard for consumers to know the short-term or long-term effectiveness and cost of treatments recommended by a provider. Furthermore, all but the wealthiest consumers cannot afford expensive procedures like extended hospitalization, so they buy insurance to protect themselves from catastrophic financial loss. The insurance carrier becomes a "third party" in the market, both a seller (of insurance) and a buyer (of health care). The economic interest of the insurer may conflict with those of both consumer and provider. This puts consumers at risk from insufficient information in relation to both providers and insurers. Consumers are also in an inadequate position to bargain over price and product in emergency situations or other situations in which mental illness itself causes an inability to have and use sufficient information to make good purchasing decisions (Frank, 1989; McGuire and Weisbrod, 1981b).

10.1.2 EXTERNALITIES

Externalities are outcomes of producing, selling, or buying services that affect the well-being of a third party or the community at large. If the third party is able to bargain effectively, these competing interests can often be worked out in the marketplace. When whole communities are affected, effective bargaining is very difficult and often takes the form of pressure on government to regulate the market. For example, using inpatient or other restrictive care sparingly appears to increase the cost-effectiveness of mental health services, since costs are contained and persons with severe mental illness have maximum freedom and maximum opportunity to improve their living and working skills. This treatment and rehabilitation approach produces an externality, however, by increasing the probability that some persons with severe mental illness will become homeless or behave in public places in ways that make citizens in general feel uncomfortable or unsafe. This externality leads to public pressure to incarcerate the people who make the community uncomfortable. In general, externalities lead communities to restrict the freedom of providers and consumers in an attempt to attain some common good (Frank, 1989; McGuire and Weisbrod, 1981b).

10.1.3 DISTRIBUTIONAL INEQUITY

Distributional inequity, or unfairness in access to mental health care, also leads communities to constrain aspects of the market that cause inequities. History seems to have shown that market competition is necessary to maintain work incentive and economic efficiency. History also suggests that political freedom and democracy force modifications in the economic system that ensure a minimum quality of life that is better than a completely free market will provide. One can see this as an ethical position about the value of human life, or take a more cynical position that the poor must have a sufficiently safe and fulfilling life so they will not revolt successfully against the rich. Thus, there is a tension between an efficient, competitive economy that allows a few to become very rich and powerful and a socially integrated and democratic community in which all citizens feel they can participate. The present rapid growth of international communication and economic interdependency is extending this tension to the worldwide community.

The community's first response to distributional concerns is to support stopgap "safety net" programs such as income entitlements, homeless shelters, and emergency health care (Rubin, 1991). The longer term response is to work toward a well-tuned economic system that provides equitable opportunity through high quality universal education and preventive health care. Movement toward this goal with regard to a specific product or service is sometimes referred to as "improved market quality," which balances efficiency, equity, and other societal goals.

10.2 RESEARCH CONTRIBUTIONS TO MENTAL HEALTH POLICY

Cost–outcome research can directly address the three market problems of asymmetric information, externalities, and distributional inequity. Asymmetric information problems are reduced by carrying out cost–outcome research and by disseminating findings to both producers and consumers. Effective dissemination requires synthesizing cumulated findings, incorporating conclusions into changed treatment guidelines, in some cases testing further the relative merits of alternate guideline configurations, and making guidelines widely available to health care organizations and directly to consumers. While informing consumers is a major task, health care newsletters, World Wide Web sources, media coverage, and point-of-diagnosis patient education techniques are improving. Cost–outcome research also contributes by identifying quality-of-care indicators that are so closely linked to effectiveness or cost-effectiveness that they can be used as inexpensive proxy measures. Then, quality-of-care research can monitor and disseminate information about the quality of care delivered by specific provider organizations, which potentially creates market pressure favoring organizations that deliver high-quality care.

Externality problems are addressed in cost–outcome research by examining unintended or unwanted effects of services and discovering how to prevent these unwanted effects in the context of cost-effective services. The societal perspective on costs identifies cost-shifting caused by an innovation, whether costs are shifted away from or onto payers who pay the cost of current usual care. For example, an innovation that saves hospital days may increase the financial and time burden on family caretakers or increase the utilization of police contacts and jail time. Similarly, cost–outcome research that takes a broad perspective on outcomes examines possible societal effects relevant to the target group, such as productive work, homelessness, substance abuse, criminal behavior, and psychological burden on family caregivers. In studying broad mental health care innovations such as capitation and contracting for mental health care, adequate information about externalities may require sampling from an eligible target population rather than restricting attention to those who seek services.

Distributional inequity is addressed in cost–outcome research by assuring that service innovations improve or maintain equitable service access as well as service cost and outcome. For example, in several of the assertive community treatment studies mentioned in the example at the beginning of this chapter, ACT services led to effective engagement of withdrawn, alienated, or disruptive clients in the service process; while under usual care conditions such patients were not engaged or quickly terminated services. In studies of capitated services, in which the provider is at financial risk for all needed care, capitation induces an incentive not to provide care when this does not lead to other high costs for the provider, regardless of the quality of life for those who are underserved. Cost–outcome research on capitated services therefore usually pays close attention to what happens to service dropouts or service seekers who never access the service they are seeking. As in studying externalities, studying equity requires research to include information on persons in the target group, whether they receive mental health services or not.

Research contributions to the problems of asymmetric information, externalities, and distributional inequity may gradually allow a shift in the focus of government policy regarding mental health care. Government may be able to reduce its inherently awkward and inflexible direct intervention in the market as the insurer, purchaser, or provider of last resort for mental health care. This would need to be replaced by effective but more flexible and ongoing influences on the market through funding and regulatory support for research and for the dissemination of research findings.

The policy questions that need to be resolved can be broad and complex. Recent managed care innovations in the United States are portrayed by some as reintroducing market forces into a health care system, correcting a situation in which government regulation had so insulated prices from competition that health care costs and health professional incomes had risen at a rate well above the inflation of general prices and wages. Specific managed care innovations, however, may involve an increase in government regulation, not a decrease. Another complexity is the debate about decentralization of policy authority. Some argue that state and local policy authority leads to greater efficiency and better ability to adapt to local needs (i.e., an improved market quality), while others argue that the trend away from national policy authority (in which consumers arguably have greater opportunity to develop political strength) allows greater corporate control of the political process and increased risk of market failure in some localities. As research accumulates on specific examples of government mental health policy innovations, it will also be valuable to review the pattern of findings for their implications for these "big picture" policy issues.

How then should cost–outcome research be focused to most usefully develop evidence about policy choices? The most direct route is to examine the effects of specific policy innovations, such as state capitation and contracting schemes for financing and managing Medicaid-reimbursed mental health services. Such research will examine whether the innovation has improved market quality, that is, whether it leads to equitable access by the target population to good quality care and to beneficial outcomes while containing costs. Over time, research at this level can discover the mix of financing and management policies that are most likely to lead to market improvement. At a more clinical level, cost–outcome research will continue to examine the relative cost-effectiveness of alternative mental health interventions in order to refine treatment guidelines and clarify the meaning of "good quality care."

The breadth of perspective in cost–outcome research is important. For example, Frank (1993) noted that there is reasonably good evidence for superior cost–outcome performance for several mental health innovations that have not been widely adopted, as in the case example at the beginning of this chapter. Adoption by local mental health programs, Frank suggests, is strongly affected by cost shifts associated with an innovation. He illustrates this with evidence that adopting assertive community treatment for severely ill patients, with its concurrent reduction of hospital and other care, can double the proportion of care provided by local funds, relieving pressure on state funds. Thus local implementation of assertive community treatment may be more likely when state funds have been allocated for assertive community treatment or state funds are under local control.

Most policy choices have not been studied and will not be studied in the foreseeable future. Existing studies may also yield inadequate evidence that findings are broadly applicable. Even in situations in which the evidence about a particular policy choice is good, the range of findings from multiple studies may not have been reviewed and critiqued sufficiently to produce a clear scientific consensus about their implications. Under these conditions, research findings are not ready to be applied with confidence to mental health policy. Obtaining policy-relevant research evidence requires closing these information gaps with regard to the most important policy choices.

The logic applied in using cost–outcome evidence also makes a difference. Frank (1993) describes two extreme positions on the use of research findings in determining insurance reimbursement policy for specific mental health treatments. At one extreme would be the insurer who proposes not to pay for a service in which research had failed to demonstrate significant benefit relative to standard treatment. An argument of this sort, though somewhat less extreme, was presented by Bennett (1996) regarding reimbursement for psychotherapy. Bennett argues that psychotherapy should be reimbursed in three circumstances: (1) when it is used as an adjunct to a treatment of demonstrated efficacy, (2) when its efficacy alone is established for a given disorder, and (3) as a "holding operation" when no effective treatment exists. Given imperfect evidence, of course, only a few very well studied services would be reimbursed, and under the proposed rule all failings in study power, design, or relevance would be used to deny reimbursement. Many medical treatments would fail this test, except for standard medications approved by the U.S. Food and Drug Administration. At the other extreme, a policy that no insurer could afford to endorse would be to reimburse every service unless there was clear evidence that it is not cost-effective relative to usual care. Borenstein (1996), arguing for less restriction in the reimbursement of psychotherapy, makes an argument somewhat like this in suggesting that "until carefully constructed outcome studies demonstrate that there are no adverse consequences of cost-based constraints on established psychiatric treatments, such constraints are not acceptable" (p. 974). Under such a rule, all weaknesses in the cost–effectiveness evidence would lead to coverage. While it is certainly defensible to reimburse services that have been shown to be cost-effective and deny coverage for services that have been shown not to be cost-effective, there is insufficient evidence to apply this decision rule to the majority of treatments. Proprietary treatments with large capital backing can attract research funding to improve their position in such a research-based marketplace, but that does not ensure that research will be funded to examine the choice points most likely to improve the efficiency and outcome of mental health care.

We will never have adequate evidence about the relative cost-effectiveness of every possible procedure. A rational approach is to develop decision guidelines based a combination of the available evidence and the consensus of expert clinicians. Such guidelines identify decision circumstances for which there is clear evidence, other circumstances for which there is clear consensus, and a third set of circumstances for which there are several plausible choices. This process is proceeding rapidly in all aspects of health care, including mental health care. An important new area of mental health services research is testing the relative cost–outcome performance of well-implemented guidelines against usual care. We will continue to need cost–outcome research on new interventions to identify their appropriate place in treatment guidelines. In some cases it may be more efficient to study the relative cost-effectiveness of alternative guidelines, rather than studying each single component.

10.3 INTEGRATING THE FINDINGS FROM MULTIPLE STUDIES

While one can always lament the lack of relevant research evidence, the body of research findings is constantly growing and there is an increasing foundation for "evidence-based" practice and policy. The situation would be much improved were existing evidence widely available in a very accessible form. This would provide a sound basis for policy advocacy and would usefully inform day-to-day clinical practice and clinical training. There are several techniques for integrating research findings. While integration is usually carried out by researchers, advanced methods for integrating findings are not usually covered in clinical research training.

A single study rarely provides clear guidance to clinicians and clinical administrators, but it can contribute to an accumulation of findings from multiple studies, as in the case example at the beginning of this chapter. The process by which this synthesis takes place is important to keep in mind in designing a study and later when reporting findings. Therefore we next compare four models for synthesizing research findings: traditional qualitative reviews, meta-analysis, clinical decision analysis and modeling, and cross-design synthesis. Each has implications for study design and reporting.

10.3.1 QUALITATIVE REVIEWS

The traditional and perhaps still the most common way to understand the accumulated meaning of multiple research studies is to examine them systematically but qualitatively. A reviewer often begins by rating the design quality of each study. Such design features might include whether the study utilized random assignment, a relevant control or comparison condition, comprehensive measures of outcome and cost, and blinding of ratings. The reviewer may note whether the study had adequate sample size and statistical power, whether the nature of experimental and control interventions was clear, whether there was adequate documentation of the faithful implementation of the intended interventions, and how well the study sample represented the target population. The reviewer may subclassify intervention types to compare results more meaningfully. Ultimately the reviewer counts how many good quality studies found statistically reliable evidence for improved effectiveness or cost-effectiveness of the innovative treatment. If a majority of studies found no significant effect, the conclusion is usually that the benefit of the innovation has not been demonstrated.

Sometimes the reviewer displays more closely the size of effect that can be ruled out by each study, taking into account the statistical power, and therefore the precision, of the studies being compared (e.g., Hargreaves, 1983; McGrew et al., 1994), but this has been rare. Qualitative reviews, usually done by subject-matter experts in a particular field, are an important tool for assessing the clinical and public policy impact of medical effectiveness research and will probably remain so. Nine of the 11 reviews cited in the case example at the beginning of this chapter were qualitative reviews (Scott and Dixon, 1995).

The qualitative approach has come under increasing criticism in recent years. Subject-matter experts have noted potential for bias in the many judgments made in reviewing research findings. Perhaps more importantly, some simple statistical facts show how misleading conclusions can be when the true effect of an intervention is relatively small. Since the statistical power of most studies is modest, many of them will fail to detect a "statistically significant effect" when the true effect in the population is small. As more and more studies are completed, the proportion with "significant" findings will remain very low, leading to the erroneous conclusion that the population effect size is zero (Schmidt, 1996). More broadly, variability in significance across studies can be related not only to sample size, but to differences in methodology, sampling, and measurement. It is hard to examine these factors thoroughly in qualitative reviews.

10.3.2 META-ANALYSIS

Meta-analysis systematically examines the variability in study findings from all relevant studies in relation to variability due to sampling error as a way to avoid the negative bias inherent in qualitative reviews (Cooper and Hedges, 1992; Dickersin and Berlin, 1992; Hedges, 1982; Hedges and Olkin, 1985; Petitti, 1994). Sampling error for the hypothesized treatment effect is reduced by combining samples across many studies. It is not uncommon for meta-analysis to find that the average effect is statistically significant even when a relatively low proportion of the individual studies show statistically significant effects. One can also construct a confidence interval estimate of the population effect size, and examine predictors of effect size, such as study quality, intervention variation, and patient sample variation (e.g., Gaffan et al., 1995; Knight et al., 1996; Bettencourt and Miller, 1996).

The term "meta-analysis" was coined by educational researcher Gene V.

Glass (1976). One of the prominent early meta-analyses was actually done on mental health care, a review by Smith and co-workers (1980) of psychotherapy outcome studies. During the 1980s, meta-analysis became a standard method for synthesizing the findings of medical effectiveness studies, and it has been widely applied in the social sciences as well (Mann, 1994). Meta-analysis can also play an important role in the design of clinical trials (Henderson et al., 1995).

There are four steps in a meta-analysis (Petitti, 1994): (1) studies with relevant data are identified, (2) eligibility criteria for inclusion and exclusion of the studies are defined and eligible studies selected, (3) data are abstracted, and (4) the abstracted data are analyzed statistically.

Meta-analysis is not without its own problems (Cook, 1992; Cooper and Hedges, 1992; National Research Council, 1992; Schmidt, 1992). The most difficult and fundamental problem is the "file drawer problem." This refers to the fact that negative results often do not get published (Sterling, 1959; Simes, 1986; Esterbrook et al., 1991). This primarily results from the failure of investigators to submit papers from their studies with negative findings, and not from the reluctance of journals to accept such papers (Dickersin et al., 1992). The effect on meta-analysis (and indeed on any review process) is to bias effect sizes upward, risking a conclusion that there are positive effects when, in fact, there are none.

In any particular review it is impossible to precisely estimate the size of the file drawer problem, but practical steps to control it are available (Petitti, 1994). There are two steps in reducing bias. The primary remedy is to make every effort to locate all relevant studies, whether published or not, and the second is to examine the observed effect sizes for evidence of lost negative studies. Studies published in a language other than English should be included if at all possible, as well as studies published over the past several decades. Several electronic databases should be searched, including dissertation abstracts. Electronic search by itself is not sufficient. One must examine all relevant studies cited in research reports and reviews, and inquire of published investigators and other experts in the field about their knowledge of unpublished studies. Archives of clinical trials are very helpful in reducing the publication bias problem in meta-analysis (Chernoff et al., 1995) and it would be valuable to pursue their construction vigorously with regard to mental disorders and mental health interventions.

A simple graphical method to estimate whether negative studies have been overlooked has been suggested by Light and Pillemer (1984). One constructs a scatter plot of the obtained studies, plotting the reported effect size on the horizontal axis and the sample size on the vertical axis. Small sample studies at the bottom of the plot should show a wide spread of effect sizes, which narrow as sample size increases, giving the plot the shape of an inverted funnel. If the base of the funnel spreads symmetrically around the narrow point at the top, this is reassuring that there has not been a biased loss of negative studies. If the plot looks more like a right triangle with a vertical side on the left, one should search more diligently for missing studies.

Statistical methods have been suggested for estimating the size of the publication bias, rather than simply its presence (Rosenthal, 1979; Orwin, 1983; Hedges, 1984; Hedges and Olkin, 1985). These methods have been criticized by Iyengar and Greenhouse (1988). Petitti (1994) recommends against these methods, and the reader is referred to her discussion.

Beyond the file drawer problem, it is obvious that meta-analysis requires as much judgment as traditional review techniques. Studies usually present findings on many different outcome measures. If meta-analysis is restricted to effect sizes for outcome measures shared by all studies, only the most common outcomes can be examined, often not ones that we would most like to know about. Kalaian and Raudenbush (1996) have suggested a multivariate model for meta-analysis that incorporates multiple effect sizes per study and allows different studies to have different subsets of effect sizes. Sometimes authors do not report findings in a form that allows effect sizes to be computed. Reviewers then have the choice of dropping studies, using approximations to estimate effect sizes, or trying to obtain original data from each investigator. Ray and Shadish (1996) have shown that methods for approximating effect sizes can produce results that are not equivalent to the use of the original effect sizes. All of these strategies may lead to eliminating studies from the analysis, which may introduce bias. Methods for estimating the effect of unreliability in meta-analysis judgments about study inclusion have been developed, but are rarely employed (Orwin and Corday, 1985).

The take-home message for investigators is to report all treatment effects so that effect sizes can be calculated. In studies in which the outcome is an event such as relapse, effect size is commonly expressed as an odds ratio. An odds ratio can be computed whenever the investigator reports the number of subjects in each group who experience each outcome. When the outcome is a quantitative measure, an effect size statistic can be computed if the investigator reports the sample size, mean outcome, and standard deviation in both the experimental and control condition. Results of regression analyses that report adjusted R^2 increments for treatment effects as well as the total variance accounted for by the model can be used to compute effect sizes. Means of each treatment group along with appropriate t or F statistics with their degrees of freedom will also allow one to compute effect sizes.

Since 1994 meta-analysis of randomized controlled trials of medical treatments has been initiated on a very comprehensive and broad scale (Bero and Rennie, 1995; Taubes, 1996). Known as the Cochrane Collaboration, after the late British epidemiologist Archie Cochrane, an international volunteer effort is searching the world literature for all of the randomized trials ever published, as well as any unpublished trials that can be located. Updated regularly and published electronically, this effort aims for nothing less than a continuous synthesis of the current state of knowledge about every available therapy, providing implications for practice and research. While critics worry that "industrial scale" meta-analysis will lack the penetrating search for errors and thoughtful discussion of results, members of the Cochrane Collaboration have put a lot of work into protocols to minimize these problems. They have developed an extensive handbook, a process of expert refereeing, software to guide data entry regarding individual studies, and a method for e-mail comment by any reader. These efforts should detect error and strengthen progressive revision of meta-analysis findings as new evidence appears. Reviews have been undertaken for nearly 100 conditions, including schizophrenia, in just the first 2 years of the collaboration.

Reviewers are selected among young investigators who are willing to make a long-term volunteer commitment to updating their review topic. This means that most reviewers are not initially seasoned subject matter experts as is typical among the authors of qualitative reviews. One hopes that as reviewers become more seasoned, and as subject matter experts contribute their comments and qualitative reviews, the quality of the Cochrane reviews will steadily improve. Reviews are published in the *Cochrane Database of Systematic Reviews*, which is available on floppy disks, CD-ROM, and the World Wide Web. The ready accessibility of these reviews in everyday clinical practice and clinical training promises to make "evidence-based medicine" an increasing reality.

10.3.3 CLINICAL DECISION ANALYSIS AND MODELING

Clinical decision analysis and modeling (Weinstein and Fineberg, 1980; Pauker and Kassirer, 1987; Petitti, 1994; Revicki and Luce, 1995) are useful for estimating the costs and outcomes associated with a new intervention compared to standard treatment. The intent is to model and simulate the practice and outcome of treatment. Various computer simulations of the probabilities of these sequential events are constructed, such as Markov state-transition models. The structure of the model and the variables making up the model are taken from the clinical literature, completed clinical trials, and expert clinical judgment, in an attempt to represent the actual treatment of patients in real-life situations. Meta-analysis is the preferred method for estimating treatment efficacy when findings from multiple studies are available. Treatment costs may be based on primary or secondary data on the use of health services or estimated on the basis of clinical judgment about practice patterns. A fully developed example of decision analysis and modeling comparing three antidepressant drugs can be seen in Revicki et al. (1995).

Modeling has some obvious advantages (Revicki and Luce, 1995). First, modeling is a relatively inexpensive and timely way to estimate the economic and clinical impact of new treatments. Second, a model identifies key variables and gaps in the research literature, which may be helpful in targeting mental health services research toward fruitful topics. Third, the approach is flexible, and can incorporate different structures and durations, from several years to a lifetime. Fourth, sensitivity analysis is used to test the model and its assumptions to determine the robustness of findings. One can first set the "base case" version of the model with the best estimate of each parameter. Then the sensitivity analysis is a series of recomputations of the model while varying parameters between their highest and lowest plausible value, to determine how such variation affects the estimated cost and outcome of each of the interventions being compared (Briggs et al., 1994). Sensitivity analysis identifies the parameter estimates that are both crucial and unreliable, so that extra attention can be focused on them in the analysis and in interpreting the findings, in order to give the reader a realistic picture of the precision of the estimates in the model.

Modeling also has serious limitations and is often met with great skepticism by clinicians and health care decision makers. Decision models may lack precision and may be subject to bias. Simplifying assumptions and decisions must always be made when constructing a model. This makes it important that the analyst clearly explain the model structure, assumptions, and methods of estimating each parameter, so that informed readers can detect likely biases in the model. In this regard, sensitivity analyses play a very important role in clarifying where in the model small changes in assumptions could have led to large differences in the results. Sensitivity analyses should reveal which parameters have large effects on overall cost or outcome estimates. Even more important, sensitivity analysis should indicate whether treatment differences in estimated cost or outcome are sensitive to questionable assumptions in the model. For example, when a controlled trial finding is used to estimate a parameter in the model, it is common to use the point estimate of the parameter. Sensitivity analysis should then explore the effects of using the upper and lower bound of the 95% confidence interval of the parameter. In addition, projections of short-term study findings to lifetime effects require assumptions about the time course of effects. Model estimates may be especially sensitive to these assumptions.

Even with extensive sensitivity analyses, informed readers may be skeptical, knowing that the assumptions of a model can often be adjusted to favor a particular result. The analyst must accept that there will be this informed and skeptical audience, and should discuss potential biases as clearly and realistically as possible. Needless to say, if the model evaluates a new pharmaceutical product or treatment device (e.g., electroconvulsive therapy machines), the financial relationship of the authors to the manufacturer and whether the manufacturer funded the analysis must be made clear.

10.3.4 CROSS-DESIGN SYNTHESIS

With the establishment of the Agency for Health Care Policy and Research in 1989, the U.S. Congress launched an "effectiveness initiative" intended to improve the quality of health care through research-based development of national guidelines for medical practice. Guidelines require results that are both scientifically valid and relevant to the conditions of medical practice. The difficulty of this ambitious task led four U.S. senators to ask the General Accounting Office (GAO) to review existing designs for evaluating medical effectiveness and suggest an improved evaluation strategy.

In response, Silberman and colleagues at the GAO (1992) proposed a method of "cross-design synthesis." They noted that two types of studies might bear on assessing differential medical effectiveness: randomized treatment trials and the analysis of large scale databases in which outcomes are observed for groups nonrandomly subjected to different treatments. It was proposed that the superior internal validity of the former and the superior generalizability of the latter allow a synthesis that can inform clinical practice.

Building on an extensive review of designs, GAO devised a strategy that extends the logic of meta-analysis. The method capitalizes on both established and lesser known techniques for assessing, adjusting, and combining the results of existing studies. These techniques are organized into four major tasks that are undertaken by a reviewer of a body of findings: (1) assessing existing randomized studies for generalizability across the full range of relevant patients; (2) assessing nonexperimental database analyses for "imbalanced comparison groups"; (3) adjusting the results of each randomized study and each database analysis, compensating for biases as needed; and (4) synthesizing the adjusted study findings within and across design categories. We will concentrate on the first task in this discussion, since it has the most bearing on the design and reporting of cost–effectiveness controlled trials.

Methods for Evaluating Controlled Trial Generalizability

Task 1 is to determine whether a cross-design synthesis is needed. When randomized study results from several studies are all generalizable to the relevant patient population, traditional meta-analysis techniques are adequate. Generalizability can be judged in two ways: (1) by the design of patient recruitment and (2) by the characteristics of the subjects actually included. Investigators must report this information fully so readers can evaluate the generalizability of their findings.

The first way to evaluate generalizability is to analyze the recruitment design. Recruitment design problems arise from: (1) specific exclusion of relevant parts of the target population in the patient selection criteria, (2) a recruitment mode (e.g., inpatients) that biases patient selection, (3) rejection by investigators of qualified patients for reasons that are not adequately described, and (4) the biased avoidance or explicit refusal of the randomized trial by patients or referring clinicians. An example of the latter from psychiatric research was a study of oral versus depot medication for schizophrenia, in which no relapse difference was found (Schooler, 1980). The investigator noted that the study could have failed if those who were likely to refuse oral medication also refused to give informed consent to enter the study. Obviously the study could have been more valuable had the investigators anticipated this problem and obtained data on the previous treatment refusal behavior of eligible patients who entered or refused the study. These issues underscore how important it is for the investigator to consider these sources of bias in study design, and especially to anticipate potentially unavoidable bias and attempt to document the nature and extent of the biased losses from the full target population.

The second phase of Task 1 is to assess the representativeness of the achieved patient sample. Even if study patients cannot be randomly selected from the relevant target population, it may be possible to identify a large sample of members of the relevant target population and compare their baseline characteristics to those of the study subjects. Baseline characteristics can be ranked in importance. The most important are characteristics known to be linked to differential effects of the treatments in question. The next most important are prognostic factors (e.g., severity of illness). Finally, numerous demographic and other patient characteristics are also potentially related to the effect that a treatment will have.

Synthesizing Research Conclusions

Tasks 2 to 4 complete the synthesis of research conclusions. Task 2, assessing database analyses for imbalanced comparison groups, shows whether cross-design synthesis is possible. Only if assessment shows that existing database analyses have sufficient internal validity will it be possible to carry out a cross-design synthesis that combines the results of controlled trials data with database analyses (e.g., see Heinsman and Shadish, 1996). Database analyses lose validity as they suffer from comparison bias, or the confounding of baseline prognosis with treatment effects. The reviewer examines the investigator's attempts to detect and deal with these potentially confounding biases, in order to judge the sources and degree of threats to internal validity.

Task 3 is to assess the results of each randomized study and each database analysis and to try to compensate for detected biases as needed. This step uses in-depth assessments from Tasks 1 and 2 to adjust each study's results and clarify the range of uncertainty associated with each study's results. For example, if a randomized trial shows biased selection of subjects who are more likely to show a differential effect of the innovation, and the degree of this bias can be estimated, then the estimated differential effect of the innovation can be reduced for subgroups like those excluded from the controlled trial. A comparable example involving a database analysis would arise if a database analysis seems to have poorer prognosis patients in the innovative treatment than in usual care, and the degree of this bias can be estimated from the baseline data. In this case the raw outcomes following the innovative treatment can be adjusted to be closer to the outcomes of usual care.

Task 4 calls for the reviewer to synthesize the adjusted results within and across the two design categories, controlled trials and nonexperimental treatment comparisons. To the extent that the adjustments made in the previous step (Task 3) are correct, all of the findings from the individual studies should now be equally generalizable to the target population and relatively unbiased by the methodological problems that the reviewer has detected. Now they can be synthesized into an overall finding or set of findings, perhaps weighting each study within the two design types by its sample size and comparing the conclusions from the synthesized controlled trials to the conclusions from the synthesized database analyses.

Cross-design synthesis obviously requires a series of complex judgments and can be as subject to bias as any other method for integrating research findings. One can imagine that in the future a routine, ongoing process of cross-design synthesis in the style of the Cochrane Collaboration meta-analyses, tempered by expert review panels and wide participation of relevant experts, will reduce the likelihood of influence by particular commercial interests or narrow clinical viewpoints while furthering "evidence-based" clinical care.

10.4 FUTURE DEVELOPMENTS IN APPLYING RESEARCH TO POLICY

Meta-analysis, modeling, and cross-design synthesis will probably assume increasing prominence in mental health research and policy. Psychiatry has a smaller number of large, relevant databases than other areas of medical care, but this will probably change with time. Study designs intermediate between randomized trials and database studies are being facilitated by the formation of large "practice research networks," including one in mental health (Zarin et al., 1996). Some large correlational studies have already made important contributions to mental health services research (Wells and Sturm, 1996). As the updated reviews from the Cochrane Collaboration become more widely known and methods like cross-design synthesis are more widely applied, their impact on research, policy, and practice should increase.

In the design of controlled cost–effectiveness studies, meta-analysis and cross-design synthesis processes call our attention to study design and reporting principles that maximize the impact of a controlled study on knowledge synthesis and policy formulation. All of the design quality factors discussed in this book play a role in strengthening this contribution, especially the investigator's careful attention to internal and external validity. In reporting findings, clear discussion of problems that remain in interpretation will help the reviewer and consumer of the results to understand the contribution to knowledge made by particular studies. Finally, controlled trial data is beginning to be archived in an accessible format across multiple studies (e.g., Chernoff et al., 1995). Organizing this process for studies of mental health care could improve the value of all methods for integrating study findings.

10.5 CHAPTER REVIEW

Two types of policy are (1) plans by government or large organizations about how to allocate support for mental health services, and (2) clinical guidelines for choosing among alternative interventions for specific mental health problems.

From an economic perspective, such policies are needed because the market for mental health services is either nonexistent or of poor quality.

Three factors impair the quality of the market for mental health care and lead to the first type of policy formation by government: asymmetric information, externalities, and distributional inequity.

Cost–outcome research can directly address these three market problems. Asymmetric information problems are reduced by discovering which services are most cost-effective, by disseminating findings to providers and consumers in the form of treatment guidelines, and by identifying quality-of-care indicators that are closely linked to cost-effectiveness. Externality problems are addressed by examining unintended or unwanted effects of service innovations and discovering how to minimize these unwanted effects in the context of cost-effective services. Distributional inequity is addressed by assuring that service innovations improve or maintain equitable service access as well as service cost and outcome. Thus cost–outcome research aims to improve market quality by discovering how to make services more effective, efficient, environmentally friendly, and equitably accessible to informed consumers from informed providers.

A single study rarely provides clear policy guidance. Policy usually flows from an accumulation of findings that are synthesized to focus on their policy implications. There are four models for synthesizing research findings: qualitative reviews, meta-analysis, clinical decision analysis and modeling, and cross-design synthesis. Qualitative reviews are still the most common, but the other three methods have important advantages. Meta-analysis is important to detect relatively small effects, the size of which can only be estimated reliably with very large sample sizes and high statistical power. By combining the results of all relevant studies, meta-analysis provides this high statistical power. Clinical decision analysis and modeling build on findings from controlled trials and meta-analyses by gathering additional ratings of practice patterns and/or outcome utilities and combining these with further assumptions in simulations to project findings to long-term effects on patients or target populations. Modeling is often the only way to estimate long-term effects, and it highlights the specific assumptions on which policy must be based when solid empirical data are lacking. Cross-design synthesis attempts to combine the good internal validity of randomized trials and the good external validity of naturalistic databases with data on treatment and outcome. It does so by examining the limits of the generalizability of available randomized trials, examining the treatment selection bias in naturalistic comparisons, attempting to adjust the observed size of effect in each study for these limitations, and then synthesizing the results from all studies to draw policy implications for particular target populations.

These methods of synthesizing research findings highlight the kinds of information that investigators need to report in order for their research findings to be interpretable. Effect sizes, sources of bias in the selection of subjects, and ways that treatment selection was confounded with prognosis should always be reported as fully as possible.

BIBLIOGRAPHY

Abdellah FG, Levine E. Work-sampling applied to the study of nursing personnel. *Nursing Research* 3:11–16, 1954.

Achenbach TM, Edelbrock CS. The classification of child psychopathology: A review and analysis of empirical efforts. *Psychological Bulletin* 85:1275–1301, 1978.

Achenbach TM, Edelbrock CS. The Child Behavior Profile: II. Boys aged 12–16 and girls aged 6–11 and 12–16. *Journal of Consulting and Clinical Psychology* 47:223–233, 1979.

Achenbach TM, Edelbrock CS. Behavioral problems and competencies reported by parents of normal and disturbed children aged four through sixteen. *Monographs of the Society for Research in Child Development* 46:1–82, 1981.

Adams ME, McCall NT, Gray DT, Orza MJ, Chalmers TC. Economic analysis in randomized control trials. *Medical Care* 30:231–243, 1992.

Aft LS. *Productivity, Measurement, and Improvement.* Reston, VA: Reston Publishing, 1983.

Aguilar-Gaxiola S, Vega W, Peifer K, Gray T. *Development of the Fresno Composite International Diagnostic Interview: Fresno CIDI 1995.* Berkeley: Institute for Mental Health Services Research Working Paper Series, 1995.

Alexander CS, Becker HJ. The use of vignettes in survey research. *Public Opinion Quarterly* 42:93–104, 1978.

Alterman AI, Erdlen FR, McLellan AT, Mann SC. Problem drinking in hospitalized schizophrenic patients. *Addictive Behaviors* 5:273–276, 1980.

American Psychiatric Association. *Diagnostic and Statistical Manual of Mental Disorders DSM-III-R.* 3rd-revised ed. Washington, DC: American Psychiatric Association, 1987.

American Psychiatric Association. *Diagnostic and Statistical Manual of Mental Disorders DSM-IV.* 4th ed. Washington, DC: American Psychiatric Association, 1994.

Anderson NH. *Foundations of Information Integration Theory.* New York: Academic Press, 1981.

Anderson S, Auquier A, Hauck WW, Oakes D, Vandaele W, Weisberg HI. *Statistical Methods for Comparative Studies: Techniques for Bias Reduction.* New York: John Wiley and Sons, 1980.

Anderson S, Hauck WW. A new procedure for testing equivalence in comparative bioavailability and other clinical trials. *Communications in Statistics—Theory and Methods* 12:2663–2692, 1983.

Andreasen NC. Negative symptoms in schizophrenia: Definition and reliability. *Archives of General Psychiatry* 39:784–788, 1982.

Andreasen NC. Scale for the assessment of thought, language, and communication (TLC). *Schizophrenia Bulletin* 12:473–482, 1986.

Anthony JC, Folstein M, Romanoski AJ, Von Korff MR, Nestadt GR, Chahal R, et al. Comparison of the lay Diagnostic Interview Schedule and a standardized psychiatric diagnosis: Experience in eastern Boston. *Archives of General Psychiatry* 42:667–675, 1985.

Anthony WA, Cohen M, Farkas M. A psychiatric rehabilitation treatment program: Can I recognize one if I see one? *Community Mental Health Journal* 18:83–96, 1982.

Anthony WA, Farkas MD. A client outcome planning model for assessing psychiatric rehabilitation interventions. *Schizophrenia Bulletin* 8:13–29, 1982.

Appel LJ, Steinberg EP, Powe NR, Anderson GF, Dwyer SA, Faden RR. Risk reduction from low osmolality contrast media. *Medical Care* 28:324–337, 1990.

Attkisson C, Cook J, Karno M, Lehman A, McGlashan TH, Meltzer HY, et al. Clinical services research. *Schizophrenia Bulletin* 18:561–626, 1992.

Audini B, Marks IM, Lawrence RE, Connolly J, Watts V. Home-based versus out-patient/in-patient care for people with serious mental illness: Phase II of a controlled study. *British Journal of Psychiatry* 165:204–210, 1994.

Babor TF, Longabaugh R, Zweben A, Fuller RK, Stout RL, Anton RF, et al. Issues in the definition and measurement of drinking outcomes in alcoholism treatment research. *Journal of Studies on Alcohol* 12:101–111, 1994.

Babor TF, Stephens RS, Marlatt GA. Verbal report methods in clinical research on alcoholism: Response bias and its minimization. *Journal of Studies on Alcohol* 48:410–424, 1987.

Bachrach LL. Overview: Model programs for chronic mental patients. *American Journal of Psychiatry* 137:1023–1031, 1980.

Bachrach LL. Case management: Toward a shared definition. *Hospital and Community Psychiatry* 40:883–884, 1989.

Barker S, Barron N, McFarland BH, Bigelow DA. A community ability scale for chronically mentally ill consumers: I. Reliability and validity. *Community Mental Health Journal* 30:363–383, 1994a.

Barker S, Barron N, McFarland BH, Bigelow DA, Carnahan T. A community ability scale for chronically mentally ill consumers: II. Applications. *Community Mental Health Journal* 30:459–472, 1994b.

Barron FH, Person HB. Assessment of multiplicative utility functions via holistic judgments. *Organizational Behavior and Human Performance* 24:147–166, 1979.

Battiato SE. Cost–benefit analysis and the theory of resource allocation. In Williams A, Giardina E, editors. *Efficiency in the Public Sector: The Theory and Practice of Cost–Benefit Analysis.* Brookfield, VT: Edward Elgar Publishing, 1993.

Beattie MC, Swindle RW, Tomko LA. *Department of Veterans Affairs Databases Resource Guide.* Palo Alto: HSR&D Center for Health Care Evaluation, 1992.

Beck AT, Steer RA, Brown GK. *Manual, Beck Depression Inventory II.* 2nd ed. San Antonio: Harcourt Brace, 1996.

Beck C, Heithoff K, Baldwin B, Cuffel B, Chumbler NR. Assessing disruptive behavior in older adults: The Disruptive Behavior Scale. *Aging and Mental Health* 1:71–79, 1997.

Bell M, Milstein R, Goulet J, Lysaker P, Cicchetti D. The Positive and Negative Syndrome Scale and the Brief Psychiatric Rating Scale: Reliability, comparability, and predictive validity. *Journal of Nervous and Mental Disease* 180:723–728, 1992.

Belson WA. *Validity in Survey Research.* Brookfield, VT: Gower, 1985.

Bennett MJ. Is psychotherapy ever medically necessary? *Psychiatric Services* 47:966–970, 1996.

Bergner M, Bobbitt RA, Carter WB, Gilson BS. The Sickness Impact Profile: Development and final revision of a health status measure. *Medical Care* XIX:787–805, 1981.

Bernheim KF, Lehman AF. *Working with Families of the Mentally Ill.* New York: W. W. Norton, 1985.

Bero L, Rennie D. The Cochrane Collaboration: Preparing, maintaining, and disseminating systematic reviews of the effects of health care. *Journal of the American Medical Association* 274:1935–1938, 1995.

Bettencourt BA, Miller N. Gender differences in agression as a function of provocation: A meta-analysis. *Psychological Bulletin* 119:422–447, 1996.

Bickman L, editor. *New Directions for Program Evaluation* 33, 1987.

Bickman L, editor. *New Directions for Program Evaluation* 47, 1990.

Bigelow DA, Brodsky G, Stewart L, Olson M. The concept and measurement of quality of life as a dependent variable in evaluation of mental health services. In Tash W, Stahler G, editors. *Innovative Approaches to Mental Health Evaluation*. New York: Academic Press, 1982.

Bigelow DA, McFarland BH, Olson MM. Quality of life of community mental health program clients: Validating a measure. *Community Mental Health Journal* 27:43–55, 1991.

Bigelow DA, Young DJ. Effectiveness of a case management program. *Community Mental Health Journal* 27:115–123, 1991.

Birchwood M, Smith J, Cochrane R, Wetton S, Copestake S. The Social Functioning Scale: The development and validation of a new scale of social adjustment for use in family intervention programmes for schizophrenic patients. *British Journal of Psychiatry* 157:853–859, 1990.

Bloom J, Hu T, Cuffel B, Hausman J, Wallace N, Scheffler R. Mental health costs under alternative capitation systems in Colorado, US. Unpublished.

Blouin A, Helzer JE. *Computerized DSM-III-R Criteria Checklist Users Manual*. Ottawa, Canada: C-DIS Group, 1992.

Bond GR. An economic analysis of psychosocial rehabilitation. *Hospital and Community Psychiatry* 35:356–362, 1984.

Bond GR, McDonel EC, Miller LD, Pensec M. Assertive community treatment and reference groups: An evaluation of their effectiveness for young adults with serious mental illness and substance abuse problems. *Psychosocial Rehabilitation Journal* 15:31–43, 1991a.

Bond GR, McGrew JH, Fekete DM. Assertive outreach for frequent users of psychiatric hospital: A meta-analysis. *Journal of Mental Health Administration* 22:4–16, 1995.

Bond GR, Miller LD, Krumwied R, Ward RS. Assertive case management in three CMHCs: A controlled study. *Hospital and Community Psychiatry* 39:411–418, 1988.

Bond GR, Pensec M, Dietzen L, McCafferty D, Grezza R, Sipple H. Intensive case management for frequent users of psychiatric hospitals in a large city: A comparison of team and individual caseloads. *Psychosocial Rehabilitation Journal* 15:90–98, 1991b.

Bond GR, Witheridge TF, Dincin J, Wasmer D, Webb J, DeGraaf-Kaser R. Assertive Community Treatment for frequent users of psychiatric hospitals in a large city: A controlled study. *American Journal of Community Psychology* 18:865–891, 1990.

Borenstein DB. Does managed care permit appropriate use of psychotherapy? *Psychiatric Services* 47:971–974, 1996.

Brekke JS. What do we really know about community support programs? Strategies for better monitoring. *Hospital and Community Psychiatry* 39:946–952, 1988.

Brekke JS, Test MA. An empirical analysis of services delivered in a model community support program. *Psychosocial Rehabilitation Journal* 10:51–61, 1987.

Brekke JS, Test MA. A model for measuring the implementation of community support programs: Results from three sites. *Community Mental Health Journal* 28:227–247, 1992.

Brekke JS, Wolkon GH. Monitoring program implementation in community mental health settings. *Evaluation and the Health Professions* 11:425–440, 1988.

Brent RJ. The role of public and private transfers in the cost–benefit analysis of mental health programs. Unpublished.

Briggs A, Sculpher M, Buxton M. Uncertainty in the economic evaluation of health care technologies: The role of sensitivity analysis. *Health Economics* 3:95–104, 1994.

Brisley CL. Work sampling. In Maynard HB, editor. *Industrial Engineering Handbook*. New York: McGraw-Hill, 1971.

Burnam MA, Wells KB. Use of a two-stage procedure to identify depression: The Medical Outcomes Study. In Attkisson CC, Zich JM, editors. *Depression in Primary Care: Screening and Detection*. New York: Routledge, 1990.

Burnes AJ, Roen SR. Social roles and adaptation to the community. *Community Mental Health Journal* 3:153–158, 1967.

Burns BJ, Santos AB. Assertive community treatment: An update of randomized trials. *Psychiatric Services* 46:669–675, 1995.

Burns BJ, Taube JE, Permutt T, Rudin SC, Mulcare ME, Harbin HT, et al. Evaluation of a Maryland fiscal incentive plan for placing state hospital patients in nursing homes. *Hospital and Community Psychiatry* 42:1228–1233, 1991.

Burns BJ, Wagner R, Taube JE, Magaziner J, Permutt T, Landerman LR. Mental health service use by elderly in nursing homes. *American Journal of Public Health* 83:331–337, 1993.

Cadman D, Goldsmith C. Construction of social value or utility-based health indices: The usefulness of factorial experimental design plans. *Journal of Chronic Disease* 39:643–651, 1986.

Cairns JA. Valuing future benefits. *Health Economics* 3:221–229, 1994.

Callahan D. Setting mental health priorities: Problems and possibilities. *The Millbank Quarterly* 72:451–469, 1994.

Campbell DT, Fiske DW. Convergent and discriminant validation by the multitrait-multimethod matrix. *Psychological Bulletin* 56:81–105, 1959.

Campbell DT, Stanley JC. *Experimental and Quasi-Experimental Designs for Research.* Chicago: Rand McNally, 1966.

Carpentier N, Lesage A, Goulet J, Lalonde P, Renaud M. Burden of care of families not living with young schizophrenic relatives. *Hospital and Community Psychiatry* 43:38–43, 1992.

Carroll BJ, Fielding JM, Blashki TG. Depression rating scales: A critical review. *Archives of General Psychiatry* 28:361–366, 1973.

Cassell WA, Smith CM, Grunberg F, Boan JA, Thomas RF. Comparing costs of hospital and community care. *Hospital and Community Psychiatry* 23:17–20, 1972.

Chamberlain R, Rapp CA. A decade of case management: A methodological review of outcome research. *Community Mental Health Journal* 27:171–188, 1991.

Chandler D, Hu TW, Meisel J, McGowen M, Madison K. Mental health costs, other public costs, and family burden among mental health clients in capitated integrated service agencies. *Journal of Mental Health Administration* 24:178–188, 1997.

Chandler D, Meisel J, Hu T, McGowen M, Madison K. A capitated model for a cross-section of severely mentally ill clients: Employment outcomes. *Community Mental Health Journal, in press.*

Chandler D, Meisel J, Hu T, McGowen M, Madison K. Client outcomes in a three-year controlled study of an integrated service agency model. *Psychiatric Services* 47:1337–1343, 1996a.

Chandler D, Meisel J, McGowen M, Mintz J, Madison K. Client outcomes in two model capitated integrated service agencies. *Psychiatric Services* 47:175–180, 1996b.

Chaudhary MA, Stearns SC. Estimating confidence intervals for cost–effectiveness ratios: An example from a randomized trial. *Statistics in Medicine* 14:1447–1458, 1996.

Chen HT, editor. *Evaluation and Program Planning* 12, 1989.

Chen HT. *Theory-Driven Evaluations.* Newbury Park, CA: Sage, 1990.

Chernoff MC, Wang M, Anderson JJ, Felson DT. Problems and suggested solutions in creating an archive of clinical trials data to permit later meta-analysis: An example of methotrexate trials in rheumatoid arthritis. *Controlled Clinical Trials* 16:342–355, 1995.

Chevron ES, Rounsaville BJ. Evaluating the clinical skills of psychotherapists: A comparison of techniques. *Archives of General Psychiatry* 40:1129–1132, 1983.

Chevron ES, Rounsaville BJ, Rothblum ED, Weissman MM. Selecting psychotherapists to participate in psychotherapy outcome studies: Relationship between psychotherapist characteristics and assesssment of clinical skills. *Journal of Nervous and Mental Disease* 171:348–353, 1983.

Chirikos TN, Nestel G. Further evidence on the economic effects of poor health. *Review of Economics and Statistics* 67:61–69, 1985.

Chouinard G, Albright P. Utility analysis of risperidone cost-effectiveness. *Journal of Clinical Psychopharmacology, in press.*

Christianson JB, Manning W, Lurie N, Stoner TJ, Gray DZ, Popkin M, et al. Utah's prepaid mental health plan: The first year. *Health Affairs* 14:160–172, 1995.

Ciampi A, Silberfeld M, Till JE. Measurement of individual preferences: The importance of "situation-specific" variables. *Medical Decision Making* 2:483–495, 1982.

Ciarlo JA, Windle C. Mental health program evaluation and needs assessment. *New Directions for Program Evaluation* 37:99–120, 1988.

Clark RE. Family costs associated with severe mental illness and substance use. *Hospital and Community Psychiatry* 45:808–813, 1994.

Clark RE, Drake RE. Expenditures of time and money by families of people with severe mental illness and substance use disorders. *Community Mental Health Journal* 30:145–163, 1994.

Clark RE, Teague GB, Ricketts SK, Bush PW, Keller AM, Zubkoff M, et al. Measuring resource use in economic evaluations: determining the social costs of mental illness. *Journal of Mental Health Administration* 21:32–41, 1994.

Cleverley WO. *Essentials of Health Care Finance.* 2nd ed. Rockville: Aspen Publications, 1986.

Cochran WG, Cox GM. *Experimental Designs.* New York: Wiley, 1957.

Cohen J. *Statistical Power Analysis for the Behavioral Sciences.* 2nd ed. Hillsdale, NJ: Lawrence Erlbaum Associates, 1988.

Cohen-Mansfield J. Agitated behavior and cognitive functioning in nursing home residents: Preliminary results. *Clinical Gerontologist* 7:11–22, 1988.

Cook TD. *Meta-Analysis for Explanation: A Casebook.* New York: Russell Sage, 1992.

Cook TD, Campbell DT. *Quasi-Experimentation.* Chicago: Rand McNally, 1979.

Cooper HM, Hedges LV. *The Handbook of Research Synthesis.* New York: Russell Sage, 1992.

Copley-Merriman C, Lair TJ. Valuation of medical resource units collected in health economics studies. *Clinical Therapeutics* 16:553–568, 1994.

Cottler LB, Robbins L, Helzer JE. Reliability of the CIDI-SAM: A comprehensive substance abuse interview. *British Journal of the Addictions* 84:801–814, 1990.

Cropper ML, Aydede SK, Portney PR. Preferences for life saving programs: How the public discounts time and age. *Journal of Risk and Uncertainty* 8:243–265, 1994.

Cullis JG, West PA. *The Economics of Health.* New York: New York University Press, 1979.

Culyer AJ, Wagstaff A. QALYs versus HYEs. *Journal of Health Economics* 11:311–323, 1993.

Danis M, Gerrity MS, Southerland LI, Patrick DL. A comparison of patient, family, and physician assessments of the value of medical intensive care. *Critical Care Medicine* 16:594–600, 1988.

Dardis R. The value of a life: New evidence from the marketplace. *American Economic Review* 70:1077–1082, 1980.

Dauwalder JP, Ciompi L. Cost-effectiveness over 10 years: A study of community-based social psychiatric care in the 1980s. *Social Psychiatry and Psychiatric Epidemiology* 30:171–184, 1995.

Deci PA, Santos AB, Hoitt DW, Schoenwald S, Dias JK. Dissemination of assertive community treatment programs. *Psychiatric Services* 46:676–678, 1995.

DeJong A, Giel R, Slooff CJ, Wiersma D. Social disability and outcome in schizophrenic patients. *British Journal of Psychiatry* 147:631–636, 1985.

Dennis ML, Fairbank JA, Rachal JV. Measuring substance abuse counseling: The methadone enhanced treatment (MET) study approach. Unpublished.

Derogatis LR. *SCL-90-R Administration, Scoring, and Procedures Manual-II.* Towson, MD: Clinical Psychometric Research, 1983.

Derogatis LR, Lipman RS, Rickels K, Uhlenhuth EH, Covi L. The Hopkins Symptom Checklist (HSCL): A self-report symptom inventory. *Behavioral Science* 19:1–15, 1974.

Dey A. *Orthogonal Fractional Factorial Designs.* New York: Wiley, 1985.

Diamond RJ. The role of the hospital in treating the chronically disabled. *New Directions for Mental Health Services* 2:45–56, 1979.

Diamond RJ. Increasing medication compliance in young adult chronic psychiatric patients. *New Directions for Mental Health Services* 21:59–69, 1984.

Dickersin K, Berlin JA. Meta-analysis: State-of-the-science. *Epidemiology Reviews* 14:154–176, 1992.

Dickersin K, Min Y, Meinert CL. Factors influencing publication of research results: Follow-up of applications submitted to two institutional review boards. *Journal of the American Medical Association* 267:374–378, 1992.

Dickey B, Cannon N, McGuire T. Mental health cost studies: Some observations on methodology. *Administration in Mental Health* 13:189–201, 1986a.

Dickey B, Cannon NL, McGuire TG, Gudeman JE. The Quarterway House: A two-year cost study of an experimental residential program. *Hospital and Community Psychiatry* 37:1136–1143, 1986b.

Dickey B, McGuire TG, Cannon NL, Gudeman JE. Mental health cost models: Refinements and applications. *Medical Care* 24:857–867, 1986c.

Dickey B, Wagenaar H. Evaluating health status. In Sederer LI, Dickey B, editors. *Outcomes Assessment in Clinical Practice.* Baltimore: Williams & Wilkins, 1996.

Dickey B, Wagenaar H, Stewart A. Using health status measures with the seriously mentally ill in health services research. *Medical Care* 34:112–116, 1996.

Dobson KS, Shaw BF, Vallis TM. Reliability of a measure of the quality of cognitive therapy. *British Journal of Clinical Psychology* 24:295–300, 1985.

Donaldson C, Atkinson A, Bond J, Wright K. Should QALYs be programme-specific? *Journal of Health Economics* 7:239–257, 1988.

Donham CS, Sensenig AL. Health care indicators. *Health Care Financing Review* 16:201–231, 1994.

Dove HG. Use of the resource-based relative value scale for private insurers. *Health Affairs* Winter:193–201, 1994.

Drake RE, Alterman AI, Rosenberg SR. Detection of substance use disorders in severly mentally ill patients. *Community Mental Health Journal* 29:175–192, 1993a.

Drake RE, Bartels SJ, Teague GB, Noordsy DL, Clark RE. Treatment of substance abuse in severely mentally ill patients. *Journal of Nervous and Mental Disease* 181:606–611, 1993b.

Drake RE, Becker DR, Biesanz JC, Torrey WC, McHugo GJ, Wyzik PF. Rehabilitative day treatment vs. supported employment: I. Vocational outcomes. *Community Mental Health Journal* 30:519–532, 1994.

Drake RE, Osher FC, Wallach MA. Alcohol use and abuse in schizophrenia: A prospective community study. *Journal of Nervous and Mental Disease* 177:408–414, 1989.

Drake RE, Teague GB, Warren RS. New Hampshire's dual diagnosis program for people with severe mental illness and substance abuse. *Addiction and Recovery* 10:35–39, 1990.

Dranove D. Pricing by non-profit institutions: The case of hospital cost-shifting. *Journal of Health Economics* 7:47–57, 1988.

Drummond MF. Allocating resources. *International Journal of Technology Assessment in Health Care* 6:77–92, 1990.

Drummond MF. Cost–benefit analysis in health and health care: Fine in practice, but does it work in theory? In Williams A, Giardina E, editors. *Efficiency in the Public Sector: The Theory and Practice of Cost–Benefit Analysis.* Brookfield, VT: Edward Elgar Publishing, 1993.

Drummond M, Brandt A, Luce B, Rovira J. Standardizing methodologies for economic evaluation in health care. *International Journal of Technology Assessment in Health Care* 9:26–36, 1993.

Drummond M, O'Brien B, Stoddart G, Torrance G. *Methods for the Economic Evaluation of Health Care Programmes.* 2nd ed. Oxford: Oxford University Press, 1997.

Drummond MF, Stoddart GL, Torrance GW. *Methods for the Economic Evaluation of Health Care Programmes.* Oxford: Oxford University Press, 1987.

Dworkin RJ, Friedman LC, Telschow RL, Grant KD, Moffic HS, Sloan VJ. The longitudinal use of the Global Assessment Scale in multiple-rater situations. *Community Mental Health Journal* 26:335–344, 1990.

Ebbesen EB, Konecni VJ. On the external validity of decision-making research: What do we know about decisions in the real world? In Wallsten TS, editor. *Cognitive Processes in Choice and Decision Behavior.* Hillsdale, NJ: Lawrence Erlbaum Associates, 1980.

Edwards BC, Lambert MJ, Moran PW, McCully T, Smith KC, Ellingson AG. A meta-analytic comparison of the Beck Depression Inventory and the Hamilton Rating Scale for Depression as measures of treatment outcome. *British Journal of Clinical Psychology* 23:93–99, 1984.

Efron B, Tibshirani RJ. *An Introduction to the Bootstrap.* New York: Chapman and Hall, 1993.

Elkin I. The NIMH Treatment of Depression Collaborative Research Program: Where we began and where we are. In Bergin AE, Garfield SL, editors. *Handbook of Psychotherapy and Behavior Change.* 4th ed. New York: Wiley, 1993.

Elkin I, Parloff MB, Hadley SW, Autrey JH. NIMH Treatment of Depression Collaborative Research Program: Background and research plan. *Archives of General Psychiatry* 42:305–316, 1985.

Elkin I, Shea MT, Watkins JT, Imber SD, Sotsky SM, Collins JF, et al. NIMH Treatment of Depression Collaborative Research Program: General effectiveness of treatments. *Archives of General Psychiatry* 46:971–892, 1989.

Ellsworth RB, Foster L, Childers B, Arthur G, Krocker D. Hospital and community adjustment as perceived by psychiatric patients, their families, and staff. *Journal of Consulting and Clinical Psychology Monograph* 32, Part 2:1–14, 1968.

Endicott J, Nee J. Endicott Work Productivity Scale (EWPS): A new measure to assess treatment effects. *Psychopharmacology Bulletin* 33:13–16, 1997.

Endicott J, Spitzer RL. What! Another rating scale? The Psychiatric Evaluation Form. *Journal of Nervous and Mental Disease* 154:88–104, 1972.

Endicott J, Spitzer RL, Fleiss JL, Cohen J. The Global Assessment Scale: A procedure for measuring overall severity of psychiatric disturbance. *Archives of General Psychiatry* 33:766–771, 1976.

Essock SM. Clozapine's cost effectiveness (letter). *American Journal of Psychiatry* 152:152, 1995.

Essock SM, Hargreaves WA, Covell NH, Goethe J. Clozapine's effectiveness for patients in state hospitals: Results from a randomized trial. *Psychopharmacology Bulletin* 32:683–697, 1996b.

Essock SM, Hargreaves WA, Dohm FA, Goethe J, Carver L, Hipshman L. Clozapine eligibility among state hospital patients. *Schizophrenia Bulletin* 22:15–25, 1996a.

Essock SM, Kontos N. Implementing assertive community treatment teams. *Psychiatric Services* 46:679–683, 1995.

Esterbrook PJ, Berlin JA, Gopalan R, Matthews DR. Publication bias in research. *Lancet* 337:867–872, 1991.

Estroff S. *Making It Crazy: An Ethnography of Psychiatric Clients in an American Community.* Berkeley: University of California Press, 1981.

Evans WN, Viscusi WK. Income effects and the value of health. *The Journal of Human Resources* 28:497–518, 1993.

Fairweather GW, editor. *New Directions for Mental Health Services* 7, 1980.

Farkas MD, Cohen MR, Nemec PB. Psychiatric rehabilitation programs: Putting concepts into practice? *Community Mental Health Journal* 24:7–21, 1988.

Fawcett J, Epstein P, Fiester SJ, Elkin I, Autry JH. Clinical Management-Imipramine/Placebo Administration Manual: NIMH Treatment of Depression Collaborative Research Program. *Psychopharmacology Bulletin* 23:309–324, 1987.

Feinstein AR. Scientific standards in epidemiologic studies of the menace of daily life. *Science* 242:1257–1263, 1988.

Feldstein PJ. *Health Care Economics.* 3rd ed. New York: Delmar Publishers, 1988.

Fenton FR, Tessier L, Struening EL, Smith FA, Benoit C, Contandiopoulos AP, et al. A two-year follow-up of a comparative trial of the cost-effectiveness of home and hospital psychiatric treatment. *Canadian Journal of Psychiatry* 29:205–211, 1984.

Finkler SA, Knickman JR, Hendrickson G, Lipkin M. A comparison of work-sampling and time-and-motion techniques for studies in health services research. *Health Services Research* 28:577–597, 1993.

Finney J, Moos R. Environmental assessment and evaluation research: Examples from mental health and substance abuse programs. *Evaluation and Program Planning* 7:151–167, 1984.

Finney JW, Moos RH, editors. *Evaluation & Program Planning* 12, 1989.

Fisher PW, Shaffer D, Piacentini J, Lapkin J, Kafantaris V, Leonard H, et al. Sensitivity of the Diagnostic Interview Schedule for Children, 2nd edition (DISC-2.1) for specific diagnoses of children and adolescents. *Journal of the American Academy of Child and Adolescent Psychiatry* 32:666–673, 1993.

Fogelson DL, Nuechterlein KH, Asarnow RF, Subotnik KL, Talovic SA. Interrater reliability of the structured clinical interview for DSM-III-R, Axis II: Schizophrenia spectrum and affective spectrum disorders. *Psychiatry Research* 39:55–63, 1991.

Foster EM, McLanahan S. An illustration of the use of instrumental variables: Do neighborhood conditions affect a young person's chance of finishing high school. *Psychological Methods* 1:249–260, 1996.

Frank R. Cost–benefit analysis in mental health services: A review of the literature. *Administration in Mental Health* 8:161–176, 1981.

Frank RG. Regulatory responses to information deficiencies in the market for mental health services. In Taube CA, Mechanic D, Hohmann AA, editors. *The Future of Mental Health Services Research*. DHHS (ADM) 89-1600. Rockville, MD: US Department of Health and Human Services, 1989.

Frank RG. Cost–benefit evaluations in mental health: Implications for financing policy. *Advances in Health Economics and Health Services Research* 14:1–16, 1993.

Frank RG, Manning WG, editors. *Economics and Mental Health*. Baltimore: Johns Hopkins University Press, 1992.

Franklin JL, Solovitz B, Mason M, Clemons JR, Miller GE. An evaluation of case management. *American Journal of Public Health* 77:674–678, 1987.

Franks DD. Economic contribution of families caring for persons with severe and persistent mental illness. *Administration and Policy in Mental Health* 18:9–18, 1990.

Frisman L, Rosenheck R. The treatment of transfer payments in cost–effectiveness and cost–benefit analysis. Unpublished.

Froberg DG, Kane RL. Methodology for measuring health-state preferences-I: Measurement strategies. *Journal of Clinical Epidemiology* 42:345–354, 1989a.

Froberg DG, Kane RL. Methodology for measuring health-state preferences-II: Scaling methods. *Journal of Clinical Epidemiology* 42:459–471, 1989b.

Froberg DG, Kane RL. Methodology for measuring health-state preferences-III: Population and context effects. *Journal of Clinical Epidemiology* 42:585–592, 1989c.

Froberg DG, Kane RL. Methodology for measuring health-state preferences-IV: Progress and a research agenda. *Journal of Clinical Epidemiology* 42:675–685, 1989d.

Gaffan EA, Tsaousis I, Kemp-Wheeler SM. Researcher allegiance and meta-analysis: The case of cognitive therapy for depression. *Journal of Consulting and Clinical Psychology* 63:966–980, 1995.

Gafni A. Willingness-to-pay as a measure of benefits. *Medical Care* 29:1246–1252, 1991.

Gafni A, Birch S. Preferences for outcomes in economic evaluation: An economic approach to addressing economic problems. *Social Science and Medicine* 40:767–776, 1995.

Gafni A, Birch S, Mehrez A. Economics, health and health economics: HYE versus QALYs. *Journal of Health Economics* 11:325–339, 1993.

Ganiats TG, Wong AF. Evaluation of cost–effectiveness research: A survey of recent publications. *Family Medicine* 23:457–462, 1991.

Garber AM, Phelps CE. *Economic Foundations of Cost-Effectiveness Analysis*. Cambridge, MA: National Bureau of Economic Research Working Paper Series, 1992.

Getzen TE. Medical care price indexes: Theory, construction and empirical analysis of the US series 1927–1990. *Advances in Health Economics and Health Services Research* 13:83–128, 1992.

Gibbons RD, Hedeker D. Application of random-effects probit regression models. *Journal of Consulting and Clinical Psychology* 62:285–296, 1994.

Gibbons RD, Hedeker D, Elkin I, Waternaux C, Kraemer HC, Greenhouse JB, et al. Some conceptual and statistical issues in analysis of longitudinal psychiatric data. *Archives of General Psychiatry* 50:739–750, 1993.

Gibbons RD, Hedeker D, Waternaux CM, Davis J. Random regression models: A comprehensive approach to the analysis of longitudinal psychiatric data. *Psychopharmacology Bulletin* 24:438–443, 1988.

Glass GV. Primary, secondary, and meta-analysis research. *Educational Researcher* 6:3–8, 1976.

Gold MR, Russell LB, Siegel JE, Weinstein MC, editors. *Cost-Effectiveness in Health and Medicine*. New York: Oxford University Press, 1996.

Goldberg D. Cost–effectiveness studies in the treatment of schizophrenia: A review. *Schizophrenia Bulletin* 17:453–459, 1991.

Goldberg D. Cost-effectiveness in the treatment of patients with schizophrenia. *Acta Psychiatrica Scandinavica* 89:89–92, 1994.

Goldberg D. Cost–effectiveness studies in the evaluation of mental health services in the community: Current knowledge and unsolved problems. *International Clinical Psychopharmacology* Suppl 5:29–34, 1995.

Goldman HH, Skodol AE, Lave TR. Revising axis V for DSM-IV: A review of measures of social functioning. *American Journal of Psychiatry* 149:1148–1156, 1992.

Goldschmidt Y, Gafni A. A managerial approach to allocating indirect fixed costs in health care organizations. *Health Care Management Review* 15:43–51, 1990.

Goldstein MK, Clarke AE, Michelson D, Garber AL, Bergen MR, Lenert LA. Developing and testing a multimedia presentation of a health-state description. *Medical Decision Making* 14:336–344, 1994.

Goldstein R. Power and sample size via MS/PC-DOS computers. *American Statistician* 43:253–260, 1989.

Goodman J, Greene E. The use of paraphrase analysis in the simplification of jury instructions. *Journal of Social Behavior and Personality* 4:237–251, 1989.

Graboyes RF. Medical care price indexes. *Economic Quarterly* 80:69–89, 1994.

Grad J, Sainsbury P. Mental illness and the family. *Lancet* i:544–547, 1963.

Grad J, Sainsbury P. The effects that patients have on their families in a community care and control psychiatric service: A two year follow-up. *British Journal of Psychiatry* 114:265–278, 1968.

Green DP, Kahneman D, Kunreuther H. How the scope and method of public funding affect willingness to pay for public goods. *Public Opinion Quarterly* 58:49–67, 1994.

Green RS, Gracely EJ. Selecting a rating scale for evaluating services to the chronically mentally ill. *Community Mental Health Journal* 23:91–102, 1987.

Greenhouse JB. Clinical trials in psychiatry: Should protocol deviation censor patient data? A comment. *Neuropsychopharmacology* 6:53–55, 1992.

Groves RM, Fultz NH, Martin E. Direct questioning about comprehension in a survey setting. In Tanur JA, editor. *Questions about Questions: Inquiries into the Cognitive Bases of Surveys.* New York: Russell Sage Foundation, 1991.

Gubman GD, Tessler RC. The impact of mental illness on families. *Journal of Family Issues* 8:226–245, 1987.

Guillette W, Crowley B, Savitz SA, Goldberg FD. Day hospitalization as a cost-effective alternative to inpatient care: A pilot study. *Hospital and Community Psychiatry* 29:525–527, 1978.

Gur RE, Mozley PD, Resnick SM, Levick S, Erwin R, Saykin AJ, et al. Relations among clinical scales in schizophrenia. *American Journal of Psychiatry* 148:472–478, 1991.

Hadorn DC, Hays RD, Uebersax J, Hauber T. Improving task comprehension in the measurement of health state preferences: A trial of informational cartoon figures and a paired-comparison task. *Journal of Clinical Epidemiology* 45:233–243, 1992.

Hahn B, Lefkowitz D. *Annual Expenses and Sources of Payment for Health Care Services.* ACHPR 93-0007. Rockville, MD: US Department of Health and Human Services, 1992.

Hamilton M. A rating scale for depression. *Journal of Neurology, Neurosurgery and Psychiatry* 23:56–62, 1960.

Hargreaves WA. Methadone dose and duration for maintenance treatment. In Cooper JR, Altman F, Brown BS, Czechowicz D, editors. *Research on the Treatment of Narcotic Addiction: State of the Art.* DHHS (ADM) 83-1281. Washington, DC: Department of Health and Human Services, 1983.

Hargreaves WA. A capitation model for providing mental health services in California. *Hospital and Community Psychiatry* 43:275–277, 1992.

Hargreaves WA, Catalano R, Hu TW, Cuffel B. Mental health services research. In Schooler NR, editor. *Comprehensive Clinical Psychology, Vol. 3: Research Methods.* Oxford: Elsevier, in press.

Hargreaves WA, Chouljian T, Coppolino C, Hughes R, Mance R, Wade J. Monitoring service implementation in controlled services trials (abstract). *Schizophrenia Research* 4:289, 1991.

Hargreaves WA, Jerrell JM, Fares S. Measuring program practices. Unpublished.

Hargreaves WA, LeGoullon M, Binder R, Reus V, Zachary R. Neuroleptic dose: A statistical model for analyzing historical trends. *Journal of Psychiatric Research* 23:199–214, 1987.

Hargreaves WA, Shumway M. Effectiveness of mental health services for the severely mentally ill. In Taube CA, Mechanic D, Hohmann AA, editors. *The Future of Mental Health Services Research.* DHHS (ADM) 89-1600. Rockville, MD: US Department of Health and Human Services, 1989.

Hargreaves WA, Shumway M. Pharmacoeconomics of antipsychotic drug therapy. *Journal of Clinical Psychiatry* 57:66–76, 1996.

Hatziandreu EJ, Brown RE, Revicki DA, Turner R, Martindale J, Levine S. Cost utility of maintenance treatment of recurrent depression with sertraline versus episodic treatment with dothiepin. *Pharmacoeconomics* 5:249–268, 1994.

Heckman J. Sample selection bias: A specification error. *Econometrica* 47:153–161, 1979.

Hedeker D. *MIXREG: A Fortran Program for Mixed-Effects Linear Regression Models.* Chicago: University of Illinois, 1993a.

Hedeker D. *MIXOR: A Fortran Program for Mixed-Effects Ordinal Probit and Logistic Regression.* Chicago: University of Illinois, 1993b.

Hedges LV. Estimation of effect size from a series of independent experiments. *Psychological Bulletin* 92:490–499, 1982.

Hedges LV. Estimation of effect size under nonrandom sampling: The effects of censoring studies yielding statistically insignificant mean differences. *Journal of Educational Statistics* 9:61–85, 1984.

Hedges LV, Olkin I. *Statistical Methods for Meta-Analysis.* Orlando, FL: Academic Press, 1985.

Heinsman DT, Shadish WR. Assignment methods in experimentation: When do nonrandomized experiments approximate answers from randomized experiments? *Psychological Methods* 1:154–169, 1996.

Helzer JE, Robins LN, McEvoy LT, Spitznagel EL, Stoltzman RK, Farmer A, et al. A comparison of clinical and diagnostic interview schedule diagnoses. Physician reexamination of lay-interviewed cases in the general population. *Archives of General Psychiatry* 42:657–666, 1985.

Helzer JE, Spitznagel EL, McEvoy L. The predictive validity of lay Diagnostic Interview Schedule diagnoses in the general population: A comparison with physician examiners. *Archives of General Psychiatry* 44:1069–1077, 1987.

Henderson WG, Moritz T, Goldman S, Copeland J, Sethi G. Use of cumulative meta-analysis in the design, monitoring, and final analysis of a clinical trial: A case study. *Controlled Clinical Trials* 16:331–341, 1995.

Hesselbrock M, Babor TF, Hesselbrock V, Meyer RE, Workman K. "Never believe an alcoholic"? On the validity of self-report measures of alcohol dependence and related constructs. *International Journal of the Addictions* 18:593–609, 1983.

Hill CE, O'Grady KE, Elkin I. Applying the Collaborative Study of Psychotherapy Rating Scale to rate therapist adherence in cognitive-behavior therapy, interpersonal therapy, and clinical management. *Journal of Consulting and Clinical Psychology* 60:73–79, 1992.

Hodges K. Structured interviews for assessing children. *Journal of Child Psychology and Psychiatry and Allied Disciplines* 34:49–68, 1993.

Holmes A, Culler S, Freund D. Recommendations for presentation of variable estimates and guideline costs. In Grady M, Weid K, editors. *Cost Analysis Methodology for Clinical Practice Guidelines Conference Proceedings.* Rockville, MD: Agency for Health Care Policy and Research, 1995.

Hoult J. Community care of the acutely mentally ill. *British Journal of Psychiatry* 149:137–144, 1986.

Hoult J, Reynolds I. Schizophrenia: A comparative trial of community oriented and hospital oriented psychiatric care. *Acta Psychiatrica Scandinavica* 69:359–372, 1984.

Hoult J. Reynolds I, Charbonneau-Powis M, Coles P, Briggs J. A controlled study of psychiatric hospital versus community treatment: The effect on relatives. *Australia and New Zealand Journal of Psychiatry* 15:323–328, 1981.

Hoult J, Reynolds I, Charbonneau-Powis M, Weekes P, Briggs J. Psychiatric treatment versus community treatment: The results of a randomised trial. *Australia and New Zealand Journal of Psychiatry* 37:160–167, 1983.

Hoult J, Rosen A, Reynolds I. Community orientated treatment compared to psychiatric hospital orientated treatment. *Social Science and Medicine* 18:1005–1010, 1984.

Hu T. *Econometrics: An Introductory Analysis.* 2nd ed. Baltimore: University Park, 1982.

Hu T. Cost–effectiveness analysis of three case management programs in mental health services. Unpublished.

Hu T, Hausman J. Cost-effectiveness of community based care for individuals with mental health problems. Unpublished.

Hu T, Jerrell J. Cost-effectiveness of alternative approaches in treating the severely mentally ill in California. *Schizophrenia Bulletin* 17:461–468, 1991.

Hu T, Jerrell J. *Services Variations and Costs of Case Management for Severely Mentally Ill Clients.* Berkeley: Institute for Mental Health Services Research Working Paper Series, 1993.

Hu T, Sandifer F. *Synthesis of Cost of Illness Methodology (Final Report).* Washington, DC: Public Service Laboratory, 1981.

Hudziak JJ, Helzer JE, Wetzel MW, Kessel KB, McGee B, Janca A, et al. Use of the DSM-III-R checklist for initial diagnostic assessments. *Comprehensive Psychiatry* 34:375–383, 1993.

Iyengar SI, Greenhouse JB. Selection models and the file drawer problem. *Statistical Science* 3:109–117, 1988.

Jacobs P. *The Economics of Health and Medical Care.* 3rd ed. Gaithersburg, MD: Aspen Publishers, 1991.

Jacoby J, McEwen T, Guynes R. *National Baseline Information on Offender Processing Costs: Source Data.* Washington, DC: Jefferson Institute for Justice Studies, 1987.

Jerrell J, Hu T. Cost-effectiveness of intensive clinical and case management compared to an existing system of care. *Inquiry* 26:224–234, 1989.

Jerrell JM, Hargreaves W. *The Operating Philosophy of Community Programs.* Berkeley: Institute for Mental Health Services Research Working Paper Series, 1991.

Jerrell JM, Hu T, Ridgely MS. Cost-effectiveness of substance disorder interventions for people with severe mental illness. *The Journal of Mental Health Administration* 21:283–297, 1994.

Johannesson M. The concept of cost in the economic evaluation of health care. *International Journal of Technology in Health Care* 10:675–682, 1994.

Johannesson M, Jonsson B. Willingness to pay for antihypertensive therapy—results of a Swedish pilot study. *Journal of Health Economics* 10:461–474, 1991.

Johansson PO. *An Introduction to Modern Welfare Economics.* New York: Cambridge University Press, 1991.

Kahneman D, Tversky A. The psychology of preference. *Scientific American* 246:160–173, 1982.

Kalaian HA, Raudenbush SW. A multivariate mixed linear model for meta-analysis. *Psychological Methods* 1:227–235, 1996.

Kamlet MS, Paul N, Greenhouse J, Kupfer D, Frank E, Wade M. Cost utility analysis of maintenance treatment for recurrent depression. *Controlled Clinical Trials* 16:17–40, 1995.

Kaplan RM. Using quality of life information to set priorities in health policy. *Social Indicators Research* 33:121–163, 1994a.

Kaplan RM. Value judgment in the Oregon Medicaid experiment. *Medical Care* 32:975–988, 1994b.

Kaplan RM, Anderson JP. The General Health Policy Model: An integrated approach. In Spilker B, editor. *Quality of Life Assessments in Clinical Trials.* New York: Raven Press, 1990.

Kaplan RM, Bush JW, Berry CC. The reliability, stability, and generalizability of a health status index. Proceedings of the American Statistical Association, Social Statistics Section, 1978.

Kaplan RM, Bush JW, Berry CC. Health status index: Category rating versus magnitude estimation for measuring levels of well-being. *Medical Care* XVII:501–525, 1979.

Kaplan RM, Ernst JA. Do category rating scales produce biased preference weights for a health index? *Medical Care* 21:193–207, 1983.

Kaplan RM, Feeny D, Revicki DA. Methods for assessing relative importance in preference based outcome measures. *Quality of Life Research* 2:467–475, 1993.

Kartzinel R, Lisook AB, Rullo B, Severe JB, Spilker B. Clinical trial implementation. In Prien RF, Robinson DS, editors. *Clinical Evaluation of Psychotropic Drugs: Principles and Guidelines.* New York: Raven Press, 1994.

Katz MM, Lyerly SB. Methods for measuring adjustment and social behavior in the community: I. Rationale, description, discriminative validity and scale development. *Psychological Reports* 13:503–535, 1963.

Kay SR, Fiszbein A, Opler LA. The positive and negative syndrome scale (PANSS) for schizophrenia. *Schizophrenia Bulletin* 13:261–276, 1987.

Kay SR, Wolkenfeld F, Murrill LM. Profiles of aggression among psychiatric patients: I. Nature and prevalence. *Journal of Nervous and Mental Disease* 176:539–546, 1988.

Keeler EB, Cretin S. Discounting of life-saving and other nonmonetary effects. *Management Science* 29:300–306, 1983.

Kelman S. Cost–benefit analysis: an ethical critique. In Gilroy JM, Wade M, editors. *The Moral Dimensions of Public Policy Choice: Beyond the Market Paradigm.* Pittsburgh: University of Pittsburgh Press, 1992.

Kessler RC, McGonagle KA, Zhao S, Nelson CB, Hughes M, Eshleman S, et al. Lifetime and 12-month prevalence of DSM-III-R psychiatric disorders in the United States: Results from the National Comorbidity Survey. *Archives of General Psychiatry* 51:8–19, 1994.

Knapp MRJ. *The Economics of Social Care.* London: Macmillan, 1984.

Knapp MRJ. Principles of applied cost research. In Netten A, Beecham J, editors. *Costing Community Care: Theory and Practice.* Aldershot, England: Ashgate Publishing, 1993.

Knapp MRJ. *The Economic Evaluation of Mental Health Care.* Aldershot, England: Ashgate Publishing, 1995a.

Knapp MRJ. Costs and outcomes: Variations and comparisons. In Knapp MRJ, editor. *The Economic Evaluation of Mental Health Care.* Aldershot, England: Ashgate Publishing, 1995b.

Knapp MRJ, Beecham J. Reduced list costings: Examination of an informed short cut in mental health research. *Health Economics* 2:313–322, 1993.

Knapp M, Beecham J, Koutsogeorgopoulou V, Hallam A, Fenyo A, Marks IM, et al. Service use and costs of home-based versus hospital-based care for people with serious mental illness. *British Journal of Psychiatry* 165:195–203, 1994.

Knight GP, Fabes RA, Higgins DA. Concerns about drawing causal inferences from meta-analyses: An example in the study of gender differences in aggression. *Psychological Bulletin* 119:410–421, 1996.

Knoedler WH. How the Training in Community Living program helps patients work. *New Directions for Mental Health Services* 2:57–66, 1979.

Knoedler WH. The continuous treatment team model: The role of the psychiatrist. *Psychiatric Annals* 19:35–40, 1989.

Koopmanschap MA, van Ineveld BM. Towards a new approach for estimating indirect costs of disease. *Social Science and Medicine* 34:1005–1010, 1992.

Koran LM, Agras WS, Rossiter EM, Arnow B, Schneider JA, Telch CF, et al. Comparing the cost effectiveness of psychiatric treatments: bulimia nervosa. *Psychiatry Research* 58:13–21, 1995.

Kraemer HC. Clinical trials in psychiatry: Should protocol deviation censor patient data? A comment. *Neuropsychopharmacology* 6:51–52, 1992.

Kraemer HC, Pruyn JP. The evaluation of different approaches to randomized clinical trials. *Archives of General Psychiatry* 47:1163–1169, 1990.

Krahn M, Gafni A. Discounting in the economic evaluation of health care interventions. *Medical Care* 31:403–418, 1993.

Krosnick JA, Alwin DF. An evaluation of a cognitive theory of response-order effects in survey measurement. *Public Opinion Quarterly* 51:201–219, 1987.

Krupnick JL, Pincus HA. The cost-effectiveness of psychotherapy: A plan for research. *American Journal of Psychiatry* 149:1295–1305, 1992.

LaFond JQ, Durham ML. *Back to the Asylum: The Future of Mental Health Law and Policy in the United States.* New York: Oxford University Press, 1992.

Laird NM, Ware JH. Random effects models for longitudinal data. *Biometrics* 38:963–974, 1982.

Lambert MJ, Hatch DR, Kingston MD, Edwards BC. Zung, Beck, and Hamilton Rating Scales as measures of treatment outcome: A meta-analytic comparison. *Journal of Consulting and Clinical Psychology* 54:54–59, 1986.

Lambert MJ, Masters KS, Astle D. An effect-size comparison of the Beck, Zung, and Hamilton Rating Scales for Depression: A three-week and twelve-week analysis. *Psychological Reports* 63:467–470, 1988.

Landefeld SJ, Seskin EP. The economic value of life: Linking theory to practice. *American Journal of Public Health* 72:555–566, 1982.

Laska EM. Clinical trials in psychiatry: Should protocol deviation censor patient data? A comment. *Neuropsychopharmacology* 6:57–58, 1992.

Laska EM, Klein DF, Lavori PW, Levine J, Robinson DS. Design issues for the clinical evaluation of psychotropic drugs. In Prien RF, Robinson DS, editors. *Clinical Evaluation of Psychotropic Drugs: Principles and Guidelines*. New York: Raven Press, 1994.

Lave JR, Pashos CL, Anderson GF, Brailer D, Bubolz T, Conrad D, et al. Costing medical care: Using Medicare administrative data. *Medical Care* 32:JS77–JS89, 1994.

Lavori PW. Clinical trials in psychiatry: Should protocol deviation censor patient data? *Neuropsychopharmacology* 6:39–48, 1992a.

Lavori PW. Clinical trials in psychiatry: Should protocol deviation censor patient data? Reply to comments. *Neuropsychopharmacology* 6:61–63, 1992b.

Layard R, Glaister S, editors. *Cost–Benefit Analysis*. 2nd ed. Cambridge, England: Cambridge University Press, 1994.

Lefley HP. Impact of mental illness in families of mental health professionals. *Journal of Nervous and Mental Disease* 175:613–619, 1987.

Leginski WA, Croze C, Driggers J, Dumpman S, Geertsen D, Kamis-Gould E, et al. *Data Standards for Mental Health Decision Support Systems*. DHHS (ADM) 89-1589. Rockville, MD: US Department of Health and Human Services, 1989.

Lehman AF. The well-being of chronic mental patients. *Archives of General Psychiatry* 40:369–373, 1983.

Lehman AF. A quality of life interview for the chronically mentally ill. *Evaluation and Program Planning* 11:51–62, 1988.

Lehman AF. Quality of life interview (QOLI). In Sederer LI, Dickey B, editors. *Outcomes Assessment in Clinical Practice*. Baltimore: Williams & Wilkins, 1996.

Lehman AF, Burns BJ. Severe mental illness in the community. In Spilker B, editor. *Quality of Life Assessments in Clinical Trials*. New York: Raven Press, 1990.

Lehman AF, Carpenter WT, Goldman HH, Steinwachs DM. Treatment outcomes in schizophrenia: Implications for practice, policy, and research. *Schizophrenia Bulletin* 21:669–675, 1995.

Lehman AF, Herron JD, Schwartz RP, Myers CP. Rehabilitation for adults with severe mental illness and substance use disorders: A clinical trial. *Journal of Nervous and Mental Disease* 181:86–90, 1993.

Lemke S, Moos RH. Personal and environmental determinants of activity involvement among elderly residents of congregate facilities. *Journals of Gerontology* 44:S139–S148, 1989.

Lenert LA, Michelson D, Flowers C, Bergen MR. IMPACT: An object-oriented graphical environment for construction of multimedia patient interviewing software. Annual Symposium on Computer Applications in Medical Care, 1995.

Lenth RV. PowerPack (Version 2.22) (computer program), 1987.

Liberman RP. Coping with chronic mental disorders: A framework for hope. In Liberman RP, editor. *Psychiatric Rehabilitation of Chronic Mental Patients*. Washington, DC: American Psychiatric Press, Inc. 1988.

Light RJ, Pillemer DB. *Summing Up: The Science of Reviewing Research*. Cambridge, MA: Harvard University Press, 1984.

Lipsey MW. Theory as method: Small theories of treatments. In Sechrest L, Perrin E, Bunker J, editors. *Research Methodology: Strengthening Causal Interpretations of Nonexperimental Data.* DHHS (PHS) 90-3454. Rockville, MD: US Department of Health and Human Services, 1990.

Lipsey MW, Pollard JA. Driving toward theory in program evaluation: More models to choose from. *Evaluation & Program Planning* 12:317–328, 1989.

Llewellyn-Thomas H, Sutherland HJ, Tibshirani R, Ciampi A, Till JE, Boyd NF. Describing health states: Methodologic issues in obtaining values for health states. *Medical Care* 22:543–552, 1984.

Loomes G, McKenzie L. The use of QALYs in health care decision making. *Social Science and Medicine* 28:299–308, 1989.

Louviere JL. *Analyzing Decision Making: Metric Conjoint Analysis.* Newbury Park, CA: Sage, 1988.

Lubeck DP, Yelin EH. A question of value: Measuring the impact of chronic disease. *The Milbank Quarterly* 66:444–464, 1988.

Luce BR, Simpson K. Methods of cost–effectiveness analysis: Areas of consensus and debate. *Clinical Therapeutics* 17:109–125, 1995.

Luft HS. The impact of poor health on earnings. *Review of Economics and Statistics* 57:43–52, 1975.

Lurie N, Moscovie IS, Finch M, Christianson JB, Popkin MK. Does capitation affect the health of the chronically mentally ill? *Journal of the American Medical Association* 267:3300–3304, 1992.

Maddala GS, Lee L. Recursive models with qualitative endogenous variables. *Annals of Economic and Social Measurement* 5:525–545, 1976.

Makuch R, Simon R. Sample size requirements for evaluating a conservative therapy. *Cancer Treatment Reports* 62:1037–1040, 1978.

Manchanda R, Hirsch SR, Barnes TRE. A review of rating scales for measuring symptom change in schizophrenia. In Thompson C, editor. *The Instruments of Psychiatric Research.* New York: Wiley, 1989.

Mann CC. Can meta-analysis make policy? *Science* 266:960–962, 1994.

Marks IM, Connolly J, Muijen M, Audini B, McNamee G, Lawrence RE. Home-based versus hospital-based care for people with serious mental illness. *British Journal of Psychiatry* 165:179–194, 1994.

Marlatt GA, Miller WR. *Comprehensive Drinker Profile.* Odessa, FL: Psychological Assessment Resources, 1984.

Marx AJ, Test MA, Stein LI. Extrohospital management of severe mental illness. *Archives of General Psychiatry* 29:505–511, 1973.

McCaffree KM. *Program Evaluation in the Health Fields.* New York: Behavioral Publications, 1969.

McFarlane WR, Dushay RA, Stastny P, Deakins SM, Link B. A comparison of two levels of family-aided assertive community treatment. *Psychiatric Services* 47:744–750, 1996.

McFarlane WR, Stastny P. *Treatment Manual for Training in Community Living.* New York: New York State Psychiatric Institute, 1987.

McFarlane WR, Stastny P, Deakins S. Family-aided assertive community treatment: A comprehensive rehabilitation and intensive case management approach for persons with schizophrenic disorders. *New Directions for Mental Health Services* 53:43–54, 1992.

McGrew JH, Bond GR. Critical ingredients of assertive community treatment: Judgements of the experts. *Journal of Mental Health Administration* 22:113–125, 1995.

McGrew JH, Bond GR, Dietzen L, McKasson M, Miller LD. A multisite study of client outcomes in assertive community treatment. *Psychiatric Services* 46:696–701, 1995.

McGrew JH, Bond GR, Dietzen L, Salyers M. Measuring the fidelity of implementation of a mental health program model. *Journal of Consulting and Clinical Psychology* 62:670–678, 1994.

McGuire TG. Measuring the economic costs of schizophrenia. *Schizophrenia Bulletin* 17:375–388, 1991.

McGuire TG, Weisbrod BA, editors. *Economics and Mental Health.* ADM 81-1114. Rockville, MD: US Department of Health and Human Services, 1981a.

McGuire TG, Weisbrod BA. Perspectives on the economics of mental health. *Journal of Human Resources* 16:494–500, 1981b.

McHorney CA, Ware JE, Lu JF, Sherbourne CD. The MOS 36-item Short-Form Health Survey (SF-36): III. Tests of data quality, scaling assumptions, and reliability across diverse patient groups. *Medical Care* 32:40–66, 1994.

McHugo GJ, Drake RE, Burton HL, Ackerson TH. A scale for assessing the stage of substance abuse treatment in persons with severe mental illness. *Journal of Nervous and Mental Disease* 183:762–767, 1995.

Mechanic D, Bevilacqua JJ, Goldman H, Hargreaves WA, Howe J, Knisley M, et al. Research resources. *Schizophrenia Bulletin* 18:669–696, 1992.

Mehrez A, Gafni A. The healthy-years-equivalents: How to measure them using the standard gamble approach. *Medical Decision Making* 11:140–146, 1991.

Meltzer HY, Cola P. Clozapine's cost effectiveness. *American Journal of Psychiatry* 152:153–154, 1995.

Meltzer HY, Cola P, Way L, Thompson PA, Bastani B, Davies MA, et al. Cost effectiveness of clozapine in neuroleptic-resistant schizophrenia. *American Journal of Psychiatry* 150:1630–1638, 1993.

Merkhofer MW. *Decision Science and Social Risk Management: A Comparative Evaluation of Cost–Benefit Analysis, Decision Analysis, and Other Formal Decision-Aiding Approaches.* Boston: Kluwer Academic Publishers, 1987.

Merson S, Tyrer P, Onyett S, Lack S, Birkett P, Lynch S, et al. Early intervention in psychiatric emergencies: A controlled clinical trial. *Lancet* 339:1311–1314, 1992.

Miller GA. The magical number seven plus or minus two: Some limits on our capacity to process information. *Psychological Review* 63:81–97, 1956.

Miller NE, Magruder KM. *The Cost Effectiveness of Psychotherapy: A Guide for Practitioners, Researchers and Policymakers,* in press.

Miller WR, Del Boca FK. Measurement of drinking behavior using the Form 90 family of instruments. *Journal of Studies on Alcohol* 12:112–118, 1994.

Miranda J, Munoz RF, Shumway M. Depression prevention research: The need for screening scales that truly predict. In Attkisson CC, Zich JM, editors. *Depression in Primary Care: Screening and Detection.* New York: Routledge, 1990.

Mishan EJ. *Cost–Benefit Analysis: An Informal Introduction.* 4th ed. London: Unwin Hyman, 1988.

Molken M, Van Doorslaer E, Van Vliet R. Statistical analysis of cost outcomes in a randomized controlled clinical trial. *Health Economics* 3:333–345, 1994.

Montgomery DC. *Design and Analysis of Experiments.* 2nd ed. New York: John Wiley and Sons, 1976.

Moore MJ, Viscusi WK. Models for estimating discount rates for long-term health risks using labor market data. *Journal of Risk and Uncertainty* 3:381–401, 1990.

Moos R, Igra A. Determinants of the social environments of sheltered care settings. *Journal of Health and Social Behavior* 21:88–98, 1980.

Moos R, Lemke S. *Multiphasic Environmental Assessment Procedure Manual.* Palo Alto: Social Ecology Laboratory, Veterans Administration Medical Center, Stanford University, 1984.

Moos R, Otto J. The Community-Oriented Programs Environment Scale: A methodology for the facilitation and evaluation of social change. *Community Mental Health Journal* 8:28–37, 1972.

Morse G, Calsyn RJ, Allen G, Tempelhoff B, Smith R. Experimental comparison of the effects of three treatment programs for homeless mentally ill people. *Hospital and Community Psychiatry* 43:1005–1010, 1992.

Morss SE, Lenert LA, Faustman WO. The side effects of antipsychotic drugs and patients' quality of life: Patient education and preference assessment with computers and multimedia. Annual Symposium on Computer Applications in Medical Care, 1993.

Morton SC, Kominski GF, Kahan JP. An examination of the resource-based relative value scale cross-specialty linkage method. *Medical Care* 32:25–39, 1994.

Moscarelli M, Maffei C, Cesana BM, Boato P, Farma T, Grilli A, et al. An international perspective on assessment of negative and positive symptoms in schizophrenia. *American Journal of Psychiatry* 144:1595–1598, 1987.

Moscarelli M, Rupp A, Sartorius N, editors. *Handbook of Mental Health Economics and Health Policy, Vol. 1: Schizophrenia.* Chichester, England: John Wiley & Sons, 1996.

Muijen M, Marks I, Connolly J, Audini B. Home based care and standard hospital care for patients with severe mental illness: A randomised controlled trial. *British Medical Journal* 304:749–754, 1992.

Mulder R. *Evaluation of the Harbinger Program, 1982–1985.* Lansing, MI: Department of Mental Health, 1985.

Mullahy J, Manning W. Statistical issues in cost–effectiveness analysis. In Sloan F, editor. *Valuing Health Care.* Cambridge University Press, 1994.

Mulvey EP, Lidz CW. Measuring patient violence in dangerousnesss research. *Law and Human Behavior* 17:277–288, 1993.

Mungas D, Weiler P, Franzi C, Henry R. Assessment of disruptive behavior associated with dementia: The disruptive behavior rating scales. *Journal of Geriatric Psychiatry and Neurology* 2:196–202, 1989.

Murphy JG, Datel WE. A cost–benefit analysis of community versus institutional living. *Hospital and Community Psychiatry* 27:165–170, 1976.

National Research Council. *Combining Information: Statistical Issues and Opportunities for Research.* Washington, DC: National Academy Press, 1992.

Netten A, Beecham J. *Costing Community Care: Theory and Practice.* Aldershot, England: Ashgate Publishing, 1993.

Nickman NA, Guerrero RM, Bair JN. Self-reported work-sampling methods for evaluating pharmaceutical services. *American Journal of Hospital Pharmacy* 47:1611–1617, 1990.

Noh S, Avison WR. Spouses of discharged patients: Factors associated with their experience of burden. *Journal of Marriage and the Family* 50:377–389, 1988.

Nord E. Methods for quality adjustment of life years. *Social Science and Medicine* 34:559–569, 1992.

Nord E, Richardson J, Macarounas-Kirchmann K. Social evaluation of health care versus personal evaluation of health states. *International Journal of Technology Assessment in Health Care* 9:463–478, 1993.

O'Brien BJ, Drummond MF, Labelle RJ, Willan A. In search of power and significance: Issues in the design and analysis of stochastic cost–effectiveness studies in health care. *Medical Care* 32:150–163, 1994.

O'Connell JF. *Welfare Economic Theory.* Boston: Auburn House Publishing, 1982.

O'Hara MW, Rehm LP. Hamilton Rating Scale for Depression: Reliability and validity of judgements of novice raters. *Journal of Consulting and Clinical Psychology* 51:318–319, 1983.

O'Hare T, Bennett P, Leduc D. Reliability of self-reports of alcohol use by community clients. *Hospital and Community Psychiatry* 42:406–408, 1991.

Oddone E, Cowper P, Hamilton J, Feussner J. A cost–effectiveness analysis of hepatitis B vaccine in predialysis patients. *Health Services Research* 28:97–121, 1993a.

Oddone E, Guarisco S, Simel D. Comparison of housestaff's estimates of their workday activities with results of a random work-sampling study. *Academic Medicine* 68:859–861, 1993b.

Oddone E, Weinberger M, Hurder A, Henderson W, Simel D. Measuring activities in clinical trials using random work sampling: Implications for cost–effectiveness analysis and measurement of the intervention. *Journal of Clinical Epidemiology* 48:1011–1018, 1995.

Olfson M. Assertive community treatment: An evaluation of the experimental evidence. *Hospital and Community Psychiatry* 41:634–641, 1990.

Olsen JA. On what basis should health be discounted? *Journal of Health Economics* 12:39–53, 1993a.

Olsen JA. Time preferences for health gains: An empirical investigation. *Health Economics* 2:257–265, 1993b.

Orwin RG. A fail-safe N for effect size in meta-analysis. *Journal of Educational Statistics* 8:157–159, 1983.

Orwin RG, Corday DS. Effects of deficient reporting on meta-analysis: A conceptual framework and reanalysis. *Psychological Bulletin* 97:134–147, 1985.

Overall JE, Gorham DR. The brief psychiatric rating scale. *Psychological Reports* 10:799–812, 1962.

Overall JE, Gorham DR. The Brief Psychiatric Rating Scale (BPRS): Recent developments in ascertainment and scaling. *Psychopharmacology Bulletin* 24:97–100, 1988.

Overall JE, Starbuck RR. Sample size estimation for randomized pre-post designs. *Journal of Psychiatric Research* 15:51–55, 1979.

Parker G, Hadzi-Pavlovic D. The capacity of a measure of disability (the LSP) to predict hospital readmission in those with schizophrenia. *Psychological Medicine* 25:157–163, 1995.

Parker G, Rosen A, Emdur N, Hadzi-Pavlovic D. The life skills profile: Psychometric properties of a measure assessing function and disability in schizophrenia. *Acta Psychiatrica Scandinavica* 83:145–152, 1991.

Parsonage M, Neuburger H. Discounting and health benefits. *Health Economics* 1:71–76, 1992.

Patrick DL, Bush JW, Chen MM. Methods for measuring levels of well-being for a health status index. *Health Services Research* Fall:228–245, 1973.

Patrick DL, Deyo RA. Generic and disease-specific measures in assessing health status and quality of life. *Medical Care* 27(suppl.3):S217–S232, 1989.

Patrick DL, Erickson P. *Health Status and Health Policy: Quality of Life in Health Care Evaluation and Resource Allocation.* New York: Oxford University Press, 1993.

Patterson DA, Lee M. Field trial of the Global Assessment of Functionining Scale—Modified. *American Journal of Psychiatry* 152:1386–1388, 1995.

Pauker SG, Kassirer JP. Medical progress-decision analysis. *New England Journal of Medicine* 316:250–258, 1987.

Perreault WD. Controlling order effect bias. *Public Opinion Quarterly* 39:544–551, 1976.

Peskin J. *The value of household work in the 1980s.* Washington, DC: American Statistical Association, 1983 Proceedings of the Social Statistics Section, 1984.

Petitti DB. *Meta-Analysis, Decision Analysis, and Cost–Effectiveness Analysis: Methods for Quantitative Synthesis in Medicine.* New York: Oxford University Press, 1994.

Phelps CE, Mushlin AI. On the (near) equivalence of cost–effectiveness and cost–benefit analyses. *International Journal of Technology Assessment in Health Care* 7:12–21, 1991.

Phillips KA, Rosenblatt A. Speaking in tongues: Integrating economics and psychology into health and mental health services outcomes research. *Medical Care Review* 49:191–231, 1992.

Piacentini J, Shaffer D, Fisher P, Schwab-Stone M, Davies M, Gioia P. The Diagnostic Interview Schedule for Children-Revised Version (DISC-R): III. Concurrent criterion validity. *Journal of the American Academy of Child and Adolescent Psychiatry* 32:658–665, 1993.

Pindyck R, Rubinfeld D. *Econometric Models and Economic Forecasts.* 3rd ed. New York: McGraw-Hill, 1991.

Platt S, Weyman A, Hirsch S, Hewett S. The Social Behavior Assessment Schedule: Rationale, contents, scoring and reliability of a new interview schedule. *Social Psychiatry* 15:43–55, 1980.

Pollack S, Bruce P, Borenstein M, Lieberman J. The resampling method of statistical analysis. *Psychopharmacology Bulletin* 30:227–234, 1994.

Powe NR, Griffiths RI. The clinical-economic trial: Promise, problems, and challenges. *Controlled Clinical Trials* 16:377–394, 1995.

Price RH, Moos RH. Toward a taxonomy of inpatient treatment environments. *Journal of Abnormal Psychology* 84:181–188, 1975.

Prochaska JO, DiClemente CC, Norcross JC. In search of how people change: Applications to addictive behaviors. *American Psychologist* 47:1102–1114, 1992.

Propst RN. Standards for clubhouse programs: Why and how they were developed. *Psychosocial Rehabilitation Journal* 16:25–30, 1992.

Przybeck TR, Helzer JE, Janka A. DSM-III-R checklist computer program (computer program). St. Louis: 1988.

Randolph FL. NIMH-funded research demonstrations of (P/ACT) models. *Outlook* 2:9–12, 1992.

Rapp CA, Chamberlain R. Case management services for the chronically mentally ill. *Social Work* 30:417–422, 1985.

Ray JW, Shadish WR. How interchangeable are different estimators of effect size? *Journal of Consulting and Clinical Psychology* 64:1316–1325, 1996.

Read JL, Quinn RJ, Hoefer MA. Measuring overall health: An evaluation of three important approaches. *Journal of Chronic Disease* 40:7S–21S, 1987.

Redelmeier DA, Heller DN. Time preference in medical decision making and cost–effectiveness analysis. *Medical Decision Making* 13:212–217, 1993.

Reed SK, Hennessy KD, Mitchell OS, Babigian HM. A mental health capitation program: II. Cost–benefit analysis. *Hospital and Community Psychiatry* 45:1097–1103, 1994.

Reihman J, Ciarlo JA, Hargreaves WA. A method for obtaining follow-up outcome data. In Hargreaves WA, Attkisson CC, Sorensen JE, editors. *Resource Materials for Community Mental Health Program Evaluation.* 2nd ed. DHEW (ADM) 77-328. Rockville, MD: US Department of Health and Human Services, 1977.

Revicki DA, Brown RE, Palmer W, Bakish D, Rosser WW, Anton SF, Feeny D. Modelling the cost effectiveness of antidepressant treatment in primary care. *Pharmacoeconomics* 8:524–540, 1995.

Revicki DA, Kaplan RM. Relationship between psychometric and utility-based approaches to the measurement of health-related quality of life. *Quality of Life Research* 2:477–487, 1993.

Revicki DA, Luce BR. Methods of pharmacoeconomic evaluation of new medical treatments in psychiatry. *Psychopharmacology Bulletin* 31:57–65, 1995.

Revicki DA, Shakespeare A, Kind P. Preferences for schizoprenia-related health states: A comparison of patients, caregivers and psychiatrists. *International Clinical Psychopharmacology* 11:101–108, 1996.

Rey JM, Starling J, Wever C, Dossetor DR, Plapp JM. Inter-rater reliability of global assessment of functioning in a clinical setting. *Journal of Child Psychology and Psychiatry and Allied Disciplines* 36:787–792, 1995.

Rice DP. *Estimating the Cost of Illness.* DHEW (PHS) 947-6. Washington, DC: US Dept of Health, Education, and Welfare, 1966.

Rice DP, Kelman S, Miller LS. The economic burden of mental illness. *Hospital and Community Psychiatry* 43:1227–1232, 1992.

Rice DP, Kelman S, Miller LS, Dunmeyer S. *The Economic Costs of Alcohol and Drug Abuse and Mental Illness: 1985.* (ADM) 90-1649. Rockville, MD: US Department of Health and Human Services, 1990.

Richardson WJ. *Cost Improvement, Work Sampling, and Short Interval Scheduling.* Reston, VA: Reston Publishing, 1976.

Roberts MJ, Kvalseth TO, Jermstad RL. Work measurement in hospital pharmacy. *Topics in Hospital Pharmacy Management* 2:1–17, 1982.

Robins LN, Helzer JE, Croughan J, Ratcliff KS. National Institute of Mental Health Diagnostic Interview Schedule: Its history, characteristics, and validity. *Archives of General Psychiatry* 38:381–389, 1981.

Robins LN, Regier DA, editors. *Psychiatric Disorders in America: The Epidemiologic Catchment Area Study.* New York: Free Press, 1991.

Robins LN, Wing J, Wittchen HU, Helzer JE, Babor TF, Burke J, et al. The Composite International Diagnostic Interview: An epidemiologic instrument suitable for use in conjunction with different diagnostic systems and different cultures. *Archives of General Psychiatry* 45:1069–1077, 1988.

Robins L, Wing JK, Wittchen HU, Helzer J, Babor TF, Burke J, et al. The Composite International Diagnostic Interview. In Mezzich JE, Jorge MR, Salloum IM, editors. *Psychiatric Epidemiology: Assessment, Concepts and Methods.* Baltimore: Johns Hopkins University Press, 1994.

Robinson JC. Philosophical origins of the economic valuation of life. *The Milbank Quarterly* 64:133–155, 1986.

Robinson JC. Philosophical origins of the social rate of discount in cost–benefit analysis. *The Milbank Quarterly* 68:245–265, 1990.

Rogers JL, Howard KI, Vessey JT. Using significance tests to evaluate equivalence between two experimental groups. *Psychological Bulletin* 113:553–565, 1993.

Rogosa D, Willett J. Understanding correlates of change by modeling individual differences in growth. *Psychometrika* 50:203–228, 1985.

Rosen A. The life skills profile: A measure assessing function and disability in schizophrenia. *Schizophrenia Bulletin* 15:325–337, 1989.

Rosenblatt A, Attkisson CC. Assessing outcomes for sufferers of severe mental disorder: A conceptual framework and review. *Evaluation and Program Planning* 16:347–363, 1993.

Rosenheck R, Charney DS, Frisman LK, Cramer J. Clozapine's cost-effectiveness (letter). *American Journal of Psychiatry* 152:152–153, 1995a.

Rosenheck R, Frisman LK, Neale M. Estimating the capital component of mental health care costs in the public sector. *Administration and Policy in Mental Health* 21:493–509, 1994.

Rosenheck R, Gallup P, Frisman LK. Health care utilization and costs after entry into an outreach program for homeless mentally ill veterans. *Hospital and Community Psychiatry* 44:1166–1171, 1993.

Rosenheck R, Neale M, Frisman L. Issues in estimating the cost of innovative mental health programs. *Psychiatric Quarterly* 66:9–31, 1995b.

Rosenheck R, Neale M, Leaf P, Milstein R, Frisman L. A multi-site experimental cost study of intensive psychiatric community care. *Schizophrenia Bulletin* 21:129–140, 1995c.

Rosenthal R. The "file drawer problem" and tolerance for null results. *Psychological Bulletin* 86:638–641, 1979.

Rosset N, Andreoli A. Crisis intervention and affective disorders: A comparative cost–effectiveness study. *Social Psychiatry and Psychiatric Epidemiology* 30:231–235, 1995.

Rounsaville BJ, Chevron ES, Prusoff BA, Elkin I, Imber S, Sotsky S, et al. The relation between specific and general dimensions of the psychotherapy process in interpersonal psychotherapy of depression. *Journal of Consulting and Clinical Psychology* 55:379–384, 1987.

Rounsaville BJ, Chevron ES, Weissman MM. Specification of techniques in interpersonal psychotherapy. In Williams JBW, Spitzer RL, editors. *Psychotherapy Research: Where Are We and Where Should We Go?* New York: Guilford, 1984.

Rounsaville BJ, Chevron ES, Weissman MM, Prusoff BA, Frank E. Training therapists to perform interpersonal psychotherapy in clinical trials. *Comprehensive Psychiatry* 27:364–371, 1986.

Rubin A. Is case management effective for people with serious mental illness? A research review. *Health and Social Work* 17:138–150, 1992.

Rubin DB. Clinical trials in psychiatry: Should protocol deviation censor patient data? A comment. *Neuropsychopharmacology* 6:59–60, 1992.

Rubin J. Paying for care: Legal developments in the financing of mental health services. *Houston Law Review* 28:143–173, 1991.

Rupp A. The economic consequences of not treating depression. *British Journal of Psychiatry* 166:29–33, 1995.

Rush AJ, Guillion CM, Raskin A, Kellner R, Bartko JJ. Assessment and measurement of clinical change. In Prien RF, Robinson DS, editors. *Clinical Evaluation of Psychotropic Drugs: Principles and Guidelines*. New York: Raven Press, 1994.

Sackett DL, Torrance GW. The utility of different health states as perceived by the general public. *Journal of Chronic Disease* 31:697–704, 1978.

Santos AB, Henggeler SW, Burns BJ, Arana GW, Meisler N. Research on field-based services: Models for reform in the delivery of mental health care to populations with complex clinical problems. *American Journal of Psychiatry* 152:1111–1123, 1995.

Schiller M, Hargreaves WA. Clozapine's cost effectiveness (letter). *American Journal of Psychiatry* 152:151–152, 1995.

Schipper H, Clinch J, Powell V. Definitions and conceptual issues. In Spilker B, editor. *Quality of Life Assessments in Clinical Trials*. New York: Raven Press, 1990.

Schmidt FL. What do data really mean? Research findings, meta-analysis, and cumulative knowledge in psychology. *American Psychologist* 47:1173–1181, 1992.

Schmidt FL. Statistical significance testing and cumulative knowledge in psychology: Implications for training of researchers. *Psychological Methods* 1:115–120, 1996.

Schobel BD. Administrative expenses under OASDI. *Social Security Bulletin* 44:21–28, 1981.

Schoemaker PJH. The expected utility model: Its varients, purposes, evidence and limitations. *Journal of Economic Literature* 20:529–563, 1982.

Schooler NR. How generalizable are the results of clinical trials? *Psychopharmacology Bulletin* 16:29–31, 1980.

Schooler NR, Keith SJ, Severe JB, Matthews S. Acute treatment response and short term outcome of the NIMH treatment strategies in schizophrenia study. *Psychopharmacology Bulletin* 25:331–335, 1989.

Schooler NR, Keith SJ, Severe JB, Matthews SM, Bellack AS, Glick ID, Hargreaves WA, Kane JM, Ninan PT, Frances A, Jacobs M, Lieberman JA, Mance R, Simpson GM, Woerner M. Relapse and rehospitalization during maintenance treatment of schizophrenia: The effects of dose reduction and family treatment. *Archives of General Psychiatry* 54:453–463, 1997.

Schwab-Stone M, Fisher P, Piacentini J, Shaffer D, Davies M, Briggs M. The Diagnostic Interview Schedule for Children-Revised Version (DISC-R): II. Test-retest reliability. *Journal of the American Academy of Child and Adolescent Psychiatry* 32:651–657, 1993.

Scott JE, Dixon LB. Assertive community treatment and case management for schizophrenia. *Schizophrenia Bulletin* 21:657–591, 1995.

Sederer LI, Dickey B, editors. *Outcomes Assessment in Clinical Practice.* Baltimore: Williams & Wilkins, 1996.

Segal DL, Hersen M, Van Hasselt VB. Reliability of the Structured Clinical Interview for DSM-III-R: An evaluative review. *Comprehensive Psychiatry* 35:316–327, 1994.

Senra C. Measures of treatment outcome of depression: An effect size comparison. *Psychological Reports* 75:187–192, 1995.

Serban G. Social stress and functioning inventory for psychotic disorders: Measurement and prediction of schizophrenics' community adjustment. *Comprehensive Psychiatry* 19:337–347, 1978.

Shaffer D, Gould MS, Brasic J, Ambrosini P, Fisher P, Bird H, et al. A children's global assessment scale (CGAS). *Archives of General Psychiatry* 40:1228–1231, 1983.

Shaffer D, Schwab-Stone M, Fisher P, Cohen P, Piacentini J, Davies M, et al. The Diagnostic Interview Schedule for Children-Revised Version (DISC-R): I. Preparation, field testing, interrater reliability, and acceptability. *Journal of the American Academy of Child and Adolescent Psychiatry* 32:643–650, 1993.

Sharfstein SS, Nafziger JC. Community care: Costs and benefits for a chronic patient. *Hospital and Community Psychiatry* 27:170–173, 1976.

Sharp C. *The Economics of Time.* New York: Wiley, 1981.

Shaw BF. Specification of the training and evaluation of cognitive therapists for outcome studies. In Williams JBW, Spitzer RL, editors. *Psychotherapy Research: Where Are We and Where Should We Go?* New York: Guilford, 1984.

Shaw BF, Dobson KS. Competency judgements in training and evaluation of psychotherapists. *Journal of Consulting and Clinical Psychology* 56:666–672, 1988.

Shemo JPD. Cost-effectiveness of providing mental health services: The offset effect. *International Journal of Psychiatry in Medicine* 15:19–30, 1985.

Shrout PE. Clinical trials in psychiatry: Should protocol deviation censor patient data? A comment. *Neuropsychopharmacology* 6:49–50, 1992.

Shumway M. The value of lost productivity due to chronic illness and disability: Implications for study of severe mental illness. Unpublished.

Shumway M, Battle C. Clinicians' preferences for schizophrenia outcomes: A comparison of four methods (abstract). *Schizophrenia Research* 15:197, 1995.

Siegel C, Laska E, Meisner M. Statistical methods for cost–effectiveness analysis. *Controlled Clinical Trials* 17:387–406, 1996.

Silberman G, Droitcour JA, Scullin EW. *Cross Design Synthesis: A New Strategy for Medical Effectiveness Research.* GAO/PEMD-92-18. Washington, DC: US General Accounting Office, 1992.

Simes JR. Publication bias: The case for an international registry of trials. *Journal of Clinical Oncology* 4:1529–1541, 1986.

Sintonen H, Alander V. Comparing the cost–effectiveness analysis of drug regimens in the treatment of duodenal ulcers. *Journal of Health Economics* 9:85–101, 1990.

Sittig DF. Work-sampling: A statistical approach to evaluation of the effects of computers on work patterns in healthcare. *Methods of Information in Medicine* 32:167–174, 1993.

Skre I, Onstad S, Torgersen S, Kringlen E. High interrater reliability for the Structured Clinical Interview for DSM-III-R Axis I (SCID-I). *Acta Psychiatrica Scandinavica* 84:167–173, 1991.

Smith K, Wright K. Informal care and economic appraisal—A discussion of possible methodological approaches. *Health Economics* 3:137–148, 1994.

Smith ML, Glass GV, Miller TL. *The Benefits of Psychotherapy.* Baltimore: Johns Hopkins University Press, 1980.

Smith R, Dobson M. Measuring utility values for QALYs: Two methodological issues. *Economic Evaluation* 2:349–355, 1993.

Solomon P. The efficacy of case management services for severely mentally disabled clients. *Community Mental Health Journal* 28:163–180, 1992.

Sorensen JL, Hargreaves WA, Friedlander S. Child global rating scales: Selecting a measure of client functioning in a large mental health system. *Evaluation and Program Planning* 5:337–347, 1982.

Spilker B, editor. *Quality of Life Assessments in Clinical Trials.* New York: Raven Press, 1990.

Spitzer RL, Endicott J, Fleiss JL, Cohen J. The psychiatric status schedule: A technique for evaluating psychopathology and impairment in role functioning. *Archives of General Psychiatry* 23:41–55, 1970.

Spitzer RL, Williams JB, Gibbon M, First MB. The Structured Clinical Interview for DSM-III-R (SCID): I. History, rationale, and description. *Archives of General Psychiatry* 49:624–629, 1992.

Spitzer RL, Williams JB, Kroenke K, Linzer M, deGruy FV III, Hahn SR, et al. Utility of a new procedure for diagnosing mental disorders in primary care. The Prime-MD 1000 study. *Journal of the American Medical Association* 272:1749–1756, 1994.

Steadman HJ, Monahan J, Appelbaum PS, Grisso T, Mulvey EP, Roth LH, et al. Designing a new generation of risk assessment research. In Monahan J, Steadman HJ, editors. *Violence and Mental Disorder: Developments in Risk Assessment.* Chicago: The University of Chicago, 1994.

Steer RA, Clark DA, Beck AT, Ranieri WF. Common and specific dimensions of self-reported anxiety and depression: A replication. *Journal of Abnormal Psychology* 104:542–545, 1995.

Stegner BL, Bostrom AG, Greenfield TK. Equivalence testing for use in psychosocial and services research: An introduction with examples. *Evaluation and Program Planning* 19:193–198, 1996.

Stein LI, Diamond RJ. A program for difficult-to-treat patients. *New Directions for Mental Health Services* 26:29–39, 1985.

Stein LI, Test MA, editors. *Alternatives to Mental Hospital Treatment.* New York: Plenum, 1978.

Stein LI, Test MA. From the hospital to the community: A shift in the primary locus of care. *New Directions for Mental Health Services* 1:15–32, 1979.

Stein LI, Test MA. Alternative to mental hospital treatment: I. Conceptual model, treatment program, and clinical evaluation. *Archives of General Psychiatry* 37:392–397, 1980.

Stein LI, Test MA. Community treatment of the young adult patient. *New Directions for Mental Health Services* 14:57–67, 1982.

Stein LI, Test MA. The evolution of the Training in Community Living model. *New Directions for Mental Health Services* 26:7–16, 1985.

Stein L, Test MA, Marx A. Alternative to the hospital: A controlled study. *American Journal of Psychiatry* 132:417–422, 1975.

Steinwachs DM, Kasper JD, Skinner EA. Patterns of use and costs among severely mentally ill people. *Health Affairs* 11:178–185, 1992.

Sterling TD. Publication decisions and their possible effects on inferences drawn from tests of significance—or vice versa. *Journal of the American Statistical Association* 54:30–34, 1959.

Stewart AL, Greenfield S, Hays RD, Wells K, Rogers WH, Berry SD, et al. Functional status and well-being of patients with chronic conditions: Results from the Medical Outcomes Study. *Journal of the American Medical Association* 262:907–913, 1989.

Stoddart GL. Economic evaluation methods and health policy. *Evaluation and the Health Professions* 5:393–414, 1982.

Sturm R, Wells KB. How can care for depression become more cost-effective? *Journal of the American Medical Association* 273:51–58, 1995.

Sugar C, Sturm R, Lee T, Olshen R, Shearborne C, Wells K, et al. Use of the SF-12 to estimate utilities in depression via cluster analysis. Unpublished.

Swindle RW, Peterson KA, Paradise MJ, Moos RH. Measuring substance abuse program treatment orientations: The Drug and Alcohol Program Treatment Inventory. *Journal of Substance Abuse* 7:61–78, 1995a.

Swindle RW, Phibbs CS, Paradise MJ, Recine BP, Moos RH. Inpatient treatment for substance abuse patients with psychiatric disorders: A national study of determinants of readmission. *Journal of Substance Abuse* 7:79–97, 1995b.

Taubes G. Looking for the evidence in medicine. *Science* 272:22–24, 1996.

Teague GB, Drake RE, Ackerson TH. Evaluating use of continuous treatment teams for persons with mental illness and substance abuse. *Psychiatric Services* 46:689–695, 1995.

Tessler RC, Gamache GM. *Toolkit for Evaluating Family Experiences with Severe Mental Illness.* Cambridge, MA: Human Services Research Institute, 1995.

Tessler RC, Killian LM, Gubman GD. Stages in family response to mental illness: An ideal type. *Psychosocial Rehabilitation Journal* 10:3–16, 1987.

Test MA. Continuity of care in community treatment. *New Directions for Mental Health Services* 2:15–23, 1979.

Test MA. Training in community living. In Liberman RP, editor. *Handbook of Psychiatric Rehabilitation.* New York: Macmillan Publishing, 1992.

Test MA, Knoedler WH, Allness DJ, Burke SS. Characteristics of young adults with schizophrenic disorders treated in the community. *Hospital and Community Psychiatry* 36:853–858, 1985.

Test MA, Stein LI. Practical guidelines for the community treatment of markedly impaired patients. *Community Mental Health Journal* 12:72–82, 1976.

Test MA, Stein LI. Community treatment of the chronic patient: Research overview. *Schizophrenia Bulletin* 4:350–364, 1978.

Test MA, Stein LI. Alternative to mental hospital treatment: III. Social cost. *Archives of General Psychiatry* 37:409–412, 1980.

Thiemann S, Csernansky JG, Berger PA. Rating scales in research: The case of negative symptoms. *Psychiatry Research* 20:47–55, 1987.

Thompson KS, Griffith EEH, Leaf PJ. A historical review of the Madison model of community care. *Hospital and Community Psychiatry* 41:625–634, 1990.

Thompson MS. Willingness to pay and accept risks to cure chronic disease. *American Journal of Public Health* 76:392–396, 1986.

Thurstone LL. A law of comparative judgement. *Psychology Review* 34:273–286, 1927.

Timko C. Policies and services in residential substance abuse programs: Comparisons with psychiatric programs. *Journal of Substance Abuse* 7:43–59, 1995.

Timko C. Physical characteristics of residential psychiatric and substance abuse programs: Organizational determinants and patient outcomes. *American Journal of Community Psychology* 24:173–192, 1996.

Torrance GW. Social preference for health states: An empirical evaluation of three measurement techniques. *Socio-economic Planning Science* 10:129–136, 1976.

Torrance GW. Preferences for health states: A review of measurement methods. *Mead Johnson Symposium on Perinatal and Developmental Medicine* 20:37–45, 1982.

Truax PA, Addis ME, Koerner K, Gollan JK, Gortner E, Prince SE. A component analysis of cognitive-behavioral treatment for depression. *Journal of Consulting and Clinical Psychology* 64:293–304, 1996.

Udvarhelyi IS, Colditz GA, Rai A, Epstein AM. Cost–effectiveness and cost–benefit analyses in the medical literature: Are the methods being used correctly? *Annals of Internal Medicine* 116:238–244, 1992.

US Department of Labor, Bureau of Labor Statistics. *Employment, Hours, and Earnings: States and Areas, Data for 1987–92.* Washington, DC: US Department of Labor, 1992a.

US Department of Labor, Bureau of Labor Statistics. *The Consumer Price Index: Questions and Answers.* Washington, DC: US Department of Labor, 1992b.

US Department of Labor, Bureau of Labor Statistics. *Using the Consumer Price Index for Escalation.* Washington, DC: US Department of Labor, 1991.

Vallis TM, Shaw BF, Dobson KS. The Cognitive Therapy Scale: Psychometric properties. *Journal of Consulting and Clinical Psychology* 54:381–385, 1986.

Veit CT, Ware JE. Measuring health and health care outcomes: Issues and recomendations. In Kane RL, Kane RA, editors. *Values and Long Term Care.* Lexington, MA: Lexington Books, 1982.

Viscusi WK. *Fatal Tradeoffs: Public and Private Responsibilities for Risk.* New York: Oxford University Press, 1992.

Viscusi WK. The value of risks to life and health. *Journal of Economic Literature* XXXI(December):1912–1946, 1993.

Viscusi WK. Discounting health effects for medical decisions. In Sloan F, editor. *Valuing Health Care.* Cambridge University Press, 1995.

von Neumann J, Morgenstern O. *Theory of Games and Economic Behavior.* Princeton, NJ: Princeton University Press, 1944.

von Winterfeldt D, Edwards W. *Decision Analysis and Behavioral Research.* Cambridge: Cambridge University Press, 1986.

Wallace CJ. Functional assessment in rehabilitation. *Schizophrenia Bulletin* 12:604–630, 1986.

Waltz J, Addis ME, Koerner K, Jacobson NS. Testing the integrity of a psychotherapy protocol: Assessment of adherence and competence. *Journal of Consulting and Clinical Psychology* 61:620–630, 1993.

Ware JE. Measuring health and functional status in mental health services research. In Taube CA, Mechanic D, Hohmann AA, editors. *The Future of Mental Health Services Research.* DHHS (ADM) 89-1600. Rockville, MD: US Department of Health and Human Services, 1989.

Ware JE. The MOS 36-item short form health survey. In Sederer LI, Dickey B, editors. *Outcomes Assessment in Clinical Practice.* Baltimore: Williams & Wilkins, 1996.

Warner KE, Luce BR. *Cost–Benefit and Cost–Effectiveness Analysis in Health Care: Principles, Practice, and Potential.* Ann Arbor, MI: Health Administration Press, 1982.

Waskow IE. Specification of the technique variable in the NIMH Treatment of Depression Collaborative Research Program. In Williams JBW, Spitzer RL, editors. *Psychotherapy Research: Where Are We and Where Should We Go?* New York: Guilford, 1984.

Wayson BL, Funke GS. *What Price Justice? A Handbook for the Analysis of Criminal Justice Costs.* Washington, DC: US Department of Justice, 1989.

Weinstein MC, Fineberg HV. *Clinical Decision Analysis.* Philadelphia: W.B. Saunders Company, 1980.

Weinstein MC, Stason WB. Foundations of cost–effectiveness analysis for health and medical practices. *The New England Journal of Medicine* 296:716–721, 1977.

Weisbrod BA. Benefit–cost analysis of a controlled experiment: Treating the mentally ill. *Journal of Human Resources* 16:523–548, 1981.

Weisbrod BA. A guide to benefit–cost analysis as seen through a controlled experiment in treating the mentally ill. *Journal of Health Politics, Policy and Law* 7:808–845, 1983.

Weisbrod BA, Test MA, Stein LI. Alternative to mental hospital treatment: II. Economic benefit–cost analysis. *Archives of General Psychiatry* 37:400–405, 1980.

Weissman MM, Paykel ES. *The Depressed Woman: A Study of Social Relationships.* Chicago: University of Chicago Press, 1974.

Weissman MM, Rounsaville BJ, Chevron E. Training psychotherapists to participate in psychotherapy outcome studies. *American Journal of Psychiatry* 139:1442–1446, 1982.

Weissman MM, Sholomskas D, John K. The assessment of social adjustment: An update. *Archives of General Psychiatry* 38:1250–1258, 1981.

Wells KB, Astrachan BM, Tischler GL, Unutzer J. Issues and approaches in evaluating managed mental health care. *The Milbank Quarterly* 73:57–73, 1995.

Wells KB, Stewart A, Hays RD, Burnam MA, Rogers W, Daniels M, et al. The functioning and well-being of depressed patients. Results from the Medical Outcomes Study. *Journal of the American Medical Association* 262:914–919, 1989.

Wells KB, Sturm R. Informing the policy process: From efficacy to effectiveness data on pharmacotherapy. *Journal of Consulting and Clinical Psychology* 64:638–345, 1996.

White-Means S, Chollet D. Opportunity wages and workforce adjustments—Understanding the cost of in-home elder care. *Journals of Gerontology Series B—Psychological Sciences and Social Sciences* 51:S82–S90, 1996.

Wiersma D, Kluiter H, Nienhuis FJ, Ruphan M, Giel R. Costs and benefits of hospital and day treatment with community care of affective and schizophrenic disorders. *British Journal of Psychiatry* 166:52–59, 1995.

Willan A, O' Brien BJ. Confidence intervals for cost–effectiveness ratios: An application of Fieller's theorem. *Health Economics* 5:297–305, 1996.

Williams A. Euroqol—A new facility for the measurement of health-related quality of life. *Health Policy* 16:199–208, 1990.

Williams A. Cost–benefit analysis: Applied welfare economics or general decision aid? In Williams A, Giardina E, editors. *Efficiency in the Public Sector: The Theory and Practice of Cost–Benefit Analysis.* Brookfield, VT: Edward Elgar Publishing, 1993.

Williams JB, Gibbon M, First MB, Spitzer RL, Davies M, Borus J, et al. The Structured Clinical Interview for DSM-III-R (SCID) II. Multisite test-retest reliability. *Archives of General Psychiatry* 49:630–636, 1992.

Willis GB, Royston P, Bercini D. The use of verbal report methods in the development and testing of survey questionnaires. *Applied Cognitive Psychology* 5:251–267, 1991.

Wimo A, Mattson B, Krakau I, Erikson T, Nelvig A, Karrison G. Cost–utility analysis of group living in dementia care. *International Journal of Technology Assessment in Health Care* 11:49–65, 1995.

Witheridge TF. The "active ingredients" in an in vivo community support program. *New Directions in Mental Health Services* 52:47–64, 1992.

Wittchen H, Semler G, vonZerssen D. A comparison of two diagnostic methods: Clinical ICD diagnoses vs DSM-III and Research Diagnostic Criteria using the Diagnostic Interview Schedule (version 2). *Archives of General Psychiatry* 42:677–684, 1985.

Woerner MG, Mannuzza S, Kane JM. Anchoring the BPRS: An aid to improved reliability. *Psychopharmacology Bulletin* 24(1):112–121, 1988.

Wolf C. *Markets or Governments.* Cambridge, MA: The MIT Press, 1988.

Wolff N, Helminiak TW. Nonsampling measurement error in administrative data: Implications for economic evaluations. *Health Economics* 5:501–512, 1996.

Wolff N, Helminiak TW, Tebes JK. Getting the cost right in cost–effeciveness analysis. *American Journal of Psychiatry* 154:736–743, 1997.

Yates BT. Toward the incorporation of costs, cost–effectiveness analysis, and cost–benefit analysis into clinical research. *Journal of Consulting and Clinical Psychology* 62:729–736, 1994.

Yates BT. *Analyzing Costs, Procedures, Processes, and Outcomes in Human Services: An Introduction.* Thousand Oaks, CA: Sage, 1996.

Yates BT, Newman FL. Approaches to cost–effectiveness analysis and cost–benefit analysis of psychotherapy. In Vandenbos GR, editor. *Psychotherapy: Practice, Research, Policy.* Beverley Hills: Sage, 1980.

Yudofsky SC, Silver JM, Jackson W, Endicott J, Williams D. The overt aggression scale for the objective rating of verbal and physical aggression. *American Journal of Psychiatry* 143:35–39, 1986.

Zarin DA, West JC, Pincus HA, McIntyre JS. The American Psychiatric Association practice research network. In Sederer LI, Dickey B, editors. *Outcomes Assessment in Clinical Practice.* Baltimore: Williams & Wilkins, 1996.

Zelman WN, Stone AVW, Davenport BA. Factors contributing to artifactual differences in reported mental health costs. *Administration in Mental Health* 10:40–52, 1982.

Zick CD, Bryant WK. Shadow wage assessments of the value of home production: Patterns from the 1970s. *Lifestyles: Family and Economic Issues* 11:143–160, 1990.

Zung WWK. A self-rating depression scale. *Archives of General Psychiatry* 12:63–70, 1965.

Zung WWK. Factors influencing the self-rating depression scale. *Archives of General Psychiatry* 16:543–547, 1967.

Zung WWK, Richards CB, Gables C, Short MJ. Self-rating depression scale in an outpatient clinic. *Archives of General Psychiatry* 13:508–515, 1965.

INDEX

Accounting data, *see also* Administrative databases
  cost estimation, 77–78, 82–83, 85
  resource utilization, 69–70
ACT model, *see* Assertive Community Treatment (ACT) model
Activities of daily living (ADLs), 136
ADLs, *see* Activities of Daily Living (ADLs)
Administrative databases
  accounting, *see* Accounting data
  billing, 60–61
  claims, 60–61, 84–85
  cost estimation, 78–79, 82–85
  health maintenance organizations, *see* Health maintenance organization
  labor force participation, 88–89
  local, 65
  Medicaid, *see* Medicaid data
  medication, 81
  payment data, 84
  resource utilization, 58, 60–61, 65–67, 69–70
  service practice, 109–111
  staff time, 58, 69–70
  system, 65
  Veterans Administration, *see* Veterans Administration databases
  wages, 88–89
Adverse event, *see* Side effects
Affective disorder, *see* Depression
Aggregate data, *see* Administrative databases; Survey data
Allocation
  random, *see* Randomization
Analytic methodology, *see* Statistics; Study design
Analysis of variance (ANOVA), 179, 183
Analytic perspective, 51–53
Analyzing cost-effectiveness, *see* Statistics
Ancillary services
  cost estimation, 81
  resource utilization, 59
ANOVA, *see* Analysis of variance (ANOVA)
Assertive Community Treatment (ACT) model, 4, 5, 97, 104, 113–115, 189–191
Asymmetric information, 192–193

Attrition, 18–19, 24, 180–182
Average cost–effectiveness ratio, 172

BDI, *see* Beck Depression Inventory (BDI)
Beck Depression Inventory (BDI), 131–132
Benefits, *see* Cost–benefit analysis
Bias, *see also* Measurement error; Internal validity; External validity
  attrition, 18–19, 24, 180–182
  refusal, 23–24
  selection, 16, 19, 180–182
Billing databases, 60–61
Blinded studies, 26–27
Bootstrap methods, 180
BPRS, *see* Brief Psychiatric Rating Scale (BPRS)
Brief Psychiatric Rating Scale (BPRS), 31–33, 130

C/E ratio, *see* Cost–effectiveness ratio
CAPA, *see* Child and Adolescent Psychiatric Assessment (CAPA)
Capital cost, 81–82
Capitation, 194, 195
Caregiver burden, *see* Measures, caregiver burden, *see also* Informal care; Family cost
Caretaking, *see* Informal care
CAS, *see* Child Assessment Schedule (CAS)
Case example
  analyzing cost-effectiveness, 165
  assertive community treatment, 97, 189
  capitation, 165
  case management, 117
  clozapine, 15, 24
  cost estimation, 75
  depression, 55, 75
  economic concepts, 39
  emotionally disturbed children, 39
  health maintenance organization, 11–12, 55, 75
  jail, 117
  measuring utilization, 55
  outcome, 147
  outcome measurement, 117
  posttraumatic stress disorder, 11–12
  preference, 147
  schizophrenia, 15, 55, 75, 97, 147

232